Social Work and Mental Health

The Value of Everything

Peter Gilbert

with Peter Bates, Sarah Carr, Michael Clark,
Nick Gould and Greg Slay

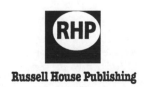

Russell House Publishing

First published in 2003 as *The Value of Everything: social work and its importance in the field of mental health* by Russell House Publishing Ltd.

This Second Edition published in 2010 by:
Russell House Publishing Ltd.
4 St. George's House
Uplyme Road
Lyme Regis
Dorset DT7 3LS
Tel: 01297-443948
Fax: 01297-442722
e-mail: help@russellhouse.co.uk
www.russellhouse.co.uk

British Library Cataloguing-in-publication Data:
A catalogue record for this book is available from the British Library.

ISBN: 978-1-905541-60-7

Typeset by TW Typesetting, Plymouth, Devon

Printed and bound in Great Britain by
CPI Antony Rowe, Chippenham and Eastbourne

Russell House Publishing

Russell House Publishing aims to publish innovative and valuable materials to help managers, practitioners, trainers, educators and students.

Our full catalogue covers: social policy, working with young people, helping children and families, care of older people, social care, combating social exclusion, revitalising communities and working with offenders.

Full details can be found at www.russellhouse.co.uk and we are pleased to send out information to you by post. Our contact details are on this page.

We are always keen to receive feedback on publications and new ideas for future projects.

Contents

Foreword

Hári Sewell

The current reality and future possibilities for social work in mental health services are becoming clearer. The profession has experienced the mutation of the Approved Social Worker (ASW) role into the one that can be undertaken by other disciplines, as well as the associated clarity that these (social work) professionals may be employed by NHS Trusts. Integration and multidisciplinary working are the order of the day. Peter Gilbert has crystallised the essential qualities of social work, which based on its history, is unique within the multidisciplinary and integrated organisational context.

In Chapter 1, the distillation of the paradigms used to understand people's experiences is insightful and the emphasis on valuing the perceptions and reality of the individual sets the tone for the book.

However, this book is not just a philosophical debate about the merits of different models for understanding and working with mental or emotional distress. It provides clear theoretical frameworks for understanding the barriers to developing the kinds of relationships that enable social workers to recognise the capacities of people who use services. See for example the model presented by Bates in Chapter 2 for understanding and working with professional boundaries.

Overall, this contemporary book provides theory, knowledge and practical hints on how to preserve and develop the unique identity of social work. Rather than proposing a professional apartheid this book celebrates the integration of perspectives and disciplines and places the value on working with those who use services as people with their own unique strengths, likes, dislikes and experiences (including issues of identity and equalities). Research and constructs are drawn from psychiatrists, psychologists and even economists – emphasising the point that social work is able to utilise the best of what is available for the good of the person using services.

This book is a timely celebration and reminder of the value of social work in mental health services. Timely in the context of the prevailing foundation trust model – with its increased focus on governance and business delivery, alongside the changes to the previous ASW role and the increasing attention given to childcare social work as a result of high profile cases that have gone terribly wrong.

Gilbert and colleagues have provided material that will equip social workers and their leaders so that as they stand shoulder to shoulder with colleagues in the advancement of modern mental health services, they will be able to do so with backs straight and heads held high.

Hári Sewell is an independent consultant; Co-founder and Chair of the Social Care Strategic Network (Mental Health); former Executive Director of Social Care and Associate Editor of the *Journal of Ethnicity and Inequalities in Health and Social Care*.

Introduction

The publication of *New Horizons* by The Department of Health (2009), to provide the new vision for mental health services, building on the *National Service Framework*, gives hope that the progress made in mental health services over the past quarter of a century will be maintained. It is also to be hoped that mental health will not be seen as some form of narrow, specialist 'mental illness' approach and service, but part of a wider and vital approach to the health of the nation as a whole. Increasingly, mental health is being seen as a crucial issue for a healthy and productive nation. The mental as well as physical health of citizens is viewed as a vital component in the regeneration of communities; and campaigns are in place to create a positive image of and focus on mental health and recovery.

Progress, however, is set against a background of cul-de-sacs in terms of policy and service development; regular moral panics; past under-investment pessimism and a workforce under considerable strain at a time when the demographic tide is running away from us. This new edition of *The Value of Everything* looks to set Social Work as one of the most vital components in a truly whole person and whole systems approach to mental health, at a time when society is becoming more complex, and when user-centred and community-centred approaches are required. The cross-government approach to personalisation, which forms a new chapter in this book, will only work if services users are enabled to gain more control over their lives and more choice in the treatment and care they receive, so that professionals work in partnership with them. At the same time it is vital that a policy which provides service users with more control, and perhaps their own budget, isn't an abnegation of society's obligation to those who are most vulnerable. At the time of writing this book the deficiencies of the health care system in the USA has come into sharp focus, with so many millions of people left really without any support, in a highly privatised approach to health and social care.

I have tried to maintain the historical and policy overview from the first book, which was appreciated by readers, and to maintain a focus on the values that social work espouses as a profession, and the value of social work in current health and social care. At the same time new chapters have been added around social inclusion, personalisation, spirituality research, the role of the social worker following new mental health legislation in 2005 and 2007, and a policy overview which takes us up to the current time.

This book considers the value of social work in light of what users and carers want from services, and the value base of the new policies of reform; the role of the social worker in different settings; and ways of taking these values and skills into these settings. I hope that it will provide a boost to the confidence of social workers by reinforcing the tremendous resource that they are to people in the greatest need in our society; and also to help partner professions and agencies to value the contribution that social work can bring.

Peter Gilbert January 2010

About the Author and the Contributors

Peter Gilbert is Professor of Social Work and Spirituality at Staffordshire University, and Visiting Professor with both Birmingham and Solihull NHS Foundation Trust and the University of Worcester. Peter was the NIMHE Project Lead on Spirituality from its inception to 31st March, 2008, and now works for the National Spirituality and Mental Health Forum. He has recently been appointed Chair of the National Development Team for Inclusion. A former Director of Social Services for Worcestershire, Peter is a qualified and registered Social Worker with 13 years of direct practice. Between 2003 and 2006 he was NIMHE/SCIE Fellow in Social Care with Professor Nick Gould, and has also been Social Care Advisor to the Sainsbury Centre for Mental Health. Peter is on the Equalities Board for the National Mental Health Development Unit Progremme and is UK advisor to Jersey Focus on Mental Health.

Peter's first career was in the Army. He was principal social worker in one of the old institutions; managed services for people with Learning Disabilities in London Borough of Merton, and people with Mental Health needs in Kent in the late 1980s and early 1990s; and was very involved in partnership working and service user and carer involvement in both Staffordshire as Director of Operations, and Worcestershire as Director of Social Services. In the 1980s he specialised in Learning Disability and Mental Health.

Having experienced an episode of depression in 2000/1 Peter is very committed to an holistic and person-centred approach.

Peter is signed up to ensuring the integration of theory with practice. He is author of *Leadership: Being Effective and Remaining Human* (2005); co-edited *Spirituality, Values and Mental Health: Jewels for the Journey* (2007) and is on several editorial boards. Having recently published guidelines for CSIP/NIMHE on Spirituality for frontline staff, and co-written a position paper on leadership and personalisation paper for SCIE, Peter is currently working on an edited handbook on Spirituality and Mental Health.

Peter Bates has led on social inclusion work for the National Development Team for Inclusion since 1999, a not-for-profit agency that provides consultancy, training and facilitation for mental health, learning disability and older person's services. He previously worked in probation, the employment service, social services, the NHS and audit. Project work has been undertaken for a range of national bodies including the National Social Inclusion Programme, Social Exclusion Unit, Mental Health and Wellbeing Division of the Scottish Government, Valuing People Support Team and Sainsbury Centre for Mental Health.

In his work with over 130 local service providers, Peter has combined a detailed knowledge of what needs to be done to make a difference, with an understanding of the realities of frontline work in hard-pressed services. He has published over 80 items in the areas of employment, disability, empowerment and inclusion including a number of landmark policy, commissioning and practice publications. He is a Visiting Research Fellow at the Faculty of Health of Staffordshire University and is constantly in demand as a lively and effective trainer.

Sarah Carr is a Senior Research Analyst at the Social Care Institute for Excellence (SCIE), currently leading on the organisation's personalisation work and advising on the policy at a national level. She recently authored *Personalisation: A Rough Guide* (2009). Before SCIE, Sarah worked for the National Institute for Social Work, Oxleas NHS Trust and the Sainsbury Centre for Mental Health, in research and information roles.

Sarah has also had a number of social care jobs including, a residential support worker at a farm hostel for homeless people in Edinburgh, a worker at a rehabilitation project for young women sex offenders and an HIV and AIDS awareness trainer in Manchester. She is currently a Social Perspectives Network Executive committee member and a member of INVOLVE, the national advisory group, funded by the Department of Health, which aims to promote and support active public involvement in NHS, public health and social care research. Sarah is also an Honorary Research Fellow at Staffordshire University.

Sarah is a long-term user of mental health services and has written on her experiences as well as general mental health practice and policy, LGB welfare and equality issues, service user empowerment and participation. She is currently involved in helping to run a service user participation programme for the Channel Island of Jersey.

Dr Michael Clark is Research Manager with the National Mental Health Development Unit and NHS West Midlands Regional Development Centre. Michael has worked in research and research management at local, regional and national health service levels. His role is as knowledge broker across research, policy and practice – actively supporting rational public reasoning across these contexts and thereby ensuring more productive synergies across them. His work in the West Midlands includes implementation of a pathways model across all mental health services in the region. He is chair of the National Improving Access to Psychological Therapies R&D Group.

Michael has written many articles and book chapters, and co-edited *Research and Development in Mental Health: Theory, Framework and Models*, and is currently working on a book on risk management and quality improvement in mental health.

Dr Nick Gould is professor of social work at the University of Bath, recognised internationally for his writing and research, and has held visiting appointments in Australia and Hong Kong. Since qualifying as a social worker over 30 years ago he has combined an academic career with maintaining involvement in mental health practice, including serving for many years as a member of the Mental Health Review Tribunal. From 2003–6 he was National Institute for Mental Health England's Fellow in Social Care (research and practice). His latest book is *Mental Health Social Work in Practice* (Routledge, 2010).

Greg Slay is Practice Development Manager – Mental Health and Lead for the Approved Mental Health Professional Service at West Sussex County Council. He has wide experience of working within and alongside mental health services. His current primary responsibilities are around mental health policy and best practice. This includes providing the overall professional leadership for the AMHP Service provided by West Sussex County Council – and where many of the AMHPs are seconded to work within Sussex Partnership NHS Foundation Trust. He

maintains his own practice base through working as an AMHP with the county's Out of Hours Service. Since 2005 he has also worked in a voluntary capacity for the Association of Directors of Adult Social Services as its national adviser on the implementation of the Mental Capacity Act's various requirements.

Acknowledgements

One of the profound aspects of social work is the creation of valued connections in achieving our goals. I find that I learn something new from someone nearly every day, and sometimes the most profound learning comes from unexpected sources.

I do need to thank my first managers in social work, Bridget Ogden and the late Jean Carruthers; and also my tutor during my Social Work qualification, Hugh England, whose book *Social Work As Art: Making Sense of Good Practice* is still a lodestone to me.

Professor Antony Sheehan was an inspiration to me when I joined the core group helping to set up the National Institute for Mental Health in England, and has remained an inspiration ever since. I would also like to thank Professor Nick Gould, my colleague in the NIMHE/SCIE Fellowship, Paddy Cooney from the South West Development Centre and leaders such as Neil Carr.

I came late into academic life, courtesy of the good offices and companionship of Professor Bernard Moss, to whom I owe a great deal; and I continue to be inspired by the leadership of Dr Christine King, the Vice Chancellor at Staffordshire University. My thanks to all my colleagues in Social Work and Advice Studies at Staffordshire University.

Since 2008 the Spirituality Project moved from NIMHE to the National Forum. My thanks to Professor Martin Aaron, Ven. Arthur Hawes, Dr Sarah Eagger, Mary Ellen Coyte, and Vicky Nicholls for their support.

It has been my good fortune to work at Birmingham and Solihull Mental Health Foundation Trust with Dr Neil Deuchar, Dr Peter Lewis, Pastor Sandra Thomas, Maddy Parkes, Dr Jo Barber and colleagues, in an innovative approach to researching the benefits of spiritual care.

Recent work with the University of Worcester has been very fruitful and I would like to thank

Professor Dominic Upton, Debbie Evans, Dr Janice Clarke, Joy Gauci, Phil Hoare and Peter Unwin.

It has been a joy to return to my home island of Jersey to do some work on service user partnership and my thanks go to Julian Clyde-Smith, Anton Skinner, Samantha Bolam, Ian Dyer and everyone in the group.

I am very fortunate to have the ongoing support of the Association of Directors of Adult Social Services and the Associates Group, and my thanks for the companionship and stimulation and support to Richard Webb and Jenny Goodall and colleagues; Richard Humphries, Brian Parrott, Cathie Williams, Jo Williams, Dame Denise Platt, Anne Williams and colleagues.

Since 2003 I have had the pleasure and privilege of coordinating and facilitating the learning set for Directors of Social Care, which is now the Social Care Strategic Network. My particular thanks to Hari Sewell, the Chair of the network, and to Ben Bano, James Sinclair, Mark Cardwell and Karen Wren. My working relationship with SCIE has been particularly helpful and my thanks to Ray Jones, Bill Kilgallon, Julie Jones and Sarah Carr.

It has been a privilege to be asked to be Chair of the National Development Team for Inclusion, and I have derived insights from working with Chief Executive Rob Greig and the Board and team.

Lastly, I would like to thank my family who have had to put up with me muttering at the computer and to Tracy Morgan who typed the manuscript and has managed to translate my handwriting into English!

From pre-publication reviews

Professor Gilbert has provided a great service to the social care community and other allied services in producing a book that is not only timely, but addresses some of the major issues in social care today. At a time when so many radical changes are taking place and professional boundaries are shifting, it is important to be reminded of the essence of what social care actually is. Among the many topics discussed and explored in this book are, the roots of social care, social work and the law , spirituality, research, leadership and service user perspectives. It is elegantly written and logically presented and I would consider it essential reading for all those embarking on social work careers, those who are already qualified and particularly for commissioners and managers of services. I found the book educational and informative and I would strongly recommend it to others.

Neil Carr OBE
CEO
South Staffordshire and Shropshire
Healthcare NHS Foundation Trust

We live in interesting times. We live in a time of great potential and of great disturbances and troubles. Like never before, it seems, we need help and we need healing. Social workers, as healing professionals, help us to help ourselves and their role, with all its challenges, is essential. In this book Peter Gilbert and his co-authors offers a fresh perspective on just what is possible. At the same time they give us some thoughts and raise questions on mental health and what it means for us as a nation and as individuals. We are challenged to make real the proposition that 'mental health is everyone's business'.

This is a book full of insights. It is challenging, it is inspiring and at the same time, it is a really good read.

Professor Christine King CBE, DL
Vice Chancellor
Staffordshire University

CHAPTER 1

No Health Without Mental Health

Peter Gilbert

Mental health is everyone's business. In 2020 mental health will be seen as an important asset for our society, one in which we all have an investment and to which we all – individuals, employers, the third and statutory sectors, local authorities, the health services and all Government departments – have an important contribution to make.

New Horizons: Towards a Shared Vision
for Mental Health. DoH, 2009

Bernadette's (her social worker's) commitment, her refusal to budge, her utter reliability, showing up week after week wherever I was, whether in hospital or out of it, her consummate patience, the sheer amount of time she was willing to offer – all these were critical in building the trust we needed to work together. But there were other important qualities – partly I suspect innate, and partly the result of years of experience. Intelligence, insight, resilience, humour . . . empathy, courage and professionalism to name just a few.

Clare Allan 'My Brilliant Survival Guide',
Society Guardian, 14 January 2009

The social work profession promotes social change, problem-solving in human relationships and the empowerment and liberation of people to enhance well-being. Utilising theories of human behaviour and social systems, social work intervenes at the points where people interact with their environment. Principles of human rights and social justice are fundamental to social work.

Revised Code of Ethics. British Association
of Social Workers, 2002

What kind of society?

The credit crunch of 2008/9 and the resulting economic crisis (see Cable, 2009) raised a whole series of issues around what a healthy society should look like. From the late 1970s onwards Britain, but more especially England, moved towards being a society caught between the rampant individualism of the USA and the more communitarian nature of Western Europe. The radical differences between the USA's concept of the relationship between the individual and society has been thrown into stark relief by the controversy surrounding President Obama's healthcare reform proposals (see Harris, 2009).

Debates about what constitutes a fair and decent society for all citizens are rife, exemplified perhaps in the recent report on the state of children in the UK undertaken by the Children's Society (see Layard and Dunn, 2009: 4) where the study compares Britain and the US with the continental countries of Western Europe. Britain and the US have more broken families than other countries, and those families are less cohesive in the way they live and eat together. The authors conclude that:

We believe there is one common theme that links all these problems – excessive individualism.

In terms of the mental health of children:

According to the Government's definitive survey, one in ten of all five to sixteen year olds have clinically significant mental health difficulties.
Layard and Dunn, 2009: 114 and Green et al., 2005

The issues of social equality and citizenship are particularly acute in the case of mental health and mental illness as, throughout history, there have been questions as to what 'madness' really means and both how to safeguard the individual and their liberty (and their property) when they are mentally incapacitated (see Chapter 8) and how to safeguard other people should there be other issues around dangerousness. When concerns about perceived dangers come to the fore, as in the early 2000s, then stigma becomes more problematic.

In August 2009 the Audit Commission warned that the recession and subsequent unemployment and social dislocation would exacerbate social problems, which would require a response from government, both centrally and locally. The World Health Organisation, Europe report on *Mental Health, Resilience and Inequalities* (Friedli, 2009) quotes the sociologist Zygmunt Bauman as stating that:

Although the risks and contradictions of life go on being as socially produced as ever, the duty and necessity of coping with them has been delegated to our individual selves.

Friedli sets out the priorities for action as:

• Social, cultural and economic contributions that support family and community life.

- Education that equips children to flourish both economically and emotionally.
- Employment opportunities and workplace pay and conditions that promote and protect mental health.
- Partnerships between health and other sectors to address social and economic problems that are a catalyst for psychological distress.
- Reducing environmental barriers to social contact.

The importance of social work in making connections between individual distress, family stresses and the wider social environment has never been so great.

Human traces

In his magisterial novel, *Human Traces*, Sebastian Faulks describes the sweep of mental health practice in the 19th and early 20th centuries, through the eyes of two fictional doctors: Jacques Rebiere and Thomas Midwinter and the latter's sister Sonia Midwinter. Through their practice and their studies they attempt to discover the essence of humanity. Rebiere moves more towards psychoanalysis, Midwinter, partly through a sudden dawning of his own early experience, begins to consider whether the hearing of voices is a natural human faculty lost as language became more sophisticated. The character Midwinter spends some of his early practice in what is clearly the county asylum for Lincolnshire, and struggles to uphold the original vision of a place of 'asylum' (from the Greek and Latin: a place of sanctuary, and safety from violence) as the founding concept sinks into warehousing. As Faulks (2006: 236) puts it:

> *Thomas passionately hoped that he would not become such a mechanical practitioner, such a clock maker, such a cobbler of the human.*

Another character in the novel, who leaves his medical studies to become a priest, has an encounter with someone suffering mental distress which leaves him profoundly altered:

> *. . . he was obliged to bear her pain: both of them were connected in some universal, though unseen, pattern of humanity. His obligation was not to diagnose her but to love her; while his greater duty was to the larger reality, the place outside time where their connection had been made, the common ground of existence into which he has been granted a privileged glimpse.*
>
> (p20)

Although progress in human affairs is always being made, the complexity of humanity always means that we have a tendency to fall as well as rise. We have a tension between individuality and social solidarity, a tension being fought out graphically in the current USA debate over healthcare. We wish for universal services, but also some measure of individual preference and choice within that. We wish to have control over our own lives but some form of safety net. As the psychologist Jonathan Haidt puts it, we are 'ultra-social animals' (Haidt, 2006) but some of that sociability now takes place by electronic means, rather than in face-to-face encounters. Globalisation has brought the world closer, but it has also made us much more like consumers and much less like citizens. Sociologist Zygmunt Bauman talks about an elite who are akin to the absentee landlords of the 18th and 19th centuries, exercising power without responsibility in a form of:

> *. . . unanchored power – a disconnection of power from obligations . . . freedom from the duty to contribute to daily life and the perpetuation of the community.*
>
> Bauman, 1998: 9

Martin Jacques writes about globalisation creating the 'illusion of intimacy' while in fact the mental distances have changed little at all (Jacques, 2006).

While a new emphasis is being placed on the 'medicine of the person', based on the work of people like Paul Tournier (see Cox et al., 2007) there is a necessary corrective that an individualised, or personalised approach (see Chapter 6 in this book), has to be balanced against concepts of family, culture and society at large. Sewell's recent work on ethnicity, race and culture in mental health stresses the cultural milieu in which we all operate (see Sewell, 2009) and Okasha in the recent publication on Tournier's work stresses that in the Islamic world view:

> *The boundaries between the person and the family are so blurred that the person cannot perceive himself as an independent self or as having a separate existence from his family.*
>
> Okasha, 2007: 111

One may immediately see how subsequent generations of families that have moved to this country may experience a considerable tension between their families' originated culture and the society they find in the United Kingdom. Zobia Arif's (2002) study of second generation Pakistani Muslims demonstrates the tensions which result. Whatever systems that we put in place to deal with the complexity of our humanity, there is always a danger that the system turns into *The System*. At the end of the day, we have to remember that we are a person face to face with another person, with the complexities and contradictions that that entails.

One of the strange aspects of mental health is a combination of its prevalence and the difficulty people have in speaking about it. Professor Lewis Wolpert, in his searing *Malignant Sadness* (Wolpert, 2006: vii) states that he is 'continually amazed how widespread depression is' because he finds that he rarely meets anyone who doesn't have some contact with depression, either their own experience, friends or family. Because Wolpert is willing to disclose about himself, he finds people open up to him. In a recent article, David Brindle, the Editor of *Society Guardian*, points out that while politicians are increasingly willing to speak about physical illness and the increased empathy they gain from the patient experience, mental illness is still a no-go area (Brindle, 2008). Much of this must be related to:

- Our desire for increased rationality as a species.
- Our anxiety that irrational decisions will be made – despite the fact that the major catastrophes of the 20th century were undertaken by small groups of people who might be classed as 'the deadly sane', who launched ideological pogroms against other human beings.
- Our evolution from small tribes where difference of various kinds would have been seen as potentially life-threatening danger.

Dr Paul Keedwell from the Maudsley Hospital suggests that depression has an evolutionary benefit because it helps us to cope with life's challenges. Wolpert reminds us that at an earlier stage in history depression was not necessarily subject to the same degree of stigma as it is today. For Aristotle, melancholy was the temperament of the creative artist, for creativity was thought to be driven by black bile. Melancholy was therefore seen as an enviable condition. Psychoanalyst, Darian Leader suggests that we have individualised sadness, and he poses the question around loss:

Is mourning more difficult today because of this erosion of social mourning rights? Mourning, I will argue requires other people.

Leader, 2008: 8

Hearing voices is usually seen as a sign of psychosis but the work by Julian Jaynes (1977) and recent work around neuroscience (see Fenwick, 2009) suggests that we are not fully cognisant of all the complexities of the human mind. Jane Taylor's fascinating recounting of her experiences (see Box 1) is a timely reminder that humanity does not have all the answers in its study of itself. This issue is also explored in a fictional sense in Sebastian Faulks' *Human Traces*.

Defining mental health

Because we tend to take good physical and mental health for granted, the debate about health and well-being tends to concentrate on aspects of physical and mental infirmity. And yet the World Health Organisation's constitution (set out in 1946) defines health as:

A state of complete physical, mental and social well-being and not merely the absence of disease and infirmity.

Quoted in McCulloch, 2006

Rankin quotes the former health promotion charity Mentality stating that mental health is:

Essentially about how we think and feel about ourselves and about others and how we interpret the world around us ... It also affects our capacity to cope with change and transitions such as life events ... Mental health may be central to all health and well-being.

Mentality, quoted in Rankin, 2005

Economist, Lord Richard Layard (2005), brought in to advise Government, has stressed that in a knowledge economy, life long learning and sound mental health is going to be increasingly vital to the economic attainment and social cohesion of the nation.

Sound mental health is therefore about:

- Emotional and spiritual resilience which enables us to enjoy life and to survive pain, suffering and disappointment.
- An underlying belief in our own worth and the worth of others.
- Interpreting the world around us as open to positive influences.
- Realising our own abilities.
- Being able and willing to contribute to society as a citizen.
- Creating a positive relationship with the world around us (see the Foresight Report, 2008).
- Sustaining mutually satisfying relationships.
- Taking control of our lives as much as possible.

Figure 1: Mental well-being and mental ill-health

MENTAL ILL-HEALTH
Diverse Perspectives

The Bio-Medical Model

Sociological Perspectives

The Human Journey

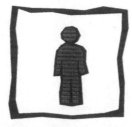

Psychoanalytic Perspectives

Legal Definitions

Cultural Perspectives

Telling Our Story

Cognitive Approaches

Religious Interpretations

Stigma

The debate over mental illness

Because of the complexities of the human mind the whole issue of what is mental ill-health is still hotly contested. While it is probably unhelpful to argue that there is no such thing as mental illness, many psychiatrists themselves are clear that the concept needs to be much more than merely regarding a human being as a purely physical entity or a quasi machine. Psychiatrist, Duncan Double states that:

> Essentially, the biomedical model of mental illness regards mental illness as a brain disease. Therefore it creates the tendency to reduce people to their biological base. Objectification of the mentally ill can make psychiatry part of the problem rather than necessarily the solution to mental health problems.
>
> Double, 2005: 56

Two other psychiatrists Patrick Bracken and Philip Thomas speak about the fact that the search for knowledge can result in what is known as 'reductionism'. They state that:

> Reductionism is the belief that all sorts of events that happen at different levels of reality can be explained in terms of (i.e. reduced to) one type of knowledge. In psychiatry, reductionism involves the assertion that as-

> pects of meaningful human behaviour (such as our worries, regrets, fears, beliefs, hopes, loves and doubts) can be fully explained in terms of 'non-meaningful' entities such as genes, neurotransmitters and ultimately atoms and molecules.
>
> Bracken and Thomas, 2005: 14

Andrew McCulloch summaries the models of mental illness as follows:

- Biological models that are concerned with the biological and chemical basis of mental illness this is what is referred to as the 'medical model'. Though many GPs and psychiatrists would use a more holistic approach.
- Social or psychological models that are concerned with life events, family dynamics and belief systems or thinking style. This encapsulates social models of disability that focus on how society reacts to disabled people, often in a discriminatory way, as well as the disability itself.
- Intuitive or spiritual explanations that see the mind as a battleground for conflicting forces: the unconscious versus the conscious, good versus evil etc. Psychoanalysis encapsulates this within modern western thinking, but belief in demonic possession is still prevalent in many societies (see Gilbert and Kalaga, 2007).

● Existential belief, which views mental illness as another valid form of human existence.
                    McCulloch, 2006: 5 (see Reed et al., 2004)

Both Jackson and Hill (2006) and Malcolm Golightley (2008, Chapter 2) provide the basic categories of mental illness and its likely effects. The most important role for the social worker is to start where the individual is and consider the person in the context of their whole situation. The phrase 'experts by experience' is often used now for people who have experienced mental health problems, and as Peter Beresford points out, the social model of disability 'draws a distinction between the (perceived) physical, sensory or intellectual impairment of the individual and the disabling social response to people seen as impaired. It highlights the oppressive nature of the dominant social response to impairment, which excludes, segregates and stigmatises . . .' (Beresford, 2005: 45). Jane Taylor describes (see Box 1) her experience of hearing voices and places that are in context.

Box 1: Whose voice should you listen to?

Jane Taylor

Hearing voices is a complicated experience. Traversing the mire of the voices is difficult enough, working out what causes them and whose explanation to accept as to why you are hearing them is virtually impossible. I should know, I heard voices for about four years. As a result I was given the almost obligatory diagnosis of psychosis and or schizophrenia, high doses of medication and was sectioned three times.

I no longer hear voices or have to take any medication – I haven't done either for 13 years now. However, I'm so intrigued by the experiences that I had during those four years, I have been compelled to try and unravel what happened.

This has taken me on quite a journey on which I have met with many others who have heard voices; spent time with them finding out what they think happened to them and where they think their voices came from. On the way I have completed an MA in Psychotherapy and as part of my MA dissertation, I conducted research in Cambodia with traditional healers who hear voices and who use them as a

---

positive tool of their trade. While in Cambodia, I also interviewed individuals from the psychiatric clinic who hear voices and have the diagnosis of psychosis or schizophrenia.

So what have I found out along the way?

There appears to be no unified theories from the world of science, psychology or theology regarding hearing voices. Also there are a variety of ways to interpret the experience of hearing voices from both an individual and a cultural perspective.

Cambodian cultural belief system is based on Buddhist and Shamanic practices, therefore it is essential for society to have traditional healers who do hear voices. These traditional healers undertake years of rigorous training and are taught techniques to control or manage the experience of hearing voices. All the traditional healers I spoke to said they would have gone mad if they had not been shown how to manage their ability to hear voices.

In Britain, over the centuries, the cultural opinion towards the phenomenon of hearing voices has ranged from being perceived as a divine gift to symptoms of an illness. De Bruijn (1993: 40) highlights the incongruence of this opinion, by noting that 'the originators of the monotheistic religions Moses, Jesus, Muhammed all heard voices not apparent to others'.

So if the current predominant religions are based upon messages that were received through the experience of hearing voices, how have we come to perceive hearing voices as pathology?

Current theories

Although psychiatry is still trying to keep 'hearing voices' to itself, its hold is slipping. Many mental health professionals and service users are pushing for the abandonment of psychiatric labels and the recognition that hearing voices is a normal, though unusual, variation in human behaviour. This body of people are gaining credence and their collective voice is creeping into scientific and psychological theories.

According to psychotherapy and psychological perspectives, voices are often triggered by an external emotional or social trauma and voices are considered to be a tool or mechanism to cope with the traumatic situation. It is thought that the events of the trauma will often be found in the content of the voices, sometimes hidden within metaphors and messages.

Lastly research has indicated that two per cent of the population hear voices whilst only a third of that percentage seeks psychiatric help.

Experts by experience

Professor Romme and Sandra Escher, who set up the Hearing Voices Network, have interviewed large numbers of people who hear voices – including both psychiatric patients and non patients. From these interviews Romme and Escher (1993: 250) discovered that 'most voice hearers were convinced that their voices came from outside themselves'. Many of the interviewees described their voices as either having a mystical nature or as part of a spiritual awakening or as 'evidence of communication with energies outside or beyond our world of sensory perception' or physical reality. Romme and Escher (1993: 250) identify this as Extra Sensory Perception (ESP). ESP is considered to be beyond normal perception or communication that occurs via the five senses i.e. hearing, vision, touch, taste, smell.

Working together with the voice hearers Romme and Escher (2002) have created a talking therapy that attempts to meet and manage the most common experiences and problems described by people who hear voices. This talking therapy includes elements of psychotherapy, psychology, various mystical concepts and therapies, reincarnation and parapsychology. This approach encourages the individual to find their own frame of reference for their experience of hearing voices, to create their own way of managing, explore where or from whom they think the voices are coming, to explore the content of the voices and to reflect on any connections between the content and the individuals' life experiences.

Coping

It has generally been thought that it is the content of the voices that leads the voice hearer to feel overwhelmed by the experience. However, recent research indicates that it is the nature of the relationship and the explanatory model that the individual uses to describe the origin of the voices that affects whether the individual copes with the experience or not. The Mental Health Foundation (quote in CSIP, 2009: 69) suggests that 'if the individual believes that the voices are in control, the individual cannot cope – if the individual believes that he or she is stronger than the voices, the individual finds ways to cope with them'.

Personal recovery

As I wrote earlier, hearing voices is a complicated experience. I've always thought that I heard voices due to multiple and separate causes and each cause or origin triggered different types of voices.

I think some of the voices I heard were literally a result of my brain or mind malfunctioning – possibly as a result of a 'chemical imbalance'. Other voices reflected emotional traumas that I had experienced during my life. Lastly, like Romme and Escher's interviewees, I too thought many of my voices came from outside myself, and possibly from entities that were from beyond this physical reality. I often wondered if I had an ability similar to a medium or shaman.

It's hard to pinpoint exactly what caused me to stop hearing voices – again I think it was a combination of factors – reflecting my hypothesis that the voices originated from a variety of causes.

The first three years that I was hearing voices were spent in a cycle of heavy doses of medication and being sectioned. Every time I was sectioned, the auditory and visual hallucinations increased in frequency, resulting in having to take higher doses of medication, which never completely eradicated the voices. On leaving hospital, it would take several months for the voices to calm down, I would begin to slowly reduce the medication, get my emotional life back in order, then have an appointment with a psychiatrist who had never met me – and then I'd be sectioned again.

A major turning point in my recovery was when I started to see only one psychiatrist, who promised that they would not section me. The stability that came with the removal of being sectioned was enormous. Having this trauma removed enabled me to become more emotionally stable, which in turn led to me hearing fewer voices.

The voices that were left were the ones that appeared to me to be coming from outside myself and coming from outside entities, and I began to tackle them in this way. I did this by literally answering them back or telling them that I was not listening to them anymore – I found swearing at them particularly successful! I began to see that I could have some power or control over the voices, as they diminished when I pushed them away.

I still today have a very clear image of the last 'person' or hallucination that was speaking to me. It was a little old lady, she wasn't threatening at all but I didn't want her hanging round my flat – and I told her this in no uncertain terms.

It is hard to know how to describe these images or hallucinations, or to know what or who they were, but for want of better words or theories I often thought that they belonged to spirits, entities, or ghosts. It was, and still is, difficult to know what to do with these kinds of experiences as they don't just challenge psychiatry or our version of sanity, they challenge western society's concept of reality. To be honest they challenged my concept of reality and I still find it hard to write about them for fear of being judged as mad, but if it makes you uncomfortable to read about, you should try experiencing it!

However, what I do know is that when I began to tackle the voices as if they were coming from spirits or entities, there were techniques that I could use to shut myself

off from them. This in turn gave me some control over them and they began to go away. Curiously, many of the techniques I used are described in Romme and Escher's book *Accepting Voices* (1993).

What I have also come to discover is that my experiences share much in common with the descriptions given by the people interviewed by Romme and Escher and with the Cambodian concept of reality and the experiences of Cambodian traditional healers.

Cambodian version of reality

Cambodia has a completely different concept of reality to western cultures. In Cambodia, due to a rich fusion of animism, Buddhist and Hindu philosophy, human experience is influenced by a belief in the existence of multiple realties that are occupied by various entities, or spirits, including the spirits of ancestors. Society puts much importance on communicating with ancestor spirits and consequently has many traditional healers who use hearing voices as a positive tool to communicate with these ancestor spirits. These traditional healers undertake years of rigorous training and are taught techniques to control or manage the experience of hearing voices.

Questions that I have been left with

I still to this day do not know if I believe in the skills of mediums, shamans, entities or spirits etc. I have no answers relating to what I heard and saw – all I've been left with are the following questions:

Did I stop hearing voices due to changing my relationship or explanatory model of the voices?

Did I have the ability to speak or communicate with entities that are beyond our physical reality?

Did outside entities have the ability to communicate with me?

Taking a traditional psychiatric model of hearing voices – i.e chemical imbalance – do mediums, shamans, traditional healers and clairvoyants hear voices because they have a 'chemical imbalance,' or perhaps more correctly a 'different' chemical balance?

Shamans regularly take drugs or use rhythmic music to change the balance of their minds to open them up to 'other realities': is this any different to a chemical imbalance?

If a shaman was taken into psychiatric care would they be considered to be delusional?

Many shamans or traditional healers across the world state their voices started after some kind of trauma. 100 per cent of the people I interviewed related the onset of their voices to a traumatic situation, as did 100 per cent of Romme and Escher's interviewees. Can trauma open you up to psychic experiences?

Many of Romme and Escher's interviewees used the same techniques that I used to make the voices stop. I do not advocate that only mediums or traditional healers should treat people who hear voices but can we learn anything from the techniques they use to control their experiences?

Whose version of reality is correct?

Conclusion

About the only solid explanation that anyone has to work with is the voice hearers' interpretations of their experiences. Research indicates these individual interpretations of hearing voices seem to share many similarities ranging from similar descriptions about the origin of the voices to different successful methods used to cope with the experience. These similarities know no boundaries and consequently are found across cultures. Descriptions provided by individuals in the west share much in common with the Cambodian cultural perception of reality and the underlying cultural concepts and classification of mental health.

Tamsin Knight (2004) who has worked as a therapist with many people who hear voices, suggests 'that hearing voices is an unusual yet normal human experience' and concludes that:

we cannot know all the answers. Perhaps we should be moving away from the idea that there is

one reality; one set of beliefs that are acceptable and another that are delusional. Instead we could accept that there is not one correct way of seeing the world; rather we all have different versions. The challenge then is to accept individuals' differences and offer them help in coping both with their reality and with living in a wider society that may not share their beliefs.

Tamsin Knight's words echo my own words, that we cannot know all the answers and there may not be only one correct way of seeing the world. Culturally there are many different ways of viewing the world and consequently multiple ways of interpreting the experience of hearing voices.

What's yours?

Jane Taylor is a psychotherapist working with refugees, asylum seekers and others who have suffered gross human rights abuses. She is also an independent consultant providing training on recovery and resilience.

Clare Allan, who has written movingly about her experiences in an inpatient unit and has also placed some of those experiences in her novel *Poppy Shakespeare* (Allan, 2006a) describes some of the dilemmas thus:

I'm not suggesting for a second that mental illness is not a reality. Anyone who's scratched all night in a corner, voices rebounding off walls around them . . . will attest to the reality of their experience. What I'm saying is that human experience – because that's what it is, nothing more, nothing less – can never be filed under neat diagnostic labels. And while diagnosis may serve some sort of purpose in helping doctors to group symptoms together and to decide on a course of treatment, they can all too easily become a replacement for genuine understanding . . . for myself, a diagnosis was validating. It was proof that my problems weren't just in my head – or proof that they really were in my head, as opposed to my having imagined them. But it was also limiting, desperately so. My life consisted of sitting in a common room, smoking. My future promised more for the same, and that's how I wanted it. My overriding fear was of being discharged.
Allan, 2006b

Calling on my own experience (see Gilbert, 2010b) in 2000/2001 I underwent a work-related episode of depression. When I eventually went to my GP, because I didn't wish to acknowledge that I was becoming ill, I was sleeping two hours a night; getting into work while the security guards were still on; losing weight at an alarming rate (to the extent that people were asking me whether I had a terminal illness) and my affect had become very flat. What helped me was a combination of factors which would probably not have worked on their own:

- A very understanding and helpful GP, who was technically astute but also able to look at the whole picture. She offered me sleeping pills and antidepressants. I was reluctant to take the antidepressants, because I didn't wish to admit to being ill. She allowed me control over this decision but left the door open for me to return, which I did do within six weeks, and the antidepressants were most helpful in stabilising my mood and giving me the strength to bring in other aspects that would be helpful to me.
  My GP was also able to understand my illness within the context of the work situation I found myself in, and was able to appreciate what strengths I might bring to the table.
- My running club which provided me with connection with nature and friends; the physical experience which provides a natural antidepressant; a sense of purpose to get out of the armchair and out of the house.
- Friendships which provided a sense of validation and a safe space for discussion of the issues.
- A place of spiritual asylum, Worth Abbey in Sussex, where I was able to go and find a place of sanctuary (see Jamison, 2006).
- A friend who placed in writing to me a powerful testimony of how she regarded my value as a person.
- Counselling which enabled me to explore issues and find a sense of resolution.
- Friends and colleagues who offered me a way back into the world of work.

Wolpert quotes the German psychiatrist Emil Kraepelin, writing in 1921, on depression:

> He [sic] *feels solitary, indescribably unhappy, as a 'creature disinherited of fate': he is sceptical about God and with a certain dull submission, which shuts out every comfort and every gleam of light, he drags himself with difficulty from one day to another. Everything has become disagreeable to him; everything wearies him . . . Everywhere he sees only the dark side and difficulties . . . Life appears to him to be aimless, he thinks that he is superfluous to the world, he cannot constrain himself any longer, the thought occurs to him to take his life without knowing why. He has a feeling as if something has cracked in him'.*
>
> Wolpert, op. cit: 2

Sharing our common humanity

Interviewed in *Society Guardian* (O'Hara, 2009) Dr Ian McPherson, former director of NIMHE and now of the National Mental Health Development Unit refers to the problem of an 'us and them' culture. McPherson was admitted as a 12 year old to a child and adolescent unit within a large psychiatric hospital on the outskirts of Glasgow. McPherson goes on:

> *I've thought early on, probably slightly naively, that having had that experience (of depression) it would actually be something that I could bring with me as well as my training. I quickly got the message – subtly and less subtly – that even in what is a fairly liberal profession there was an implicit distinction between people who are patients and people who are professionals. For a long time, that made it very difficult for me, as it did for many others, to talk about. We need to get all (professionals) to be able to feel, 'yes they've got a mental health problem, but it doesn't make them any different'.*
>
> O'Hara, op. cit.

While the march of history should have brought us a greater mutual understanding, the lessons of the mass movements of the 20th century demonstrate how easy it is for groups of human beings to create outsiders. The Nazi concentration camps and gas chambers saw the murder of many people with a mental illness or a learning disability, and homosexuals and others seen as 'outsiders', as well as Jews, Slavs and other races designated as enemies inside or outside the state (see Burleigh, 2006).

Chief Rabbi, Jonathan Sacks, reminds us that the 'basis of our humanity' is that in essence we are all the same. Recent research has shown conclusively that the human race stemmed from Africa, and any study of our own DNA demonstrates both the complexity and the common nature of our inheritance. I had my DNA tested recently and found that my patrilineal origins were Anglo Saxon; but my matrilineal origins, within recorded history, go back to the land between the Tigris and the Euphrates – a tribe who emigrated along the Mediterranean coast, which is why my maternal grandmother was Portuguese. But while we all have shared humanity, to quote Sacks:

> We are embodied creatures. We feel hunger, thirst, fear, pain. We reason, hope, dream, aspire.

> But essentially we are also unique individuals:

> Each landscape, language, culture, community is unique. Our very dignity as persons is rooted in the fact that none

of us – not even genetically identical twins – is exactly like any other.

Sacks, 2002: 47

So, in the field of mental health, we need to hold these two aspects of humanity together. At different times our drivers may come from our sense of ourselves as an individual; our family; a cultural group we were brought up in; or a formed group which we have joined. In Box 2, Zobia Arif outlines some of the tensions for 2nd generation British Pakistanis living in the UK.

Hari Sewell in his *Working with Ethnicity: Race and Culture in Mental Health* considers the interaction of race, culture and ethnicity (Sewell, 2009). As human beings we all make initial assumptions when we meet people, usually unconsciously. We need to be aware of that. Recently I met an Asian doctor who talked to me about being a practising Hindu. My mental assumption was that she came from India, but in fact her family, while they had originated in India centuries ago, more recently were amongst large numbers of people from the Indian subcontinent who had been moved by the British to work in the West Indies. So her cultural background was much more complex than my initial mental assumption had indicated. Khan and Waheed (2009) identify the issue of 'acculturative stress' as immigrants of different generations try to grapple with multiple possible identities (see Box 2).

Box 2: Issues of Identity

In 2002 I wrote a dissertation titled 'Islam and Identity among British Pakistani Youth'. The sample group were British-born Muslims whose parents originated in Pakistan but had migrated to England in later life.

My study aimed to investigate the relationship between three concepts: Culture, Identity and Religion, and how this impacted on their perception of themselves, i.e. their identity.

I found that for the majority of participants there had to be a compromise between the two cultures (i.e. British and Pakistani). Sometimes this meant that the individual felt more enriched being subject to two different cultures and feeling that they had the best of both worlds. Conversely at times the same individual would feel torn between these

cultures, with their parents representing one set of mores to them at home, and then the wider society that they live in representing a different one. A lot of my participants felt that the situation they then face with their family is confusing and difficult, as they feel that their parents do not understand them, and they do not understand their parents.

There was also a sense that one had to adapt to ways of the wider society, but such experiences could also lead to discrimination and rejection as their ethnicity is clearly visible, so no matter how hard one tried to become 'British' one still looked 'Pakistani'. The study was undertaken post 9/11 and Islam was widely discussed in the light of this, especially in the context of discrimination and rejection. Many of the participants felt that the media were portraying Muslims as terrorists and that the wider society believed this. However, instead of rejecting their faith, as something that draws negativity to oneself, the participants appeared to cling more closely to it, seeing it as 'a way of life', and also demonstrating a need to independently seek knowledge about it rather than what their parents, who also biased their religion with cultural references, told them. It seemed to me that while ethnicity can only be attributed to certain backgrounds, religion is more universal. So any person, regardless of their origin, can be a Muslim, but a Muslim cannot be labelled to a particular ethnicity. This idea fitted more favourably with my participant group. I found that the majority of participants did not feel that a single identity justified who they were. A dual identity such as British Pakistani was most favourable with the religion, Islam, being an integral way of life.

Zobia Arif Senior Social Worker

Whatever the arguments about the benefits and challenges of 'Multiculturalism' (see e.g. Modood, 2007) we are de facto a society of many cultures and identities, many of them interlocking and even contradictory. Where we become overly involved in one identity, be it national, religious

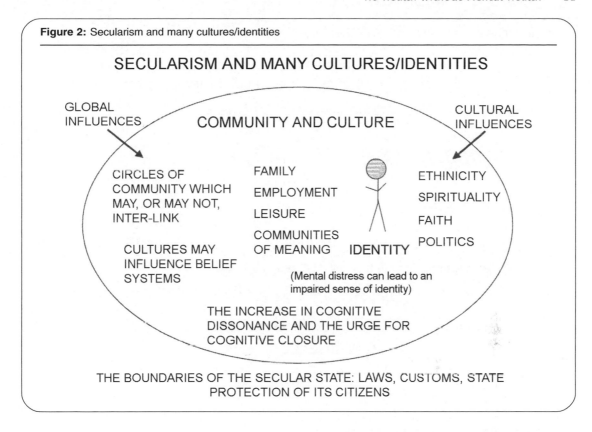

Figure 2: Secularism and many cultures/identities

SECULARISM AND MANY CULTURES/IDENTITIES

GLOBAL INFLUENCES

COMMUNITY AND CULTURE

CULTURAL INFLUENCES

CIRCLES OF COMMUNITY WHICH MAY, OR MAY NOT, INTER-LINK

FAMILY

EMPLOYMENT

LEISURE

COMMUNITIES OF MEANING

ETHINICITY

SPIRITUALITY

FAITH

POLITICS

CULTURES MAY INFLUENCE BELIEF SYSTEMS

IDENTITY

(Mental distress can lead to an impaired sense of identity)

THE INCREASE IN COGNITIVE DISSONANCE AND THE URGE FOR COGNITIVE CLOSURE

THE BOUNDARIES OF THE SECULAR STATE: LAWS, CUSTOMS, STATE PROTECTION OF ITS CITIZENS

or other, then this can turn that identity into a dangerous obsession which sees out groups as 'them' and dehumanises those who are in effect our human kin. Amartya Sen, Nobel prize winner in economics, puts it thus:

> *The intricacies of plural groups and multiple loyalties are obliterated by seeing each person as firmly imbedded in exactly one affiliation, replacing the richness of leading an abundant human life with the formulaic narrowness of insisting that any person is 'situated' in just one organic pack.*
>
> Sen, 2006: 20

Figure 2 considers the interaction of cultures and identities, and the possible impact of the 'spoiled identity' of mental ill-health:

There are particular issues of discrimination around specific groups. Dr Kwame McKenzie has written about the continual difficulties faced by people from ethnic minorities, especially perhaps young men from second or third generation Afro-Caribbean communities (see McKenzie, 2007). Lisa Appignanesi's book: *Mad, Bad and Sad* (Appignanesi, 2008) demonstrates the particular challenges that women have faced from mental

health systems through the ages (see also Carlisle, 2009). Current work with ethnic minority communities, demonstrates that there is often a mutual misunderstanding between cultural communities and statutory services. And this is true for many other minorities, for instance gay and lesbian people, dilemmas and discrimination captured so cogently by Sarah Carr who writes that:

> *To me, the medical model of homosexuality to which I was subjected during my treatment was actually harmful and eventually I found it less damaging to continue coping with my distress by self harming.*
>
> Carr, 2004: 170 (and this was only in the 1990s)

Joanna Bennett is sceptical as to whether current approaches are dealing adequately with the discrimination faced by minority groups (Bennett, 2009). At the time of the publication of the *Delivering Race Equality in Mental Health* plan (DoH, 2005) in conjunction with the independent enquiry into the death of her brother David (Rocky) Bennett, Dr Joanna Bennett made the statement:

> *Let's just get humanity right!*

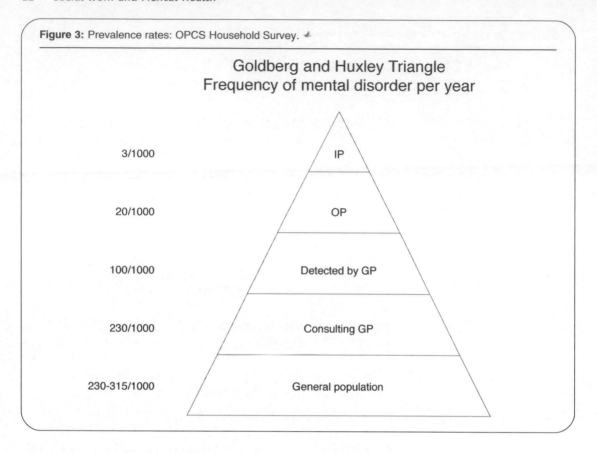

Figure 3: Prevalence rates: OPCS Household Survey.

Goldberg and Huxley Triangle
Frequency of mental disorder per year

3/1000	IP
20/1000	OP
100/1000	Detected by GP
230/1000	Consulting GP
230–315/1000	General population

Incidence of mental illness and mental distress

- One in four people will experience some kind of mental health problem during a year.
- 10 to 25 per cent of the general population seek advice from their GP.
- Two to four per cent of the above will have a severe mental illness, while a smaller number will experience severe and enduring mental illness (see NHSC, 2009).
- Estimates for the latter vary from 0.3 to 1.5 per cent of the population.
- One in ten children has a recognised mental disorder.
- 90 per cent of young offenders and people in prison have mental health needs.

Neuroses

About 10 to 30 per cent of the population suffer from anxiety or depression. It is common to talk very loosely about 'being depressed' these days, but a lowness of mood, stemming from personality type, the organic make-up of the individual, or life pressures or traumas or major changes, can lead on to a clinical condition:

- More than one in ten people are likely to have an anxiety disorder which severely affects their everyday lives, at some stage during their life.
- 13 per cent of the adult population are calculated to experience a phobia, while around 2.5 per cent are likely to have an obsessive compulsive disorder.
- One in ten people are likely to have some form of depression at any one time, while one in twenty people will have a serious or 'clinical depression'.
- Sabba Moussavi's major survey for the World Health Organisation (Moussavi et al., 2007) found that after adjustment for socio-economic factors and health conditions, depression had the largest effect on worsening mean health scores compared with other chronic conditions.

As Lewis Wolpert points out, it is very rare when one gets to know a person that depression has not in some way affected their lives or those closest to them.

Psychoses

Recent Department of Health statistics show an incidence of five to six per thousand, but the number of men from the Afro-Caribbean community who were diagnosed as having a psychosis is much higher. Likewise, the disproportionate use of compulsory orders in relation to young Afro-Caribbean men has been recorded (Cope, 1989). This is still a major issue (see Sewell, 2009; Keating, 2009; Bennett, 2009).

Schizophrenia

Estimates vary from one to four per cent of the population who may experience schizophrenia.

There is a good chance of people making a good recovery with some form of treatment; two thirds may experience repeat episodes with a need for some support from specialist agencies in between; and 10 to 15 per cent will have a severe and enduring mental illness. Early intervention is vital.

Manic depression or bi-polar mood disorder

Approximately one in a hundred adults will experience manic depression. 20 per cent of people who have a first episode do not have another one.

Personality disorder

54 men per 1,000 and 34 women per 1,000 have a personality disorder (of whom a very small percentage may have dangerous behaviours).

Substance misuse

Hazardous drinking (25 per cent) and illicit drug use (five to 15 per cent) are major causes and complications in mental disorder. The current recession is creating pressures on people's lives, with The Times recording that the Audit Commission reports that:

> *Britain faces a surge in drug addiction, alcoholism and domestic violence as the second wave of the recession and rising unemployment take a grip.*
>
> *The Times*, 12 August 2009: 1

Gender differences

Research demonstrates considerable gender differences, but some of these variances may stem as much from presentation and diagnosis as the reality of the illness:

- 18 per cent of women were found to have had a 'neurotic disorder' such as anxiety, depression, phobias and panic attacks, compared with 11 per cent of men (Carlisle, 2009). The gender differences are less apparent in the later stages of middle age, and are reversed in people aged over 55 years.
- Men are three times more likely to have a dependence on alcohol, and twice as likely to be dependent upon drugs.
- Women are more likely to consult their GP while experiencing anxiety, depression or phobias.
- Men tend to experience psychotic illnesses at an earlier stage in their lives. The response to treatment is often poorer, and the incidence of people with severe and enduring mental illness, following a psychotic breakdown, is much higher among men.
- Some ethnic minorities are reluctant to seek professional assistance due to stigma (see Keating, 2009).

Black and ethnic minorities

One of the major issues in this area is that of cultural perception (see Fernando, 1995 and 2007). Afro-Caribbeans are twice as likely as Caucasians to be diagnosed with a mental illness, and are three to five times more likely to be diagnosed and admitted to hospital for schizophrenia.

> *The reality is I see myself as 'normal' but a lot of people don't see me as normal. I see other people who have similar experiences as me but they are not seen as mentally ill . . . I often question if it's my culture, gender and/or age that gets a negative reaction.*
>
> Black service user

Joanna Bennett quotes the Mental Health Act Commission's first one-day census as revealing that African-Caribbean people are three times more likely to be admitted to hospital, and up to 44 per cent more likely to be detailed under mental health legislation. 'Black and mixed heritage service users report a far worse experience of hospital care than other ethnic groups' (Bennett, 2009: 57). This is a growing area of research (see Gupta and Bhugra, 2009).

Case Example 1

Hadley is a young Afro-Caribbean man who suffered his first psychotic episode while a student at university, and was compulsorily admitted to hospital. His mother, sister and extended family have been very supportive of Hadley, but the lack of initial understanding and information about the condition, and concerns about their own safety, meant that by the time of the first hospital admission, relations were extremely strained.

The social worker's involvement came at a time when it looked as though the young man would become increasingly isolated and could become homeless. An appreciation of the social and cultural factors as well as those specific to Hadley's mental illness, meant that the worker was able to increase the tolerance within the family of Hadley's behaviour, help him feel less isolated and stigmatised – the problem had primarily arisen initially due to discrimination he had experienced as a young, black, male, mentally ill student – and secure him appropriate accommodation following good collaboration with housing and welfare rights agencies.

Intensive work, good networking skills, and an ability to understand the complexities of the cultural context, meant that family relationships were repaired and renewed, and that when Hadley experienced periodic recurrences of his illness, services were able to intervene quickly, and in a way acceptable to the user himself.

Stanley and Manthorpe, in their trawl through the mental health enquiry reports, comment that in the case of Christopher Clunis, there was 'a tendency for professionals to resort too readily to the stereotype of the young, black man as a drug abuser in their assessments of him' (see Stanley and Manthorpe, 2001; Ritchie et al., 1994).

Mental health in children and young people

There is increasing concern around the diagnosis of autism and behavioural disorders in children and young people, and also the rise in depressive illnesses at an earlier age. One study found a large number of girls with serious depression who were not in contact with specialist services.

- Ten per cent of children and young people are estimated to have mental health problems that require professional intervention.

Mental health in older people

Mental distress and mental illness is often not well identified by professionals, as it is assumed that the memory, energy and buoyancy of people will decline as they age.

In fact, the situation is very complicated with many older people making use of the time they have to engage in activities they have always wanted to do, travel etc., while at the same time increased social mobility in personal and geographical terms has meant many more people living alone and a long way away from their extended families, often leading to problems of isolation.

- It is estimated that 15 per cent of people over 65 have depression, with an estimated five per cent having severe depression. There is a correlation between depression in older people and living alone.
- Dementia affects one per cent of people between 60 and 65 years, five per cent of people over 65 and 10 to 20 per cent of people over 80 years old.
- Contrary to popular opinion, suicide is a major risk amongst older people, with social isolation being an important factor. Chronic physical conditions can also lead to older people taking their own lives (see Tadros, 2004).

Suicide and mental health

Although the reduction of suicides is a target in the National Service Framework, mental ill-health is not a precondition to committing suicide.

Recently, suicide has moved from being the second most common cause of death amongst under 35 year olds to the most prevalent.

- The numbers of male suicides (and deaths that are undetermined but may be suicide) rose

Figure 4: The numbers of people in different sectors of the mental health service.

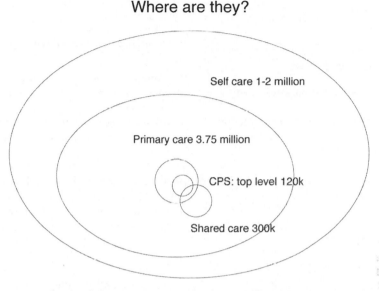

Where are they?

Self care 1-2 million

Primary care 3.75 million

CPS: top level 120k

Shared care 300k

- A quarter of people with 'common' disorders and 85% of those with severe conditions receive treatment

- 630,000 are in daily contact with services

- Between 30-50% of people with severe conditions are only in contact with the GP

sharply between the late 1970s and the 1990s. The NIMHE suicide prevention strategy brought the general suicide rate down to 7.5 per 100,000 of population in 2007 (its lowest recorded level) but the current recession is likely to see an increase in suicides.
- Despite the caveat above, a high proportion of people who take their own life have a mental illness.
- Living circumstances, childhood experiences, social networks, employment and housing are all major determinants.
- Since the 'Credit Crunch' the rate of suicide has risen again.

Health inequalities

- Depression increases the risk of developing heart disease and having strokes.
- It has an adverse effect on outcomes from asthma, arthritis and diabetes.

- In the case of schizophrenia, standard mortality rate (SMR) is twice the average.

Social and economic inequalities

On the whole, people with a mental health need experience a number of social and economic inequalities, some of which may be cause and others effect:

- A higher proportion are separated or divorced and living alone.
- On average, they have fewer educational qualifications.
- They are less likely to own property.
- Psychoses are more prevalent in the inner cities.

Inequalities in the workplace

- Mental ill-health affects approximately one in five workers.

- Six out of every seven people with a severe mental illness are unable to secure work.
- Those who have been diagnosed as having a mental illness experience greater difficulty in getting insurance, pension cover etc.

The costs to the economy

- £11.8 billion is a cost to the nation in lost employment.
- The total cost to the economy is estimated at £77.4 billion, while in 2006 £600 million was spent on medication (Sainsbury Centre for Mental Health, 2003).
- It is estimated that around one third of GPs' time is taken up by mental health problems.

Working in partnership

Mental illness is not a personal failure. In fact, if there is a failure, it is to be found in the way we have responded to people with mental and brain disorders.

WHO, 2001

In Sebastian Faulks' novel *Human Traces*, the psychiatrist Thomas Midwinter is asked by his future wife whether he had ever experienced any of the same symptoms as the patients he treated. Thomas discloses that in adolescence and early adulthood he had heard a voice:

'I have never even told myself about it', said Thomas, 'I have never let it into my conscious mind. It just moved in at that moment, when you asked me.'

'But you were aware of it?'

'I was aware of it very clearly, but only at a certain level of awareness, not at all levels.'

'And you did not question yourself about it?'

'No. It felt like everything that happens to you: it felt like nothing. I discounted it because it had happened to me personally and was therefore valueless. Of no interest.'

Faulks, 2006: 417

Now perhaps attitudes are changing. Increasingly doctors like Cathy Wield in her *Life After Darkness* (Wield, 2006) and Liz Miller, who was a successful surgeon when bipolar disorder hit her (O'Hara, 2008) are talking publicly about their experiences. Miller writes that:

The thing is, in medicine we live on this myth that illness is for other people. Doctors don't get ill. Illness is for the patients. And so I swallowed it – the whole medical thing . . .

In the past, I prided myself on my brain. I could get by on my wits. And suddenly your mind goes, and it actually

gets to the core of who you are. It says something about you as a person. You ask yourself: 'why me?' . . .

Every time I was alone, I wept. The thing about mental illness is the awful isolation. You think you are the only person there. You are so ashamed of it. There's the external stigmatising behaviours from society, but there's also the internal shame. How could you let yourself do this? I was so ashamed.

Personally I have found that disclosing my own experience of mental ill-health in public fora has freed up other people to talk about their issues, and has created a general sense of working in partnership rather than an 'us' and 'them' mentality. The States of Jersey Mental Health Services and the Jersey Mental Health Charity, Jersey Focus for Mental Health, are currently engaged on a service user partnership programme which involves a group of 20 people who are service users or providers, with a significant number with the lived experience of mental distress (see Bolam, Carr and Gilbert, forthcoming).

I recently had the pleasure of being at the graduation ceremony of BA students in social work. It was a particular pleasure to be there this year as one of the students had written to me when she commenced her studies saying that she had felt that, in a state of mental distress at the beginning of the course, perhaps she didn't have a right to be studying social work and experiencing depression. Hearing me speak about my own experience of mental distress in the induction lecture had given her the confidence to continue and complete her studies. As Ian McPherson puts it, his own illness:

. . . gives no unique insights into mental health conditions in general, but, what it has done is allow me to understand what it feels like to be seen as separate, or that person over there with a mental illness.

O'Hara, 2009

Human beings are complicated creatures; and the society we live in is ever more complex. Mental distress is a feature of being human, and at the end of the day we have got to 'get the humanity right'.

Discovery and recovery

We are learning that those of us with psychiatric disabilities can become experts in our own self-care, can regain control over our lives and can be responsible for our own journey of recovery.

Degan, 1992, quoted in Repper and Perkins, 2009

In her recent autobiography of her life and her time at High Royds, Psychiatric Hospital, near Bradford, Jean Davison (2009) describes how in the 1960s she had gone to her GP feeling low in mood and confused about life, perhaps not surprisingly for an 18 year old. Later, seeing a psychiatrist she is admitted as a voluntary patient to the old county asylum. Assessment, and the diagnosis of schizophrenia, has little relevance to the questions around the meanings of life which she is struggling with in late adolescence:

> *I couldn't see the point in taking tablets that made me too tired to talk or do anything. There was so much inside me that needed to come out. I wanted to be understood. I **needed** to talk.*
>
> Davison, 2009: 9

A leader in service user-led research Jan Wallcraft quotes survivor and trainer Ron Coleman as acknowledging that 'the system' cared for him in physical terms, but:

> *The psychiatric system, far from being a sanctuary and a system of healing was . . . a system of fear and continuation of illness for me . . . the system had no expectation of me recovering, instead the emphasis was on maintenance . . . what they did not do was consider the possibility that I could return to being the person I once was.*
>
> Coleman, 1999: 5, quoted in Wallcraft, 2005: 200

The 2007 publication by CSIP, The Royal College of Psychiatrists and SCIE (2007) traces the origins of the recovery movement back to the Quaker inspired Retreat in York at the turn of the 18th century, set up by the Tuke family. The document points out that personal stories alongside more systematic analysis, have been important in developing an approach which fosters hope and a sense of control over our own lives as opposed to mere maintenance, and despair of ever regaining a sense of ourselves. Recounting our own narrative is important for the individual's identity but also a vital part of leadership in developing services (see Chapter 11 in this book). Professor Bill Fulford and Kim Woodbridge and their development of 'values-based practice' (see Fulford and Woodbridge, 2007) stress that services must start where the individual service user is; and that within mental health services, oppression has often happened when providers of services have been absolutely convinced of their own rightness of approach without ascertaining where the person they are meant to be caring for actually is. Like all words 'recovery' can have its meaning twisted. Just as 'personalisation' (see Chapter 6) can denote personal control and choice, it can also point to the state abrogating its responsibility to individual citizens. Recovery can probably best be described as a journey, an ongoing process of discovery and pilgrimage (see Gilbert, Boodhoo and Carr, 2008).

The principles of recovery are around:

- The personal journey.
- Relating to life as a journey, so that recovery is not specific to mental health challenges but is a common human condition – this relates to Paul Keedwell's work on the evolutionary importance of depression (Keedwell, 2008).
- Recovery is not so much an end product or result but a **continuing** journey.
- As building a meaningful and satisfying life as defined by the person themselves (autobiographies such as Davison, 2009, Wield, 2006 and Jamison, 1997 aid our understanding here). It is not a professional intervention and can and does occur without professional interventions, but to do with taking back control of our lives. Governments talk about choice, but often people are confused by an overemphasis on choice, and what they are asking for is a sense of control.
- A partnership between service users and service providers (see Wallcraft, 2005; Repper and Perkins, 2009; SPN, 2007; Fisher, 2008).

Wallcraft's research into the factors which help recovery does not throw up any surprises. They are the factors that usually help us to find a satisfying life. Positive relationships; employment which is satisfying and provides financial security; being able to grow and develop; a reasonable place to live; discovering the treatments and therapies that suit oneself; having the confidence to return to helpful professionals when a crisis recurs; developing one's cultural and/or spiritual perspective (Wallcraft, 2005: 207).

There has been a danger throughout the history of mental health services, that professionals 'colonise' the approaches which service users and carers value. The over-professionalisation of human relationships (see Perkins, 2008) and the medicalisation of the human emotions which occur throughout life, can increase our dependence on the system. We need to rekindle a beacon of hope.

CHAPTER 2

Thinking About Professional Boundaries in an Inclusive Society

Peter Bates

Introduction

In this chapter, the terms 'person' and people' will generally be used in place of terms like 'client', 'patient' or 'service user'. Other people will be identified by their designation. Thus, the professional relationship exists between the 'person and the worker'. Mental health services exist at the confluence of many competing forces, values and ideologies. For social workers, one such junction occurs when attempts to 'fix the person' by offering talking therapies meet efforts to 'fix the community' by negotiating respectful, fair access to a job, a home and a social life. At the same crossroads, concerns about self-determination meet safeguarding obligations. Social workers who have trained in therapeutic interventions meet their colleagues who are drawing on the profession's community development roots to assist employers, educators and leisure providers to respond positively to people with mental health difficulties. The crossing-point is noisy with social work talk about recovery and the clamour that ensues when something goes wrong.

Elsewhere, I have set out some of the basic skills that social work staff need to promote recovery and inclusion (NSIP, 2007; Bates, 2008) and so this chapter considers safeguarding in the context of community life. All too often, the risk assessment process suggests a deterministic universe and an atomised society in which the behaviour of individuals is as predictable as that of snooker balls. Here we glimpse an altogether more complex and fascinating world. In particular, we explore the role of the professional and the implications for socially inclusive practice and our understanding of, and participation in, the wider community.

The chapter is divided into six sections, each of which explores a pair of competing priorities. These are set in opposition to one another to form the 12-point *Boundary Clock* (Figure 5). All metaphors have limited value and can carry unwanted freight. This clock has no hands, no

power source, no machinery – it is simply a face with 12 observation points. The image of a 12-person jury might work just as well, although it suggests crime and punishment. Individual case studies can then be placed on the 'clockface' and the 12 vantage points used in turn to generate ideas for shaping practice in an individual situation. As each of the 12 is merely an entry point to the clockface area, the issues that arise inevitably overlap here and there, but the 12 points frame a systematic discussion. We begin with the 12 o'clock and 6 o'clock pair and then move clockwise.

Artificial and single versus natural and multiple

Maintaining professional distance is rather like bottling a vacuum

In recent decades, psychoanalytic traditions which assert that the worker has a responsibility to maintain 'professional distance' from the person have ballooned to encompass all professional groups in any kind of contact, including social work. As a result, some workers withhold information about their personal lives or home. This allows the social worker to enjoy off-duty time in a different social setting, keeps professional status untarnished by any awkward leakage of personal information, and improves safety for the worker and their family in the event that the person feels aggrieved. The single-strand relationship helps to keep transactions between the person and the worker free of distortion.

Q1: Is guidance available from your professional body or employer that directs you in how to respond to the potential of a dual relationship? If this guidance is not routinely followed in your service, how should you deal with this?

This type of relationship is deliberately unlike a natural friendship. It does not follow the usual

Figure 5: The boundaries clock

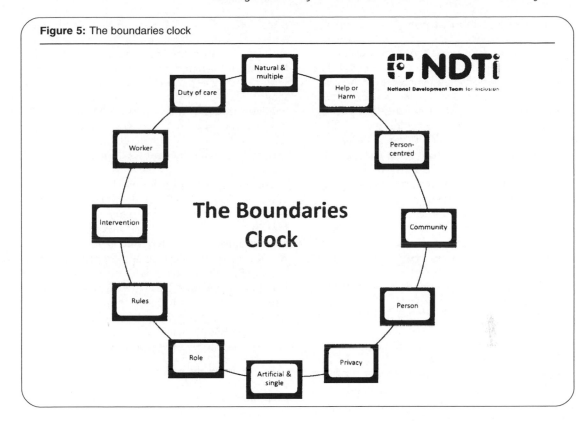

rules in which shared activity leads to gradual, mutual disclosure, but rather is an artificial, single-strand transaction.

Whilst the 'artificial and single' position is neat, it is often problematic:

- Social workers serving in isolated rural communities or working with minority groups are very likely to have a dual relationship through sharing a place of worship, neighbourhood or cultural centre.
- Forward-looking mental health services are deliberately employing substantial numbers of people who have used services themselves (Seebohm and Grove, 2006) and so professional-client relationships are jumbled up with co-worker relationships.
- The UK policy of Personalisation (HM Government, 2007) has increased the number of people who employ their own social care staff as personal assistants or brokers, blending the professional-client relationship with employer-employee relationships.
- Neighbours with shared concerns about their environment form community enterprises and

projects to improve things, and these activities may throw together social workers and their clients as co producers of a cohesive society.
- Since 2004, English mental health policy (ODPM, 2004) promotes socially inclusive lifestyles and so increases the chances that staff will introduce people to social environments that they themselves use when off-duty.

Several traditions within social work, mental health and elsewhere positively affirm the development of natural and multiple relationships, or what some authors (Galbreath, 2005) have called dual relationships. This term is sometimes used in a narrow way to refer to sexual relationships between staff and the people they support. Here it is used generically. Social work was born in the settlement movement where workers lived alongside those they helped, community development workers immerse themselves in their patch, anthropologists live in the communities they study; researchers with lived experience of mental health difficulties gather good data precisely because they disclose their shared history in the interview context; peer support workers find that people with mental health issues make a better recovery because they meet staff who have made the same journey themselves. Indeed, several authors suggest that multistrand relationships may increase the efficacy of therapy (Lazarus and Zur, 2002; Gabriel, 2005). Rather than pessimistically expecting social workers to exploit the vulnerability of the people they are paid to support, such options thread safeguarding through these multi-layered relationships.

Social workers and the agencies that employ them need to position their practice on the *Boundaries Clock* between these two viewpoints.

Help or harm versus role

Josie wanted to volunteer and asked for someone to accompany her the first time. When her social worker mentioned it to the team manager, she was refused permission and told it was not her role.

Many people enter social work to help others. Three forces threaten this ambition: restructuring of services has left many social workers assessing (eligibility, risk, service quality, outcomes) rather than providing help; as the years go by, people sometimes forget why they came into the business in the first place as bureaucratic demands, pressure of work and career aspirations take over from compassion; and thirdly, working out what is helpful in the long run is both complex and ambiguous.

Take, for example, Josie's basic need for support. Was there anybody else in the team who could accompany her? Will Josie expect the worker to accompany her every week? Does the shared activity symbolise a change in the nature of the relationship with the worker? It is not always easy to know whether our help will turn out in the end to cause harm.

Defining harm can be difficult too. Mental health social workers deprive people of their liberty, curtail help in order to promote independence and refuse to help some in order to release scarce resources for others. Some people report that they only got started on their personal recovery journey when they gave up their reliance on helpers and took some personal responsibility. Withdrawing help may be the only way to persuade some people to reconnect with their community-based roles and relationships.

On the opposite side of the *Boundaries Clock* lie a number of issues that are related to the worker's

role. Here we ask what is appropriate for someone in this job role to do. We are rightly concerned with power being abused, intentions being misinterpreted, with setting a precedent, with changing expectations, and with what others may think. Word may get out that workers are available in the evenings for social engagements, but Josie's worker may also worry whether going along the first time will help in the long run, or fear that others in her team will question her actions.

The literature on professional boundaries (Pope and Keith-Spiegel, 2008) refers to the 'slippery slope' by which staff unwittingly slide from informal acts of kindness into favouritism, over-disclosure, exclusive friendship and sexual relationships. The slope image suggests helpless inevitability rather than responsibility, and has led some agencies to ban trivial actions in an effort to prevent slippage. So, in Josie's case, going to the voluntary work site could lead in time to undue intimacy and abuse of power, and so it is safest to ban it – just in case.

Q2: Do your supervision sessions and staff meetings provide opportunities to discuss boundary crossings, admit mistakes, find creative solutions and celebrate success?

Whilst some staff find relief in receiving and obeying clear messages about the limits of their role, others include many hidden acts of kindness in their day to day work (Freud and Krug, 2002). In this complex arena, some clarity about the appropriate use of the social work role and the kind of help that a social worker can offer saves time and helps with the appropriate use of limited resources.

Person-centred versus rules

We got a memo round telling us not to kiss clients!

As the first decade of the 21st century draws to a close, English social work is in turbulent waters. The government's personalisation agenda has brought social care to the brink of its biggest change since the introduction of the Welfare State, and meanwhile, the twin concerns about safeguarding vulnerable people and holding staff to account for their productivity have substantially increased the rules. Whilst personalisation should open up more room for creative responses that fit the individual, some workers are reporting that anything up to 90 per cent of their time is spent at the computer and in meetings, rather than face to face with people in need.

In mental health, the growing adoption of recovery as an organising concept for services has focused attention on personal meaning, self-directed support and advance directives, all of which reinforce the primacy of each person's idea of what 'wellness' or 'flourishing' means for them. Similarly, some services are exploring how well-being, social inclusion and community engagement could reshape their provision, and this has the potential to take services further into person-centred approaches. Government promotion of personal budgets is one aspect of this, as more and more people take up the offer of funding to arrange their own support and buy whatever will work for them.

Q3: How do your rules change if the person is in crisis, in 24 hour care, is especially vulnerable, poses additional risks or is discharged from your service? How do the rules apply to staff who are off-duty, to volunteers, students, or to colleagues who work in another team or in the administration department?

Opposing person-centred approaches – on the other side of the *Boundaries Clock* – lie rules. The Sexual Offences Act 2003 prohibits sexual relationships between people who are unable to give consent and the staff who support them, and a vast amount of the literature on professional boundaries has been devoted to preventing this abuse. Rules about confidentiality, gifts, handling money or medication have protected people from accident, exploitation or accusation. Indeed, the careful analysis of issues that is explained as well-made rules are introduced helps the individual social worker to apply rigour to their response to individual situations.

Sadly, not all actions labelled 'person-centred' are truly individualised, and not all rules are well-made. Custom and habit narrow the spectrum of options under consideration, and rules overreach their designated field until what works in one place is forced into others, where the fit is poor and staff feel straitjacketed. Did the regulator wish to ban erotic kissing or habitual greetings in the French community? Was one person's inappropriate conduct managed by producing a rule for all – a common but cowardly response that sidesteps the uncomfortable issue of challenging the individual.

The interaction between person-centred approaches and rules is perhaps at its sharpest as people move away from the control of the mental health system. Rules that are entirely appropriate within the secure forensic inpatient setting, for example, need to be gradually relaxed as people are supported to move out into community living and learn to cope with its demands. One such inpatient environment has a ban on access to the internet that prevents people with predatory sexual appetites from viewing unsuitable material. Unfortunately, this rule is inflexible and applies to everyone, and so rehabilitation staff fear that they will be punished if they assist people to visit an internet cafe, purchase a personal computer or attend the college library. For the people concerned, their inclusion in modern society and prospects for community living, and therefore the long-term safety of all, are compromised.

Community versus intervention

After 20 years using mental health services, they have employed me. The job is great, but, just because I now get to be called 'staff' and they are 'service users', I am expected to finish with all my old friends.

At their best, communities have their own ways of keeping everyone safe and balancing individual freedom and corporate responsibility. Take, for example, the success of the Circles of Accountability pioneered by the Mennonite church in Canada. They offer friendship and informal support to notorious sex offenders after their discharge from prison. The Circle's uncompromising approach to information-sharing and zero tolerance of re-offending is maintained alongside the offer of companionship and community participation, so that ex-offenders do not have to hide their history or remain isolated and under-occupied. They have taken the general statement that bored, isolated, excluded and vulnerable people with few positive social roles are at most risk and most risky (DoH, 2008) – and turned the diagnosis into a prescription for informal, powerful community action.

In general, large, diverse and interlinked networks improve quality of life and protect people from abuse through well-meaning conversation, mutual support and advocacy (Pugh, 2007). For example, recent research on hate crimes against people with disabilities, makes a very powerful plea for community empowerment to have a safeguarding focus integrated within it (Home Office, 2008).

But until recently, mental health services have paid insufficient attention to people's community roles and relationships. All too often, admission to inpatient psychiatric care wreaks havoc to role and relationship networks, as people lose their jobs, marriage and friends that could have been retained if the service just paid some more attention to these matters. The day to day ways in which mental health services are delivered increase the strain on community roles as people have to take time off work to attend outpatient appointments and are encouraged to join the mental health community at the expense of their other connections.

Along with the undoubted benefits of personalisation comes the risk that informal relationships will be colonised and disrupted, as people invite their friends to become their paid assistants. Both the person and their new assistant can forfeit forever the elusive benefit that comes from those people who freely choose to be in their lives rather than being there by contractual obligation. Or perhaps, after all, it is possible to maintain a friendship whilst also being paid. If this is so, then the traditional argument that social workers need to avoid any social contact with the people they support is also defeated and we need to move on to a new discourse about how to deliver safe and effective interventions to people with whom we share common citizenship.

Opposing this point on the *Boundaries Clock* sits the value of a deliberate social work intervention. Creating a respectful, confidential and empowering relationship with someone who has learnt to mistrust authority figures or who is experiencing high levels of suspicion or social anxiety demands a high level of skill and it can be vital to set aside complicating factors to make enough space for the work to be done.

Q4: How does the relationship between the social worker and the person change as they move away from the 'counselling room' intervention, into informal contacts in the corridor, casual greetings in the street and shared participation in community life?

The forces that oppose each other on this aspect of the clock face are to do with emphasis and priority. When someone is lonely and the social worker suggests that they join a group provided by the mental health service, they have selected an intervention option in contrast with the community alternative of assisting the person to find a friendship circle outside the mental health service. When someone needs support to attend the gym and the service considers a personal assistant rather than asking about current or potential friends, fitness instructors at the gym or fellow-members of the running club, they have chosen an intervention option rather than a community option.

Perhaps most importantly, whenever the mental health service writes a risk management protocol that applies to its own activities and staff but that offers no framework for how to negotiate that risk with the gym staff or with friends, they direct staff towards an intervention rather than a community solution.

Person versus worker

During a training course on safeguarding, staff were instructed how to behave when off duty, such as when in the pub with friends. If a person came in who used the mental health service, staff were told that they should leave the building immediately.

One of the distinguishing marks of a professional helping relationship is that it is generally one-way. The worker is there for the person's benefit, and not the other way round. For social workers, the focus is often on particular kinds of benefit, such as when the worker assesses mental illness or capacity. Social care workers often have a broader remit and find themselves assisting, not just with care and support, but social interaction, hobbies and interests. But the time is still for the person rather than for themselves. It has been suggested that workers who have a rich and satisfying personal life are less likely to bring their own needs forward in their encounters with the people they support.

Q5: Judgements about professional boundaries, safeguarding and a life in the community are smarter when the person's viewpoint is in the centre. What have you done to ensure that they take the lead in maintaining an appropriate relationship?

Workers have rights too. Staff should not find themselves excluded from their own leisure venues by Draconian regulations, as in the example above. Care workers often wonder if they have a right of veto should the person they are supporting wish to undertake activities that they themselves would not select, whether it is assisting people to overeat or smoke, obtain pornography or join an extreme political party. The worker's rights are recognised on the Boundaries Clock.

Between the two extremes lie many subtleties:

- The social worker who occasionally discloses personal matters models the to and fro of ordinary conversation, slows the process by which continuous receiving of help can lead to unhealthy self-absorption and raises hope levels (Psychopathology Committee, 2001).
- The worker who invites people to social activities that they themselves are involved in may abuse their power to further their own personal, religious, political, business or social interests – but banning these connections closes off whole sections of community life to people who need support to participate.
- Whilst 'it is never appropriate to terminate a therapeutic relationship with the intention of pursuing a social or sexual relationship' (CHRE, 2008) staff may be quite willing to disclose information about their personal experiences or share off-duty leisure activities with the people they support – or they may prefer to maintain their personal privacy.

In deciding the right course of action for a service or with an individual, these competing needs should be acknowledged.

Duty of care versus privacy

When we arrive at work each day, we have to record every contact we had whilst we were off-duty with anyone who uses mental health services.

In order to keep everyone safe, it is sometimes necessary for social workers to use the Mental Health Act or the Mental Capacity Act to take action that over-rides the person's preferences. Mechanisms that restrict the opportunities available to certain offenders and the limits of the principle of confidentiality add to the duty of care that social workers must exercise in order to keep both the person and the community safe in the long term. In the example above, it is easy to imagine circumstances where a particular 'sighting' would quite properly be reported and action taken. Perhaps the person has a typical pattern of relapse in which a period of flamboyant disinhibition with strangers (seen by the worker on this occasion) is usually followed

by taking irresponsible risks with traffic, and, in this circumstance, prompt action would clearly be indicated.

Duty of care is not always played out in consistent ways. In one circumstance, the hospital accident and emergency team provided assistance to someone who admitted to carrying a weapon, and who said that they would feel entirely justified in using it if anyone caused them any trouble. The hospital staff notified the person's GP that the person rarely visited, feeling a duty of care to their health colleagues, but did not speak to the college that the person attended five days a week.

Q6: How should information pass between the mental health service and community organisations – the university, an employer, the local darts team or faith-based group? Consider the potential for two-way flow of information.

In general, English information-sharing protocols for social care have been negotiated with the 'usual suspects' – police, schools, health, criminal justice – but do not address the ways in which information might be appropriately shared with the person's employer, family, friends or social club. It is certainly easier to strike a deal with large, monolithic organisations that have similar sanctions against staff who misuse information, but keeping people safe in an inclusive world demands meaningful connections with the plethora of formal and informal groups and organisations that make up society.

Across the clock face lies the range of human rights that we condense here to the single word 'privacy'. The Human Rights Act enshrines in law the person's right to run their own life, participate in the community and build a home free from surveillance or interference from the state. The person can refuse medical treatment and has a right to see any records kept about them, which should only be made if they are necessary and proportionate. The state can only get involved to 'assist in diagnosis and treatment or to protect health, morals or the safety and freedom of others', and this involvement needs to be individual, proportionate and the least intrusive option.

In the example given at the top of this section, the local policy to record every contact with everyone using the service was not individual, proportionate, least intrusive or necessary for diagnosis, treatment or safeguarding. If people are told that staff are routinely using all informal and off-duty contacts as an added surveillance platform, or they read in their records that this has been taking place, then it is likely to influence their selection of social environment, and even communicate a message that the community 'belongs' to staff. Meanwhile, staff are never allowed to be off-duty. This is a very different situation from the off-duty worker who freely chooses to serve as a formal volunteer, who spontaneously assists a homeless person in the street, or who reports their concern about child abuse next door.

Conclusion

The *Boundaries Clock* reveals weaknesses in the policies of many social work employing organisations (Doel et al., 2009). It does not provide easy answers, but rather offers a framework for reviewing a wide range of issues that ultimately influence the shared citizenship of the worker and the person. Individual circumstances can be placed on the clock face and then – through discussion with the person, their family and friends, colleagues from social work and other disciplines, and reference to guidance from professional bodies and elsewhere – a judgement can be taken in the light of all 12 viewpoints. The outcome will influence the opportunities open to individuals to retain or recover their place in a diverse and cohesive community.

CHAPTER 3

The Roots of Social Policy

Peter Gilbert

It's about people who happen to use mental health services being treated as people.

New Horizons, DoH, 2009

At the beginning of the twenty-first century theoretical debates and political disagreements remain at the centre of discussion about the way that social policy should be developed, and these are underpinned by ideologies of welfare that provide very different understandings of the ways in which welfare and well-being should be identified and addressed within modern society.

Alcock, 2008: 183

Margaret Thatcher's well-known, and oft-quoted comment that there is no such thing as society, strikes at the heart of all we know about how individuals, families, neighbourhoods, groups, communities and nations work, and have worked, throughout history.

The striking and potent photo exhibition: *One in Four*, part of the Department of Health's 'Mind Out for Mental Health' campaign (February 2002) where public figures have 'come out' and spoken about their episodes of mental distress, speaks volumes about them as people, about changing attitudes to mental health, but also the enduring suspicion of and perceived shame of mental ill-health.

I've suffered from depression all my life . . . The real big one happened about thirty years ago when I suddenly started to lose confidence in my abilities as an actor and as a consequence, gave up the business. Then my daughter was born and it got much, much worse. I had agoraphobia and claustrophobia and couldn't even get out of the door to go shopping . . . There wasn't really anyone there for me at that time. It wasn't so much a lack of sympathy as a lack of understanding . . . After about a year, I remember waking up one morning and thinking 'I can't stand living in this circumscribed way any longer' so I threw the pills down the loo and ran round the block out of frustration and rage. It was the start to getting better and getting back to work.

actress, Stephanie Cole, Mental Health Today, March 2002

I have recently been undertaking some independent work with voluntary organisations on an island community. Service users made it clear that stigma was a major issue within the restricted population, where it was felt people had access to knowledge about other people's business more readily. Sometimes, small can be 'claustrophobic' as well as 'beautiful'! On the other hand, the island had many advantages. A unique system of government, laws, social institutions, welfare and culture, where policy and legislation can be influenced by a wide range of opinion-formers in an inclusive way, which is much more difficult in a larger nation state.

The size and sense of identity on the island means that its service delivery in all the areas essential to well-being: employment, housing, leisure, social groups, faith communities etc., can be worked upon in such a way that front line service delivery is sensitised to the needs of vulnerable people (see Bolam, Carr and Gilbert, 2010).

I quite agree that influencing what they call 'the top people' is the first step to make things work for you, but it's no good if that change of heart doesn't reach down to the people you meet face-to-face.

service user talking about welfare benefits

It is even more essential that professionals and professional bodies work creatively and harmoniously together. Significantly, the island has brought health and social care together in one agency, with the Community Division clearly determined to encapsulate a social perspective.

Stigma

Societies, their proportions, identity, history, culture and values, clearly influence how the most vulnerable citizens (and whether the society regards particular groups as fellow citizens at all is crucial here) are regarded and related to; and, as Mahatma Gandhi stated 'A civilisation or society must be judged by the care it gives to its weakest and most under-privileged members' (quoted in Gilbert and Scragg, 1992).

The late Roy Porter, the social historian, in his book: *Madness: A Brief History* (Porter, 2002: 62–3) revisits Irving Goffman (Goffman, 1970) who spoke about stigma as the creation of 'spoiled identity' and the disqualification of persons from full social acceptance.

Individual and groups partake of this stigmatisation because:

- Our insecurities demand we distance ourselves from those who are different from us: health (physical or mental), race, colour, creed, foreign nationals, gay/straight, outsiders etc.
- Placing some people into a metaphysical 'ghetto' makes us feel as though we are whole, the 'in crowd', secure, successful etc.

The American novelist, Ursula Le Guin, has a beautifully wry look at these issues in her short story, *S.Q.*, where an American government takes the advice of an influential psychologist and introduces a 'sanity quotient'. Very soon, far more people are in the institutional camps, for those who have 'failed' the sanity quotient, than are outside it! At the end of the novel, the psychologist himself is committed and his personal assistant runs America single-handed! (Le Guin, 1984).

Porter's work demonstrates the effect of societal perceptions and values on how people with a mental illness are responded to, and that a traditional, progressive ('Whiggish') approach to history is far too sanguine. Kathleen Jones, in her seminal work: *A History of the Mental Health Services*, writes that:

> It is important to recognise that the way in which the mentally ill ... are defined and cared for is primarily a social response to a very basic set of human problems ... How do we define (mental health)? What forms of care should the community provide? Who should be responsible for administering them? What is liberty, and how can it best be safeguarded? All societies have these problems. How they answer them depends on what they are, and the *values* they hold.
>
> Jones, 1972: xiii (my emphasis)

Historical trends

History is not a fashionable subject but it is a vital way of identifying patterns, themes and cycles of social activity. In Britain there could be said to be five common strands to the responses to the challenges which human groups face:

- Some balance of public and private provision is normally to be found.
- There are compromises as to whether the services are organised centrally or at a more local level.
- There are constant debates as to whether treatments should be delivered personally, at

home for instance, or whether recipients should be treated in institutions.
- Whether there are likewise decisions to be made about making provision in cash or kind.
- The liberty of the individual versus their safety and that of the public is a constant issue.
adapted from Midwinter, 1994

It is well worth keeping these things in mind as public policy in Britain tends to oscillate abruptly between extremes.

Public versus private

The legislation introduced by the Earl of Shaftesbury in the mid 19th century was partly as a reaction to the abuses of the private madhouses (see Parry-Jones, 1972) but the county asylums moved from being, as Jones wrote, 'the system to the System' (Jones, 1972: xii). The dead hand of an overwhelming public monopoly, with minimal oversight and support, spawned as many problems as it solved. Autobiographies such as Jean Davison's (2009) and novels like Sebastian Barry's *The Secret Scripture* (Barry, 2008) capture the tendency of human services to revert to an institutional approach (see Diagram 11 in Chapter 4).

The current political battles over the mixed economy are in part a reaction to the American-style laissez-faire economics of the 1980s, as exemplified in the struggle President Obama is having to get his healthcare bill through Congress.

Central versus local

Health and social care are prime examples of the tendency to gyrate between control from the centre, with clarity of direction, but loss of local initiative; and local autonomy and specificity , which can result in the 'post code lottery' often complained about by public and politicians alike.

When Aneurin Bevan launched the new National Health Service in 1948, he remarked that if a bedpan fell on a hospital floor the noise would resound in the Palace of Westminster (Jenkins, 1996). A later Secretary of State for Health, proclaimed, somewhat differently:

> I do not believe a million strong services can be run from Whitehall. Half a century of experience shows us that this approach limits local leadership and stifles local initiative ... Where our first term in office was concerned with

putting a national framework in place, this second term is about introducing new incentives, encouraging greater local innovation and stimulating more patient choice.
speech to the Allied Health professions and Health Care scientists, National Leadership Conference, 13 March 2002

The move towards 'Foundation Trust' status denotes increasing independence for providers of healthcare. But, battles between the Department of Health and Monitor (the Foundation regulator) in 2009 demonstrate that central/local tensions are still evident. The childcare crisis around the death of 'Baby Peter' in Haringey, and the Mid Staffordshire General Hospital scandal, both in 2009, show that when local problems arise there is a call for more central control.

Local authority social services are much more likely to be framed by local choices, driven by political or interest group decisions. Reviews and inspections often find considerable response to locally expressed need, but the downside is that citizens who move from the city of 'Seamouth' to the market town of 'Blankton' cannot understand why the range and depth of services is so different in the two local authorities.

National Service frameworks; the infrastructure of new national institutions for regulation and quality improvement (especially those with local centres) and the development of major charitable policy institutes, bring with them a chance that the pendulum will cease to oscillate so violently and a balance between national strategy and local innovation and responsiveness can be accomplished.

Treatment at home or in institutions

It would seem axiomatic to state that the former is now the dominant paradigm. The 'Personalisation' agenda, the Recovery movement and the roll out of *New Horizons* should see an accent on more user choice and control and early intervention. But, as Sarah Carr points out in Chapter 6, there are tensions inherent in the new approach (see Dowson and Greig, 2009).

All the evidence points to a need to support, sustain and improve people's living and social skills in the environments in which they live, but there are always financial and other incentives, and societal pressures, which have led by example to an increase in the number of looked-after children and in some areas a decline in home care, as opposed to the residential solutions, in the care of older people, including

those with mental health needs (evidenced by the Audit Commission to the Commons Health Select Committee, 2002).

In Mental Health, much of the investment in the old county asylum/psychiatric hospitals, which as historians have pointed out was a major capital and revenue commitment, were siphoned off into other NHS services or savings, which has left the public often suspicious of community-based solutions. 'Care in the Community' became a term to denote neglect rather than care in all the TV soaps during the 1990s. But when the then Secretary of State for Health announced that community care had failed, many would say that it had never been tried! There is a chance now to turn the concept into reality.

Social work is the profession which looks at the individual in their family and social environment and tries to marshal the resources in those communities to meet the needs of the individual.
mental health services manager

Social work is about people and the identification of the areas which impact on their ability to lead an ordinary life despite their illness.
social worker in mental health services

Cash versus kind

The legislation and policy guidance around direct payments and personalisation in all its forms (see Chapter 6 in this book) is the latest version of this theme, with its aim to empower those who need services to decide and purchase for their specific requirements.

Information on welfare rights is one of the main issues on which service users' value social work assistance (see Macdonald and Sheldon, 1997).

Liberty versus safety

The philosophical basis of English jurisprudence places a very high emphasis on the liberty of the individual citizen. Philosophical writing such as that of Locke on liberty, is however, counterbalanced by Hobbes, who argued for a ceding of some freedom of the individual into the power of the state in order to secure their individual and collective safety.

Mental Health is an area where the dichotomy between liberty and safety is most keenly felt. Again, Jones's work is particularly helpful here in

Figure 6: An historical path – local authority responsibilities.

Monasteries and leper hospitals: the first welfare state

1325   *De Praerogativa Regis*
Edward II's law distinguished between people with a mental illness and learning disabilities. It legislated for protection of property and 'to provide for their necessities'.

1388   Poor Law
Distinction between vagrants and those who were physically or mentally incapable.

Acts of 1531 and 1536
Towns and Parishes to procure alms ' . . in such good and discreet ways for the poor, impotent, lame, feeble, sick or disfigured people, being not able to work, may be provided, helped and relieved'.

1563   Compulsory poor rates.

1601   Elizabethan poor law
• Definition of County/Parish administration
• Deterents against 'sturdy beggars'
• Compassion for those unable to fend for themselves
• Workhouses

Seesaw between 'outdoor relief' and institutional care and control

1774   Act regulating private madhouses

18th/19th Centuries: industrial revolution
Community dislocation
Cycles of unemployment: strain on social systems

1782   Gilbert's Act – Unions of parishes
Professional 'guardians'

1798   Speenhamland System of outdoor relief

1808   Country Asylum Act: growth of major institutions

1834   Poor Law Amendment Act
• Interaction between central and local government
• Workhouse test of 'less eligibility'
• Workhouse: better clarification but move from refuge to house of correction.

1870s   Onwards
LAs in forefront of care of vulnerable people, education and community health services

1960s   Onwards
Move away from institutions to community care.

1970s   Formation of LA Social Services Departments.

2000+   Childrens and Adult Services separated – and then rejoined?

demonstrating how political campaigns, cause célèbres, literature, philosophical thought and financial considerations shape law and practice not in a straight line but rather a series of overlapping circles!

The pendulum is still swinging with the concerns over the diagnosis of dangerous people with severe personality disorders having influenced, some would say over-influenced, the work towards the reframing of the 1983 Mental Health Act in 2007 (see Stanley and Manthorpe, 2001, and the Sainsbury Centre for Mental Health Executive Briefing No. 14, March 2001, and Chapter 8 in this book).

Defining community

Lastly in this section, it is vital that we are very careful in our definitions of 'Community'. Words and concepts tend to have a time-limited and limiting lifespan. A word is used, and indeed often overused, because it has a positive 'feel' to it, and promoted because it can be spoken of almost as a 'good' in itself. Because of lack of definition, and over-utilisation, the word then falls into desuetude or disgrace. Community, especially in the phrase 'Care in the Community' has attracted this special status, and then the resulting opprobrium.

This has most unfortunate consequences because community and its companion words: common (as in the common good), communion, communication, commonwealth etc., have a strong provenance in English language and practical philosophy, and we don't actually have anything better to denote what we mean by groups of people bound together by some form of common interest (see below).

With the growth of communitarian ideas, and a belief that in aspects of education, crime and disorder and the care of vulnerable people, positive communities play a vital part in balancing the interests of individuals, groups and the state at large (see Gilbert and Parkes, forthcoming).

In Peter Bates' ground-breaking publication, *Working for Inclusion* (Bates, 2002, see also Bates in Chapter 2 of this book) Alyson McCollam and Julia White give the following definitions of community:

- Communities based on geographical areas or neighbourhoods where people live.

- Communities which centre on shared interest or identity (ethnicity, sexuality, faith etc.).
- Areas of shared experiences and feelings leading to 'a sense of community', in addition to the social networks and patterns of behaviour that sustain them.
- Fellowship of interests e.g. those of intellect, philosophy, faith or profession, which reach across geographical boundaries.

Issues that remain are:

- Communities that are created for administrative convenience may receive very little ownership from the citizens they exist to serve. Examples of this would be some of the local authority areas such as Cleveland and Avon, set up in the 1970s and since dismantled under the last round of local government reorganisation. Primary care groups in county areas, which served groups of people around district council boundaries, have since been absorbed into primary care trusts, serving much larger areas, akin to the old district health authority areas, and may now have more clout but less ownership.
- Choice versus ascribed belonging: people may decide to be part of a community. McCollam and White point out that people with mental health needs are increasingly regarded as part of the wider disability movement but may not perceive themselves as such.
- *Being* in a community versus *being active* in a community: people who live in an area do not necessarily wish to become active. On the other hand, someone who joins a local pressure group, political party etc., may do so in order to campaign on a specific issue or issues.
- The 'acculturative stress' (Khan and Waheed, 2009) experienced by many people moving between communities and cultures.
- Positive groups have their dysfunctional counterpart in gangs. Because human beings are ultra-social animals the social aspect can act for good or ill.

Events in Northern Ireland, especially those recent happenings in West Belfast around access to schools, and the riots in Oldham and Bradford should caution us as to any romanticised notion of community. Communities can be mutually antagonistic towards each other and can also be closed as well as open and inclusive. 'A distinguishing feature may be the extent to which communities can combine a capacity to maintain

Figure 7: Care in the community and community care.

Care in the Community

Concern over private madhouses

Issues of liberty/treatment/safety

1808 County Asylum Act

1845 Lunatics Act
      Appointment of lunacy commissioners

1900s Eugenics movement

1930 Mental Health Treatment Act

1955 Onwards • Reduction in in-patient beds
              • Rehab policy
              • New drugs
              • Reaction against institutions
              • Cost saving/cost shunting

1959 Mental Health Act

1961 Enoch Powell's speech on closing institutions

1975 White Paper 'Better Services'

1983 Mental Health Act

Late 1980s - Pendulum swings back
             to care and safety issues

1994 Ritchie Report (Clunis)

1996 Mental Health (Patients in the
     Community) Act 1995

Concerns over dangerous people with
      severe personality disorder

2000 White Paper on reform of the 1983
     Mental Health Act

Community care

1948 National Assistance Act

1979 Incentives to enter private residential care

1986 Audit Commission Report

1988 'Agenda for Action' (Griffiths)

1989 White Paper 'Caring for People'

1900 (1993) NHS and CC Act

'Needs led' vs. 'scarce resources'

1995 (1996) Carers (Recognition and
             Services) Act

1996 Eligibility criteria on continuing
     health care

1996 Community Care (Direct Payments) Act

Disparities in N.H.S./social care funding

Decline in residential and nursing care
        provision

'Care in collision?'
• Public concerns
• Structural changes
• New infrastructure and increasing resources -
but building on uncertain foundations

internal cohesion with a capacity to be outward looking and sustain links that can reach outside' (McCollam and White, in Bates, 2002).

It is also worth defining the two major uses of 'community' in recent Social and Health Care policy:

- **Community Care** – means planning and providing the services and support which people who are affected by challenges of ageing, mental illness, learning disability or physical/sensory disability need to be able to live as independently as possible in their own homes, or in 'homely' settings in the community, through the operation of the *National Health Service and Community Care Act 1990* (implemented 1st April 1993).

- **Care in the community** – the movement of vulnerable adults from long-stay institutions to services – or an absence of services – in community settings. This policy commenced with legislation such as the *1959 Mental Health Act* and the new direction on care given by the Ministry of Health in 1961/62.

I started the chapter with the famous quotation from Margaret Thatcher. In the autumn of 2002, the Conservative Party rode back from this proposition and declared that there is indeed an entity called 'society'. Recent pronouncements in fact express concern about a 'broken society'.

Images of deviance and difference; policy and legislation; models of care; community relationships, don't take place in a vacuum. Individual health and well-being takes place within a wider context in which we are all a part. As Plato pointed out, at a time when humankind was attempting to define civil and civilised life, there is an inner principle, a goal of social and individual life working itself out in society.

CHAPTER 4

Mental Health – At the Heart of Reform

Michael Clark and Peter Gilbert

By 2015, mental well-being will be a concern of all public services.

SCMH and partner agencies, 2006

Mental health: a priority

Drivers for change come from coalitions of implementers of power who recognise and express dissatisfaction with the status quo. Concern over the abuses in private 'madhouses' created the impetus to commence the tide of reforming legislation in the 19th century. The failures of the British Army in the Boer War brought about a national debate concerning education, public health, diet and fitness. Pollution and disease spreading to housing areas of all classes in Victorian England led to public health campaigns and the municipalisation of public utilities.

The fact that so many people with mental illness and learning disabilities were removed from their communities and placed in institutions, symbolically as well as geographically separate from existing centres of population (see Jones, 1972 and 1993; Porter, 2002; Wright and Digby, 1996; Gilbert and Scragg, 1992) meant that services were:

- stigmatised
- separated from community services and networks of all kinds
- poorly resourced
- under-influenced by developments elsewhere in health and social care

It is important to remember, however, that the old 'asylums' (from the Latin and Greek words for safety and sanctuary) were a massive investment in public services by our 19th century ancestors.

When the institutions were re-labelled as 'hospitals', following the NHS Act of 1946 (implemented 1948) it gave rise to a comforting belief that health care generally, and medical care in particular, was of a high quality. Anybody having worked in one of the hospitals (like Peter) however, and all the feedback from community

staff regarding the health of patients assessed once they were discharged from a medium or long stay in hospital, tends to show that this was anything but so.

So many of the old institutions have now closed that it is sometimes difficult to convey to new students in medicine, nursing, social work and therapies, the true nature of institutional care. Those who have experienced them will immediately recognise the meaning of the then Minister of Health Enoch Powell's speech in 1961 when he initiated the forthcoming Hospital Plan and the beginning of the closure of the long stay hospitals:

> *This is a colossal undertaking, not so much in the physical provision which it involves as in the sheer inertia of mind and matter which it requires to be overcome. There they stand, isolated, majestic, imperious, brooded over by the gigantic water tower and chimney combined, rising un-mistakable and daunting out of the countryside – the asylums which our forefathers built with such immense solidity. Do not for a moment underestimate their power of resistance to our assault.*

quoted in Jones, 1972: 321–2

For those readers who wish to gain an insight into the old asylums/hospitals, then *The Dark Threads*, Jean Davison's memoir of High Royds Hospital (Davison, 2009), Rutherford's *The Victorian Asylum* (2008) and Sebastian Faulks' fictional representation of psychiatric and psychoanalytic approaches in the 19th century in his *Human Traces* (Faulks, 2006) provide moving and eye-opening accounts.

As Powell so powerfully puts it, it is cultural rather than physical change that is so hard both to initiate and to sustain. Arguably, despite various structural reforms, this cultural change remained a challenge for mental health many years after Powell spoke. Our perennial challenge is that innovation quickly leads into the cul de sac of stagnation, especially if services become risk averse (see Figure 8).

Following the election victory in 1997, mental health was made one of the Labour Government's three stated priorities for the NHS, along with cancer and heart disease. This focus on mental

Figure 8: Empowerment vs institutionalisation

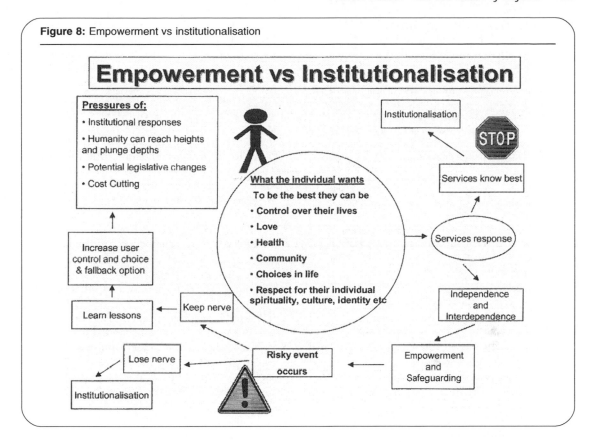

health was in part due to a realisation that, in an age where the economic strength of the workforce lies in the creativity and intelligence of each individual (see Goleman, 1996; Scott, 2000; Layard, 2005), sound mental health and rapid recovery from mental distress is in the nation's interest, as well as the individual's. It is the same scale of realisation and political imperative as that over physical health during the Boer War when the effect of poor physical capacity on the Army and industrial production became evident. More recently, the Government report Foresight Mental and Wellbeing Project (2008) and the Improving Access to Psychological Therapies (IAPT) work, IAPT building on the campaigning of the LSE's Lord Richard Layard (see Layard, 2005), have stressed the links between mental capital and individual and societal performance. This is developing into a perspective on public mental health potentially to compare with the improvements in physical health brought about by a public health perspective. All of which provides hope of a further cultural breakthrough in how mental wellbeing is conceived, managed and prioritised.

Box 3: Public mental health and well-being

Public mental health is an emerging body of knowledge, drawing on a wide range of research including neuroscience, epidemiology, and clinical research, spanning the whole life course from pre-birth to death. It includes consideration of factors at the levels of individuals, families, neighbourhoods, communities and society. As can be imagined, understanding such wide ranging, dynamic and interlocking research is complex, and several definitions, models and frameworks have been used to simplify and understand the implications of the evidence.

Whilst being well implies the absence of illness, this may undervalue the importance of the quality of life without illness. Well-being is a broader concept intended to capture this dimension and convey its importance as a concept for individual and societal attention.

Well-being and mental health have been defined as:

> *[wellbeing is a] positive physical, social and mental state; it is not just the absence of pain, discomfort and incapacity, it requires that basic needs are met, that individuals have a sense of purpose, that they feel able to achieve important goals and participate in society.*
>
> DEFRA

> *A dynamic state, in which the individual is able to develop their potential, work productively and creatively, build strong and positive relationships with others, and contribute to their community. It is enhanced when an individual is able to fulfil their personal and social goals and achieve a sense of purpose in society.*
>
> Foresight 2008

Well-being includes a consideration of *resilience* as a protective factor against adverse risks, with the concept being defined as 'the process of withstanding the negative effects of risk exposure, demonstrating positive adjustment in the face of adversity or trauma, and beating the odds associated with risks' (Bartley, 2006: 4). Such a view potentially adds to understanding well-being and intervening to improve it for individuals and communities by focusing on assets, rather than solely on more stigmatising negative deficits or risks.

For Keyes (2007) there is a need to move beyond simply thinking that an absence of mental illness means that a person is mentally healthy. He argues for thinking of mentally healthy as flourishing – a more complete mental functioning, which society ought to aim at for all, asserting that flourishing people do better than those who are moderately mentally well or those languishing on a range of indicators including number of days off sick.

Reasons to be cheerful during the Labour Government's covering the 1990s and early 2000s included:

- Mental health was one of the Government's three main health priorities.
- A National Director for Mental Health was appointed at the Department of Health, with significant civil service support for mental health. This Director continues in place into a new era of mental health policy (*New Horizons*) providing huge continuity and leadership for mental health.
- There continues to be recognition that while specific attention has to be given to those with severe and enduring mental illness, holistic and 'whole systems' approaches are required to radically improve the health of the nation. There is commitment to social inclusion, social justice and recovery approaches to working with people's experiences of mental health problems.
- The first National Service Framework (NSF) for a major service in the UK was for mental health, published in 1999 as a 10-year operational plan to reform mental health care.
- The NHS Plan published in 2000 set targets for new mental health services and a plan of increased investment in them. This and the NSF transformed the system of mental health care.
- Further major developments and work, which linked policy and practice, such as IAPT, policy guidance in many areas including personality disorder, and a refocused Care Programme Approach (CPA).
- Commitment to involvement of service users with potential to challenge policy and service delivery at a national, regional and local level. The introduction of NSF 'Framework Champions'. Added to which are policy and legislation changes for greater personalisation of health and social care in general, such as direct payments, designed to empower individuals in creating their own service around their specific needs (see Chapter 5).
- A greater involvement of carers; an approach accelerated following the implementation of the Carers' (Recognition and Services) Act of 1995. The needs and desires of users are distinct from their carers, but there is great benefit in looking at where their needs are congruent and where they are divergent, and being explicit about both an individual and a policy level. Local authorities and their productive links with voluntary and charitable organisations may reasonably be said to have led on this ahead of the NHS.
- Considerable attention given to workforce issues, through the work of the Workforce Action Team, in terms of numbers (more of them now) and how they work (New Ways of Working in Mental Health).

- A framework which connects and involves users, carers, practitioners, managers, researchers and policy makers at national, regional and local levels, such as through Local Implementation Teams (LITs), Framework Champions, and development centres (national and local). The creation of the National Institute for Mental Health in England (NIMHE) which connected research, policy development, good practice and development within a 'Whole Systems' approach. Its successor body (after a spell in which NIMHE was in the Care Services Improvement Partnership) is the National Mental Health Development Unit, established in 2009. It is a positive to have a successor body, with potential to champion mental health and incorporate, and build on, the lessons from NIMHE.
- The strength of the mental health charities, the Mental Health Network of the NHS Confederation and independent policy centres within the United Kingdom and their ability to appropriately both stand together with and stand to one side of statutory bodies. This is a strength in continuing the reasoned public policy deliberation and evolution to greater social justice.
- Major investment in mental health services, with growth in early intervention, crisis resolution and home treatment, primary care, assertive outreach, and work in prisons and training.
- New Mental Health and other legislation (see Chapter 8) around equalities, human rights and mental capacity, etc.
- An underpinning set of values and a recognition of the needs of special attention to equalities, outcomes and race, gender, culture and faith, sexual orientation etc.
- International recognition of the importance of mental health, such as the assertion that mental health is 'central to the human, social and economic capital of nations and should therefore be considered as an integral and essential part of other public policy areas such as human rights, social care, education and employment (WHO Europe, 2005: 3).

Reasons to be cautious:

- There is a seemingly ceaseless process of huge structural change going on in the NHS, including 'Shifting the Balance of Power' moving the locus of commissioning to primary care trusts, reforming Trusts and Strategic Health Authorities and changes to funding flows. Recent surveys (Crump, 2009) demonstrate that the general public is confused as to the shape of NHS structures and who does what for whom! (see Figures 10 and 11)
- Structural reform meant the creation of large mental health trusts, including Foundation Trusts, and the transfer of general community staff to PCTs. This may increase stability of services and the focus on mental health but could lead to their isolation from local communities and mainstream influences within the NHS and local authorities.
- The creation of care trusts in some localities and other transfers of local authority staff and functions to the NHS run the risk of a marginalisation of social care expertise and perspective, and a loss of the connectedness within mental health provision of the social inclusion, regeneration, education and citizenship agendas.
- 'There seems to be little understanding (in local practice) that the social situation of a person has so much impact on their mental health. There is no point in giving someone medication if they live in condemned accommodation with no heat or water. Medical input is actually a very small part of the overall treatment plan of the client presenting with mental health problems' (quotation from a social worker in a community team). Despite national priority being given to social exclusion/inclusion it is not always clear that it has translated into local planning and practice.
- The movement of social work and social care staff to mental health trusts may encourage a re-emergence of a 'biomedical model' of care and neglect of the social elements which make up the predominant proportion of the concerns of those who use the service (see Chapter 5). As one social worker in a mental health setting said:

  It is essential that social workers remain able to provide person-centred and social explanations for a range of behaviours which may otherwise become diagnostic categories.

- System reform in mental health continues, such as moves to Payment by Results and strengthened commissioning. More change, though arguably necessary, may be demoralising and needs to be managed carefully. Values, knowledge and skills may become submerged.

- The laudable approach to frameworks in education, health and social services has sometimes been seen as an oppressive increase in managerialist ideology and bureaucratic procedures, resulting in loss of professional autonomy and in direct contact with users and carers.

> *We have to fill in the multi-disciplinary forms which are long but useful for users and ourselves in care planning, but then we have to duplicate it all on the local authority forms!*
>
> Social worker in a CMHT, 1996

- Fears over the 'democratic deficit' in which local Trusts are not accountable to their communities and a de-coupling from the democratic process.

The developing policy agenda

From 1997, in line with management thinking, the Department of Health set in place a policy and practice framework through:

- White Paper, *Modernising Mental Health Services* (1998c).
- *The National Service Framework for Mental Health* (September 1999).
- The Mental Health chapter in the *National Health Service Plan*.
- *The Mental Health Policy Implementation Guidance* (2001).
- *The Journey to Recovery* (November 2001).
- *Making it Happen: A Guide to Delivering Mental Health Promotion* (May 2001).

In addition, there was a stream of guidance papers on specific mental health issues, and a range of performance targets. In short, a comprehensive programme was undertaken to codify and disseminate best practice in mental health care and to seek to improve care by central performance management. This centralist approach is breaking down, with moves to devolve decision making for operationalisation of services to the lowest NHS level, with performance management by Strategic Health Authorities for each region, and the Department of Health co-producing policy and vision with the NHS and other stakeholders.

At the time of writing, the NSF for Mental Health is coming to an end and there is a consultation process called New Horizons (DoH 2009b) to agree a new, shared vision for mental health. This promises much in terms of maintaining the high priority nationally of mental health, social values to drive service improvement including social inclusion, and an emphasis on the mental wellbeing of individuals and communities.

Box 4: New Horizons

During the summer of 2009 the Government began a consultation on New Horizons, a visionary policy for mental health. The intention was to publish the new policy toward the end of 2009.

The twin aims of New Horizons are to be:

- improving the mental health and well-being of the population
- improving the quality and accessibility of services for people with poor mental health

In his foreword to the consultation paper, Louis Appleby, the National Director for Mental Health, identified that a number of key themes were already emerging, namely:

- prevention and public mental health – recognising the need to prevent as well as treat mental health problems and promote mental health and well-being
- stigma – strengthening our focus on social inclusion and tackling stigma and discrimination wherever they occur
- early intervention – expanding the principle of early intervention to improve long-term outcomes
- personalised care – ensuring that care is based on individuals' needs and wishes, leading to recovery
- multi-agency commissioning/ collaboration – working to achieve a joint approach between local authorities, the NHS and others, mirrored by cross-government collaboration
- innovation – seeking out new and dynamic ways to achieve our objectives based on research and new technologies
- value for money – delivering cost-effective and innovative services in a period of recession
- strengthening transition – improving the often difficult transition from child and adolescent mental health services to

---

adult services, for those with continuing needs.

The consultation has a vision for mental health:

> In 2020 most adults will understand the importance of mental well-being to their full and productive functioning in society, to their physical health, and to their ability to make healthy lifestyle choices. They will also understand some of the factors that affect their mental well-being, and will have developed their own everyday ways for taking care of it. Children will increasingly be taught in school about the importance of mental well-being and how to nurture and preserve it, and a range of local services will support their well-being so that problems are detected early. Mental health needs will be identified at an early stage so that, for example, treatment and support can be provided while the individual is an adolescent, thus reducing the chances that mental health problems will continue and adversely affect their adult life.

> In 2020 physical health and mental well-being will be seen as equal priorities, and the links between them recognised as key to maintaining physical and mental health. Lifestyle and well-being services will be widespread. Psychological and family treatments will be available to all who could benefit from them. Drug treatments will be individually tailored so they have fewer adverse effects. Services will use innovative technologies to promote independent living and the effectiveness of treatment.

Added to this are commitments to personalised services, equalities, reducing stigma and increasing understanding, high quality care for all, recovery based services and working on the basis that there is no health without mental health.

Coupling mental health policy development with those powerful elements for potentially positive reform in the general policy framework for health and social care offers opportunities for improvements in mental health care. The

emphasis on personalisation and choice is one example (see Chapter 6). The emphasis on quality of care and outcomes and on local leadership for improvement and innovation written in to High Quality Care for All (DoH 2008b) and its one-year on review (DoH 2009b) are other examples. The proposed move to payment by results in mental health is another structural reform, alongside moves to improve commissioning (World Class Commissioning) that may provide improvements.

On the whole a positive policy picture emerges, but the lesson of the NSF is that the detail of operationalisation into local services can still be a challenge, on top of which we have to consider significant current political and economic turmoil which will have a major impact on service improvement – but it is now clear in which direction we are travelling.

Mental health within a wider context

If we accept that individuals live and work within a variety of relationships, networks and environments, then we must increasingly orientate ourselves towards a holistic and 'whole systems' approach.

As Peter Bates puts it in his introduction to the SCMH pack on social inclusion:

> *The more work we gathered together the more it became clear that social inclusion was not merely an attractive goal for mental health services – it was **imperative**.*
> SCMH, 2002: 3, our emphasis. (See also Chapter 2 in this book)

Mental Health services, because of the individualised, medical approach enshrined in the UK since the mid/late nineteenth century (Bracken and Thomas, 2005) still tend to concentrate on individual pathology. But the individual originates from a social context and some form of family or substitute family context; may well live with a partner; as part of an extended family; and be or have dependants.

Assessment, treatment, care, support and rehabilitation has to take place within a context of neighbourhoods, groups and communities, and the policies of public health, regeneration, place shaping; political priorities (both national and local) will have a major impact on the meaning individuals have in their lives, and the environment in which they try and function.

A considerable cause for optimism as we write this is the increasing concern within political and

Figure 9: The individual in society

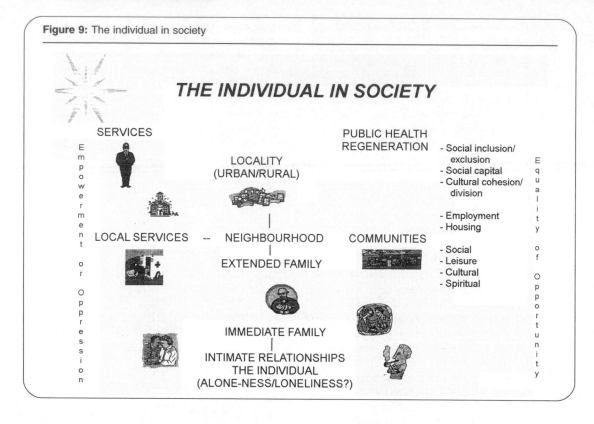

social discussion with wellbeing, inequalities and their social determinants. From the international perspective (e.g. the World Health Organisation Commission on the Social Determinants of Health (CSDH) (2008)) through to the English national level (e.g. DoH, 2009c) there is greater awareness of the social determinants of illness/health across the life course. The CSDH argued that health inequalities resulted from:

> ... *a complex system operating at global, national, and local levels which shapes the way society, at national and local level, organises its airs and embodies different forms of social position and hierarchy. The place people occupy on the social hierarchy affects their level of exposure to health-damaging factors, their vulnerability to ill health, and the consequences of ill health.*
>
> Marmot, 2007: 1156

In addition, the Foresight report (2008) on mental capital and mental well-being has also helped to raise awareness to the importance of these subjects and their determinants across the life course. Placing mental health within this arena of debate and public policy making may well reap dividends to address the health inequalities associated with mental illness.

Coupling mental health care with a strengthened inequalities and social determinants policy thread has the potential to raise up the inequalities faced by those with mental health problems. Combining this with a wellbeing perspective potentially has the power to lift the mental and physical health of wider sections in society. At the time of writing this is a compelling potential.

And how might this be operationalised at the level of services? It is clear that *open discussion* between professionals, their colleagues, and service users and carers is central, as the refocused CPA makes clear (DoH, 2008b: 7) and further adds as its principles:

> *The approach [CPA] to individuals' care and support puts them at the centre and promotes social inclusion and recovery. It is respectful – building confidence in individuals with an understanding of their strengths, goals and aspirations as well as their needs and difficulties. It recognises the individual as a person first and patient/ service user second.*
>
> *Care assessment and planning views a person 'in the round' seeing and supporting them in their individual diverse roles and the needs they have, including: family; parenting; relationships; housing; employment; leisure;*

education; creativity; spirituality; self-management and self-nurture; with the aim of optimising mental and physical health and well-being.

Stanley and Manthorpe, in their review of the major mental health enquiries, comment, in the case of Stephen Laudat: 'Mainstream agencies often fail to accept the contribution that can be made by families and communities' (Stanley and Manthorpe, 2001: 89).

And again:

The enquiry team examining the care of Anthony Smith identified the failure of the team to address his problems of unemployment and housing which were likely to contribute to a relapse ... the focus was on treating the illness rather than the patient in the round.

quoted in Stanley and Manthorpe, 2001: 92

Social work is about people and identification of the areas which impact on their ability to lead an ordinary life despite their illness.

Social worker

It was with increasing recognition that social and environmental aspects of mental health were increasingly important, and a growing concern that the medical model might be inappropriately reasserted, that led to the formation of the Social Perspectives Network in the autumn of 2001. Work within the Network redefined the social model in mental health and set out the following characteristics of it:

- It is based on an understanding of complexity of human health and well-being.
- It emphasises the interaction of social factors with those of biology and microbiology in construction of health and disease.
- It addresses the inner and outer worlds of individuals, groups and communities.
- It embraces the experiences and supports the social networks of people who are vulnerable and frail.
- It understands and works collaboratively within the institutions of civil society to promote the interests of individuals and communities and can also critique and challenge where these are detrimental to these interests.
- It emphasises shared knowledge and shared territory with a range of disciplines and with service users and the general public.
- It emphasises empowerment and capacity building at individual and community level and therefore tolerates and celebrates difference.

- It places equal value on the expertise of service users, carers and the general public but will challenge attitudes and practices that are oppressive, judgemental and destructive.
- It operationalises a critical understanding of the nature of power and hierarchy in the creation of health inequalities and social inclusion.
- It is committed to the development of theory and practice and the critical evaluation of process and outcome.

Duggan with Foster and Cooper, 2002

SPN has run a series of workshops on pertinent themes. The reports can be accessed on their website.

The ancient code of Hamurabi (1728–1686 BC) stated that you cannot separate the illness from the patient. Some centuries on, it is clear that one cannot separate the illness from the individual, the family, the community or the health of the nation.

Changing structures

We have already noted above some aspects of the structural reforms mental health care has operated within. 'Form follows function' is a useful dictum, though should not be over-emphasised and there sometimes appears to be an obsession with structural change as the way of resolving a range of challenges. In fact, of course, there is usually an excellent rationale for any reconfiguration of organisational structures. In the NHS for example:

- Area Health Authorities – with their coterminosity with county councils made a great deal of sense in the 1970s.
- District Health Authorities – created 'to bring the NHS closer to the people'.
- The purchaser/provider split (as opposed to the purchaser/provider *separation* in local authorities) – 'to bring the discipline of the market into the NHS'. Whilst further related reform is underway (e.g. Foundation Trusts, payment by results, world class commissioning, practice based commissioning) it often seems to be a case of 'playing shops' with an increase in paper exchange resulting in little discernible change in behaviours nor improvement in services.
- Primary Care Groups (PCGs) – set up to involve GPs – benefited from the experience of

Figure 10: The accelerating velocity of structural change in the NHS

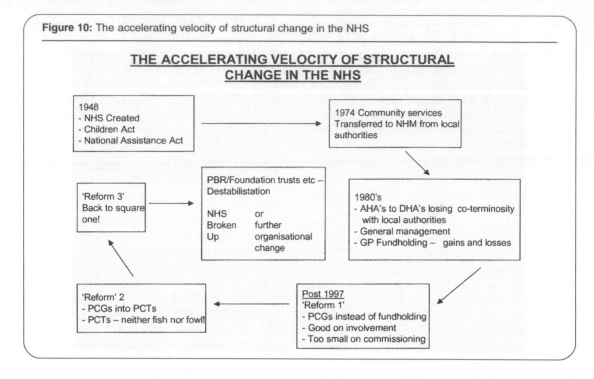

fundholding and total purchasing projects, and create synergies with district councils and their environmental health responsibilities.

• Primary Care Trusts – to form larger commissioning bodies with a primary care focus, but with a possibility of losing the local responsiveness created by PCGs.

• Care Trusts to bring the NHS and social care together and tear down 'the Berlin wall' between these two major agencies. The model is based on that which is said to work well in Northern Ireland, except that a closer examination shows an all too familiar pattern in the Province of domination by acute hospitals and neglect of some vital social care perspectives (see Campbell and McLaughlin, 2000).

All these models have a great deal of merit in themselves. But there is an insistent restlessness which leads to headlines such as 'April again? Time for another reorganisation' (*Health Service Journal*, 4 April 2002) and the impression of a search for a structural 'nirvana'.

Reorganisations in terms of structural change or mergers in public or private organisations tend to: 'Suck up a lot of management time, and that's not just manager managers but clinical managers as well', Matt Tee, Communications Director, for the then Commission for Health Improvement (CHI) (quoted in *Health Service Journal*, 14 February 2002).

Encourage people to look inwards rather than outwards: 'There is a heightened risk that the eye gets taken off the ball of service delivery', Tim Matthews, former Chief Executive of St. Thomas's Hospital, who steered through its merger with Guys Hospital in 1993 (quoted in *HSJ*, 14 February 2002).

In fact, there is no structural 'Emerald City'. In the end, like Dorothy, we have to stop relying on the Wizards of Oz, or Whitehall, and work more co-operatively together on a common agenda, forged through discussion and co-operation. Ultimately, it is *people* who drive positive change, not structures.

'You have to keep re-asserting the local authority agenda.' Member of a community mental health team for older people, quoted in SSI/Audit Commission, Dec. 2001.

In this diagram the source of power and decision-making 'A', makes rulings and sends out instructions. Limited discussion and modification is made by senior managers at 'B', but real power remains with the central caucus. Middle managers at 'C' have no real power to influence events and are the rotating arm of the module or the chain attached to the hammer, and

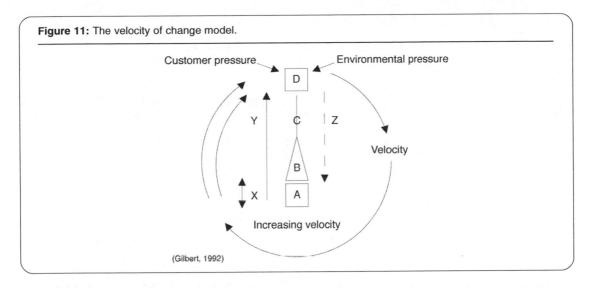

Figure 11: The velocity of change model.

(Gilbert, 1992)

can therefore only try and keep in touch with both staff and higher management. Staff at 'D' are subject to the full velocity of change with all the sense of potential helplessness and disillusion which that implies.

The real interchange of ideas only takes place at 'X' with the directive proceeding along line 'Y'. Disinformation, and environmental and customer pressures has a modifying effect at the customer interface 'D', and this is fed back slowly along line 'Z'. The time-lag and the power energy at the centre means that 'A' is already generating new ideas that have to be passed down the line and implemented before the first batch have been properly bedded down. The middle management process tends to get stretched and collapsed like a piece of elastic and often loses its coherence and creativity.

Mental health services are moving towards various forms of integration. When in 1996 Somerset Health Authority and County Councils reviewed their mental health services, the experiences of users led them to set up a Joint Commissioning Board and combined service provision (see Gulliver, Peck and Towell, June 2000, August 2000, February 2001). Chris Davies, then Director of Social Services for Somerset, has remarked that he attracted some criticism from fellow social services directors at the time for 'handing services from the local authority to the NHS'. But Davies felt strongly that with mental health services being only about eight per cent of the social services budget, the social care perspective, broader local authority agenda and

public health issues were better championed by an integrated approach rather than continued separation, even though the provision of service in effect went into a health agency. It was perhaps helpful that the first chief executive of the Somerset Partnership Trust was someone with a social work training and background.

Since the mid nineties, arrangements like Somerset have become increasingly more common through the flexibilities under Section 31 of the 1999 Health Act, and on 1 April 2002, three care trusts, focusing on users with mental health needs, were launched in Manchester, Bradford and Camden and Islington.

In the eastern region, a working group looked specifically at 'adding value to mental health partnership organisations through the successful integration of social care' (Modernisation Taskforce Report, 27 February 2002). The partnership members recognised that 'service users and carers value services that are influenced significantly by the 'social model of disability/disadvantage', comparing such services very favourably against any experiences that they consider to be over-influenced by a traditional 'medical model'. Progressive medical practitioners recognise this and thus it is vital to understand and benefit from:

- Understanding the NHS inheritance. The NHS's familiarity with internal integration issues both organisationally and clinically.
- The importance of social perspectives especially within the wider agenda of

Table 1: Distinctive strength of the mental health social care tradition

- Specialist social work responsibilities since 1959 and accumulated experience.
- Needs-led assessment and care management since 1993, and their contribution to the holistic implementation of the care programme approach.
- An emphasis on the preferences and choices of individual service users and carers (sometimes summarised as 'the social work approach'). The most recent example is facilitating this through 'direct payments'.
- Specific developments in recognition and support for carers – including the separate assessment of carers' needs.
- Support for advocacy services.
- Initiatives in involving service users and carers (or their representatives) in consultation and service planning.
- Service developments in social care support for people with mental health problems.
- Strong associations with the 'social model' of disability/disadvantage and the overall social inclusion agenda.
- Positive record on anti-discriminatory services and promoting the needs of ethnic minority communities and disabled people etc.
- Part of the wider council tradition of community development.
- Good links with employment, leisure and – especially – housing services through being part of local authorities.
- A strong tradition of staff supervision and training.

community capacity building, employment, housing and social groups.

The working group identified a number of specific valued elements the social care tradition brings to mental health.

'It is noticeable', says the document, 'that many of these characteristics seem essential to achieving National Service Framework standards'. They remain central to improvement beyond the NSF.

The series of evaluation articles on the Somerset experience, which have run in *Managing Community Care* (see Gulliver, Peck and Towell, op. cit.) show that, despite clear leadership from the top, structural integration and the concomitant development of inter-professional co-operation to produce better outcomes for service users and carers requires considerable ongoing application (see also Bogg, 2008). While 'the most consistent aspiration voiced by senior managers and local politicians for the formation of the combined trust, was the creation of a 'seamless service' supported by 'shared culture', the staff surveys picked up some lack of certainties around organisational identity and strategic direction; some uncertainty around professional roles and personal skills; and increased pressures. On the positive side, there appeared to be greater cohesion amongst the staff group; increased clarity about the teams' task; a greater appreciation of each other's professional roles and being involved in joint assessments; and an appreciation of the greater variety of work.

Within this mixed picture, with progress clearly being made, the authors make the point

that: 'Co-location and revised management arrangements may not in themselves be sufficient to develop "shared culture" and enhance "shared working", and that the trust may have to adopt some further strategies for change' (Gulliver et al., 2001). These issues of organisational culture have also been picked up by members of the Social Care Strategic Network (SCSN) such as Robb's observations on integration (see Robb and Gilbert, 2007).

Change is a long-term process. Changing the structures is relatively easy; changing the culture takes time and attention. John P. Kotter, in his incisive article on why efforts to transform organisations can so easily fail, suggests that 'declaring victory too soon' and not 'anchoring changes in the organisation's culture', are two major reasons for failure (Kotter, 1995). Gilbert produced a ten-point change process, adapted from Kotter's eight point scale, and others, including Proehl's consideration of public sector organisations, and this has the following stages:

1. Determining the need for change.
2. Establishing a sense of urgency.
3. Creating the guiding coalition.
4. Developing a vision and strategy.
5. Communicating the change vision.
6. Working with the human factors.
7. Empowering broad-based action.
8. Generating short-term wins.
9. Consolidating gains and producing more change.
10. Anchoring new approaches in the culture.

Gilbert, 2001, adapted from Kotter, 1995, and Proehl, 2001

'On an encouraging note, the Manchester Care Trust, with its history of partnership previous to April 2002, has seen a reduction in emergency hospital admissions over a three month period, down from 16 per cent to eight per cent, a 22 to 30 percent increase in the number of clients with intensive care needs supported in the community rather than in residential placements, and a halving in waiting times to see a consultant' (George, April 2002). Increased involvement of service users and carers in the planning and delivery of services is also quoted as an advantage in the Manchester Model as is their participation in training programmes, including those for psychiatrists. In the inner city of Camden and Islington 'the main advantage is seen as the care trust's ability to make social inclusion its "core business"' (George, April 2002).

The study by Macdonald and Sheldon in Westminster in the late 1990s reinforced the need for a social perspective:

Of the 92 clients interviewed, 85% survived on income support. A further seven (8%) received invalidity benefit . . . Most (71%) lived in rented accommodation; with a further 21% in hostel accommodation. 87% were unemployed. Socio-economic factors are known to play a significant part in the ability of clients to cope with mental illness and the pressures which they signify are good predictors of the need for services and their influence on relapse rates.

Macdonald and Sheldon, 1997

At the end of the day, the acid test for structural change has to be improved outcomes for service users and carers.

For the last three years she has been there whether it is for practical issues, medical issues, or just a shoulder to cry on. I feel there have been times when, without the support and understanding of the social worker, I would not have coped. It has been a lifeline to me and has helped me make progress through some very difficult experiences.

Leeds Consumer Survey, January, 1997

There is a great deal to feel encouraged about in mental health services today. As the National Service Framework comes to the end of its operational life we can see over its life a dramatic investment in and re-modelling of mental health care. The new policy framework of New Horizons and the NHS Next Stage Review provide a permissive space for all stakeholders in mental health to locally lead improvements in services and holistic outcomes for users and carers.

However, it is also too easy for managers, practitioners, those involved in governance and services as a whole to become side-tracked or pre-occupied by factors which are not the core issues for the service: e.g. structures, targets which are not well focused, inter-disciplinary rivalries etc. The leadership role for practitioners and managers is to keep their sights set firmly on core values and core goals.

CHAPTER 5

Society is us! – The Service User's and Carer's Views

Peter Gilbert

I first went to see Dr Russo on the pretext that I wanted some sleeping tablets, although what I really wanted was to talk. I thought asking for these would help me by by providing me with an easier starting point. But ten minutes later, I left his surgery with a prescription for a small supply of sleeping tablets and the comment that I shouldn't need them at my age.

Jean Davison, *The Dark Threads*, 2009

A cultural shift within mental health services is required: professionals must change their attitudes towards working with families. Carers ask for professionals to respect their expertise and knowledge.

DoH, 2006, quoted in Repper, 2009

When I think what he said on Tuesday – 'leave the medication to me. I'll make the decisions on that. That's why you chose me as your psychiatrist'. ---- off, Graham, it should be a partnership. We have to arrive at decisions with negotiation. He doesn't have to take the drugs. If I'm not in agreement, when this section is lifted, I won't co-operate. This all sounds very childish. Perhaps it's just Graham's attitude which makes me cross but then he puts me in a powerless position. I hate all psychiatrists, all registrars, all nurses, cleaners, cooks, managers, community psychiatric nurses and Virginia Bottomley.

Linda Hart, *Phone at Nine Just to Say You're Alive*, 1997

The system hasn't ever been designed around the patient, whereas almost every business these days is having to design itself around whatever you call them – customers or clients or whatever.

Derek Wanless, author of The Wanless Report on the NHS, 2002

The one thing that would have made a difference, I think, would have been someone to talk to (on admission to psychiatric hospital). That was what I was always wondering, when I went into hospital: would there be someone to talk to? But I used to shut myself off. Maybe if depression had been explained to me earlier . . .

Annemarie Randall, *The Observer*, 7 April 2002

Without medication, we would both put our heads in the gas oven. We couldn't cope at all without social workers with all the stress and problems in our lives.

Service user quoted in Macdonald and Sheldon, 1997

It is difficult for front line staff to walk around with a lot of performance indicators in their heads. In inducting new staff when I was chief executive of a trust, I would simply ask them to have in their heads the constant question: 'would this service be good enough for me or my family?'

Christina Pond, formerly NHS Leadership Centre (conversation with author)

I don't remember his name or have ever seen him since the thirty minutes he spent with me fifteen years ago but his message of hope he gave me has never left.

Service user, quoted in *Developing a Recovery Platform for Mental Health Service Delivery for People with Mental Illness/Distress in England*, 2002

Only connect

Having worked in both learning disability and mental health services, I find it fascinating that issues of citizenship and empowerment appear to be much more firmly embedded in the culture of the former than in the latter. In many ways there appears to be a greater belief in the developmental progress that people with learning disabilities can make than in the field of mental illness where the recovery movement is having to combat considerable prejudice, both latent and overt.

All the recent Mental Health policy documents, since the Mental Health White Paper, *Modernising Mental Health Services* (DoH, 1998) emphasise that services must be built on:

- The legal and civil rights of service users and carers.
- The innate dignity of each individual.
- Respect for cultural and ethnic diversity.
- The centrality of user involvement in the care planning and delivery process.
- Accessibility of services and choice.
- Partnership and support for carers.
- Working in partnership to produce the right outcomes for people, based on their existing support networks – both personal and community.
- Respect for staff and their needs as the service can only fundamentally exist in relationships between people.

One of the 'Ten Essential Shared Capabilities' for all staff is to provide 'service user centred care'

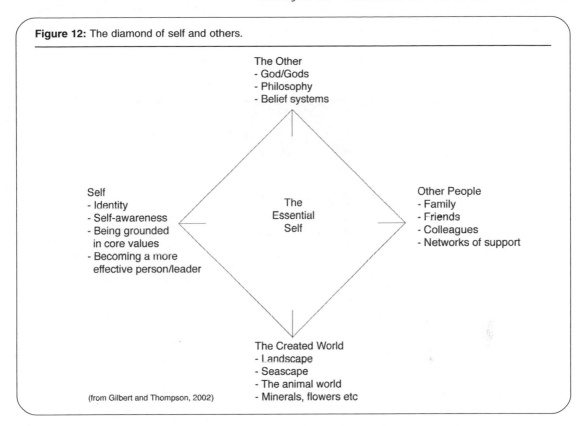

Figure 12: The diamond of self and others.

The Other
- God/Gods
- Philosophy
- Belief systems

Self
- Identity
- Self-awareness
- Being grounded
  in core values
- Becoming a more
  effective person/leader

The
Essential
Self

Other People
- Family
- Friends
- Colleagues
- Networks of support

The Created World
- Landscape
- Seascape
- The animal world
- Minerals, flowers etc

(from Gilbert and Thompson, 2002)

(see Hope, 2008) which assists the user to identify and utilise their strengths to achieve their goals and aspirations.

Mutual learning must not only be a task but a **value** held through all stages of service provision. Feedback must be mutual, not excluding service users and carers, individual service provision, general comments about services that promote constructive comments and complements. An environment must cultivate feedback as integral to developing responsive service delivery.

The longer I live the more I believe that real life is about our connectedness with other people, with 'the other' (whatever that is, and it means many different things to different people) and other aspects of life. My own social work tutor's (Hugh England, see England, 1986) favourite literary quote was from E.M. Forster's *Howard's End* 'Only connect . . . and human love will be seen at its highest. Live in fragments no longer.'

Mental distress and mental illness is so often about a disconnection, false connections or an over-concentration on one aspect of our lives. As a runner, for example, I know that dedicating a certain amount of time to the sport helps my general fitness and alertness; gives me a 'high' through the release of endorphins; connects me to the landscapes and seascapes I'm running through; and provides a bond with other runners. I am also aware that it can become an obsession; the need for 'a fix', the minutiae of race times, over-competitiveness etc.

The actress Nicola Pagett in her moving description of a manic depressive illness writes that:

Everything was unbearably, unutterably beautiful. I didn't need my husband any more. There were the cameras to talk to and the radio people to take care of me . . . I've always known what love is ever since I was small. I've always known it was for better or worse but I forgot. I pushed them away, those who love me, my husband and my daughter. I hardly spoke to them and when I did, it was brusque, clipped. They weren't real, I couldn't see them, there was something in the way and they wouldn't let me listen to my music. It didn't seem loud to me.

Nicola Pagett, *Diamonds Behind my Eyes*, 1998

To really engage with service users, and their carers and supporters, we need to be mindful of the 'whole person' within a context of family, neighbourhood and community; their history,

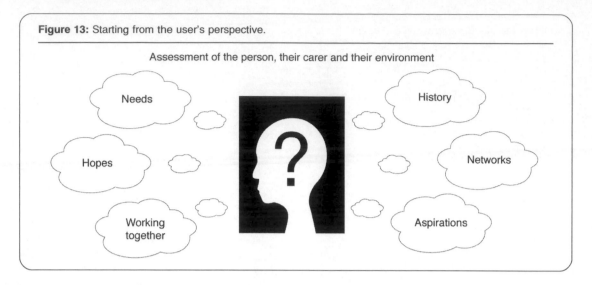

Figure 13: Starting from the user's perspective.

Assessment of the person, their carer and their environment

Needs

History

Hopes

Networks

Working together

Aspirations

hopes, fears and aspirations; and the strengths and needs they bring to the table:

> *Quite simply, social workers have the wider view, which is particularly important for those having difficulty in engaging with services and society.*
> consultant psychiatrist with special expertise in working with people with personality disorders

> *The value of social work in the provision of modern mental health services must be a particular understanding of people in the context of their lives and communities.*
> Director of Social Care in a mental health NHS trust (from a nursing and health policy background)

The word 'assessment' comes from the Latin, 'assidere' – 'to sit beside' someone, and it is only by getting alongside of the person we are trying to serve that we can release their own innate capacity to find themselves, regain control over their lives and move forward on their previous road or in exploring fresh avenues.

There may be a tendency to think that empowerment is all about middle class aspirants who have suffered some temporary disruption in their lives, but participation and self-fulfilment are crucial aspects wherever we start the journey, whatever path we are on and wherever we are going to.

Case Example 2

Arnold had a diagnosis of severe and enduring mental illness. He had become very socially isolated, with a history of non-compliance with social and medical

---

intervention, and many previous admissions to hospital.

In looking at the whole picture of Arnold's life: his style of life in an isolated rural community, with little formal education and no friends, meant that he lacked confidence and self-esteem.

Following discussion with Arnold, and in liaison with his carer, and colleagues within the multi-disciplinary team, the social worker involved a community support worker who began weekly visits to support Arnold in his daily living skills and also worked with him in attending a social drop-in centre. As Arnold's confidence built up, shopping trips were added and other social activities. A separate assessment of the needs of Arnold's carer was completed under the Carer's (Recognition and Services) Act 1995, and support was established with the local carer support service.

The close and regular input from the community support worker has enabled Arnold to engage with services more positively, increase social contacts, develop self-confidence and new skills, so that he can continue to live in the community without further hospital admissions to date; and it is has also ensured support for the carer so as to prevent a breakdown of that vital relationship.

Case Example 3

For many years it was considered the day hospital was vital to me staying alive. Having constant observation was a comfort to those that supported me. I learned very quickly that I was someone that people had little hope that I could self-direct and participate in a life outside a 'treatment facility'. This very quickly became entrenched as part of my identity, which helped only to contribute to what I understand they call 'revolving door syndrome'.

As coincidence helps change direction, I have been prescribed exercise after a serious operation. I enjoyed exercising and for the first time in a long while I didn't have to identify myself as a mentally ill person. I contacted a trainer to help me when I had trouble motivating myself. I soon found that it was more effective for my mental well-being to replace day hospital with gym sessions. At the gym, I could divert my internal attention to external drive and goals. I reconnected with my ability to achieve at what I put my mind to. I found I could manage many distressing symptoms this way.

Besides my trainer becoming one of my closest friends, she is the person who supports me but does not allow excuses for my illness. **This has been so liberating.**

taken from *Developing a Recovery Platform*
6 March 2002

Another myth is that of the inevitable separation of users and staff, as though the former are in the swamp and the latter are far removed on well-intended hillside parkland. On the contrary, many members of staff have experienced a form of mental illness and, of course, most will have experienced a period or periods of mental distress. The trouble is that often service environments do not welcome this kind of sharing. But Dr Mike Shooter (June, 2002) as incoming President of the Royal College of Psychiatrists, spoke movingly on the radio of his depression while in his final year as a medical student, and how vital it was that significant people in his life gave him hope and encouragement. Crucially, his medical supervisor believed that this episode would strengthen his ability to be an effective doctor rather than hinder it. Recently Ian McPherson, as the head of the newly formed National Mental Health Development Unit, told *Society Guardian* that, while his own experience of mental ill-health, as a teenager and again as an adult, 'gives no unique insights' into mental health conditions in general, what it has done is to 'allow me to understand what it feels like to be seen as separate or that person over there with a mental illness' (O'Hara, 2009).

Whether we have suffered from a mental illness or not, we are all likely to have experienced episodes of mental distress through trauma or life crises. We need to get and keep in touch with what is vulnerable in ourselves – and not be frightened of it – so as to be able to work alongside others in distress.

To see ourselves and other people in a holistic way, it is helpful to view the various facets of our humanity.

- Social/emotional needs:
  - relationships; loving and being loved
  - security
  - acknowledgement and expression of feelings
  - kinship
  - friendships
  - community involvement
  - empathy
  - appreciation of creation
- Mental or cognitive needs:
  - opportunities for fresh thinking
  - reading, and reflection on the texts
  - planning ahead
  - creative writing
  - visualising positive futures
  - professional development
  - films and plays
- Spiritual needs:
  - recommitting to core values
  - gaining a meaning for life
  - exploration of 'being' and 'becoming'
  - meditation and contemplation
- Physical needs:
  - a healthy diet
  - physical fitness
  - a sense of well-being and being better able to cope with the stresses of work
  - gaining a sleep and awake time balance
- Creative needs:
  - using our senses
  - exploring new ways of working/leisure

– developing creative hobbies
– Life-long learning
    From Gilbert and Thompson, 2002: 106–7

Maslow's well known work on 'needs' places these in a hierarchy from the most basic to the most profound.

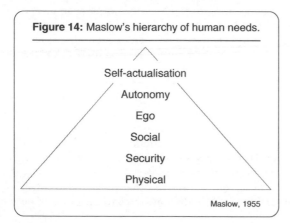

Figure 14: Maslow's hierarchy of human needs.

Self-actualisation

Autonomy

Ego

Social

Security

Physical

Maslow, 1955

The basic physical needs are food, water, shelter etc., the components of survival, security and safety needs come into play when our physical needs are satisfied and we seek a protection against danger and deprivation. Once we feel secure in ourselves and secure against external threat, we can move into contact with other people in search of friendship, intimacy and a sense of belonging to individuals and groups. Belonging in itself is not usually enough, we are then driven to becoming valued by the people and groups of people we are interacting with in a search for ego strength and esteem. As we become stronger as individuals, we look towards asserting our own individualism and autonomy; and this may well lead on to self-actualisation – a desire to fulfil our potential and talents, even though this sometimes is to the detriment of some of our more basic needs. The recent interest in the explorer Ernest Shackleton in books, films and documentaries is partly a consideration of what drove the Antarctic explorer to place so much at risk to achieve self-actualisation, and his use of the hierarchy of needs in the people he led to attain goals, preserve their safety and keep them together as a team. (See Maslow, 1955, and Cooper and Makin, 1984; for a fascinating insight into Shackleton see Morrell and Capparell, 2001).

Whilst the immediate work with a user may focus on their need to address a place to live, food, treatment and safety; any planning must engage with emotional needs and with aspirations which make life worth living. Mere existence is not enough! On the other hand, sophisticated treatment is ineffective unless it also addresses people's basic needs to live and have a meaningful occupation.

From the identification of need, we move to, as Spicker (1995) puts it: 'if people are to make an effective demand for welfare, they have not only to exercise their formal entitlements but also to overcome a series of practical obstacles'.

In all the roles I fulfilled in various social services departments, the desires of users and carers for more and better information was a constant. 'Knowledge is power', as the saying goes, and despite the fact that most statutory agencies have moved on a long way from the: 'don't let us produce any information otherwise they'll all want some(!)', information is a frequent clarion call. This is particularly true in the case of black and ethnic minorities where the issues are manifestly more complex. One Asian woman caring for her elderly mother with a long history of depressive illness told me that a very well produced leaflet from the London Borough of . . . had come through their front door. It was in the right language but unfortunately the mother could speak the language but not read it, and the daughter could neither speak nor read it fluently. One major element of conscious and unconscious racism in our society is our inability or unwillingness to inform individuals and communities of their rights and their right to services (see Sewell, 2008 and Keating, 2009).

Spicker, in his thematic approach to social policy, quotes Kerr in outlining a number of stages that service users have to go through:

- People must feel a need, or at least they must want to have what is being offered.
- They have to find out that the service exists. Even when they have identified their need for something, they may not realise that a service actually exists.
- They have to know that they are likely to receive it. A service which is for 'poor people' is not certain to be taken up by people who do not think of themselves as 'poor'.
- They have to feel that the service or benefit is worth claiming. Sometimes the service is so inflexible that it causes more problems than it solves.
- There are the beliefs and feelings of potential recipients, and as we have seen above, the issue of reciprocity is very important.

- People need to have a sense as to whether the service being offered is likely to help them through a period of time, not just immediately, but that the service may help them over a period of time, or can be adjusted as their needs change. (From Spicker, 1995.)

> *You don't get the information from the staff ... You either have to rely on other patients to tell you the information, which you might not want to, rely on, or just ignore the whole problem altogether ... I would have found it much more helpful if someone had actually sat down with me and explained whatever happened to me, how I had got to hospital, what they thought was wrong with me and how they envisage life going for me.*
> Service user quoted in *Mental Health Foundation*, November 1999

When I was admitted to hospital for a sinus operation, the ward sister sat down with all of us admitted on the same day and explained step by step exactly what was going to happen in terms of care, pre-treatment, the operation and after care. She used simple diagrams and was very happy to field questions. All of us felt much more reassured and in control in an alien environment, and an additional outcome was that we were all very supportive of each other during the whole process.

Working with 'informal' carers

While service users and carers may have differing perspectives the carers view is a vital ingredient of care, and issues around partnership and confidentiality need to be resolved. Family or 'informal' carers are a major resource. It is estimated that around 1.5 million people are involved in caring for a relative or friend with a mental illness; and the saving to the Treasury by informal caring runs into billions of pounds.

Legislation for carers really came on the scene with the 1995 *Carers (Recognition and Services) Act*, and a growing raft of legislation and policy documents (e.g. DoH, 2002) have added detail. As the Department of Health guidance of 2002 puts it: 'providing help, support and advice to carers can be one of the best ways of helping people with mental health problems'. Standard 6 of the NSF focused on carers' needs, and the CPA identifies a number of key action points:

- Identify carers of people with mental health problems.
- Provide carers with the information they need in order to help them to provide care.

- Listen to what carers have to say.
- Consider whether carers are providing regular and substantial care.
- Assess carer's needs.
- Co-ordinate with carer, service user and other agencies to meet Standard 6 of the NSF.
- Formulate carer's care plan.
- Review annually, or if circumstances change significantly.
- Consult with carers about the services they receive.
- Involve carers in the planning and development of services.
> Repper et al., 2008 and Repper, 2009

Writing about her husband, Malcolm (now sadly deceased) who had early onset dementia, Barbara Pointon says that:

> *I have come to realise that despite all Malcolm's obvious mental and physical attrition, his spirit still shines through, several of his carers have remarked upon Malcolm still 'being there' ... As for me, it can only stiffen my determination to strive for quality of life and quality of dying for my husband.*
>
> *And amazingly, Malcolm is equally sensitive to me if I'm not feeling well, or trying to deal with a crisis-I can tell from his eyes and feel a psychic connection. To stand stripped of everything the world values and see each other as we really are is a very precious and humbling experience, and one which I would never have encountered were it not for the ravages of dementia. Paradoxically, Malcolm's 'losses' have turned into 'gains'.*
> Pointon, 2007: 119

The Westminster Study

Geraldine Macdonald and Brian Sheldon's 1997 study of people with a mental illness in Westminster and their relationship with their social workers, gives a very clear picture of loss and deprivation in a London borough with high social mobility.

As quoted earlier in this book, 85 per cent of the clients interviewed survived on income support. A further eight per cent received invalidity benefit, and five users reported receiving occasional income from other sources such as training courses. Most (71 per cent) lived in rented accommodation, with a further 21 per cent in hostels. 87 per cent were unemployed, 'socio-economic factors are known to play a significant part in the ability of clients to cope with mental illness and the pressures which they signify are good predictors of the need for services and their influence on relapse rates' (Macdonald and Sheldon, 1997).

Of the kinds of problems they experienced, it was the range of interpersonal and social issues which challenge us all, but become especially hard to overcome when allied with recurrent or

Table 2:   The incidence of problems cited by respondents

Problem	N*	%*
Mental state	64	25
Financial difficulties/problems	41	16
Family relationships	25	10
Housing/accommodation	24	9
Social isolation	24	9
Practical problems	22	8
Medical	16	6
Unemployment/boredom	13	5
Living circumstances	11	4
Other	20	8
Total	**260**	**100**

*Respondents often cited more than one problem. Percentages are of the sample interviewed.

chronic illness, and when living in an area where social problems are exacerbated.

The authors remark that '. . . many recurrent problems were social and financial in nature and not *directly* related to the mental condition of the clients'. It is worth noting that while people's mental state was a high preoccupation with the users interviewed, medical issues featured fairly low on the list. It is very evident that the multi-faceted nature of the challenges facing this group and need to broker solutions with a wide range of agencies and community groups were something which played to a specific strength of social work.

Service users were overwhelmingly positive about the work that social workers undertook with them:

- Clients valued the opportunity to discuss and clarify their worries and fears, and examine ways of overcoming them.
- The actual support from a social worker appeared as the most often quoted source of positive services. Next in order of perceived significance were day centres or drop-in facilities, followed by practical help, advocacy and accommodation.
- Most respondents perceived social workers treating them with dignity and respect.
- 60 per cent of those interviewed 'recognised the

pivotal role of social workers in providing and co-ordinating services' (Macdonald and Sheldon) though a number felt that their psychiatrist was the central figure.
- Service users appear to feel that the contact they had with social workers was appropriate to their needs.

This kind of feedback is mirrored in the Leeds Survey (Leeds, 1997) where 92 per cent of users who responded identified 'the service of talking, listening, and counselling, as being provided by their social worker'. 75 per cent of respondents considered talking, listening and counselling as being the most beneficial service provided by the social worker.

The next highest figure in this category is advice on benefits. Social workers were seen as dealing with requests adequately (87 per cent) being helpful (96 per cent) and being punctual and reliable (82 per cent).

These services are superb, they help you a lot and without them you'd be sunk.
service user in the Westminster Survey

I find my social worker excellent, reliable, reassuring, punctual, helpful and genuine.
   Always friendly and reliable – always contacts me if unable to see me on the day planned. Good liaison between social worker and doctor.
   Living alone, this service is more than important to me having an understanding person to listen to me and give advice in absolute confidence.
service users in the Leeds Survey

The Westminster Survey was not entirely positive, however. Problems identified were:

- Structural gaps between general practitioners and social workers.
- A significant number of service users did not feel that their social workers understood the nature of their problems, or disagreed substantially about their priority. As one service user put it 'He wants to make a life as he sees it. He's not very sympathetic. He speaks in a soft voice to cover up his bad temper and this makes me bad tempered after speaking to him. We are not able to talk'. On the other hand, where differences in perspective were dealt with in a genuine manner, then this was appreciated: 'He doesn't always agree about my voices, and says, "no, it's your sicknesses". I can talk to him about it. I feel quite comfortable discussing differences of opinion with him'.

Figure 15: What service users want.

A place of my own

Near shops, church, pub, leisure centres etc.

Acceptance in my neighbourhood

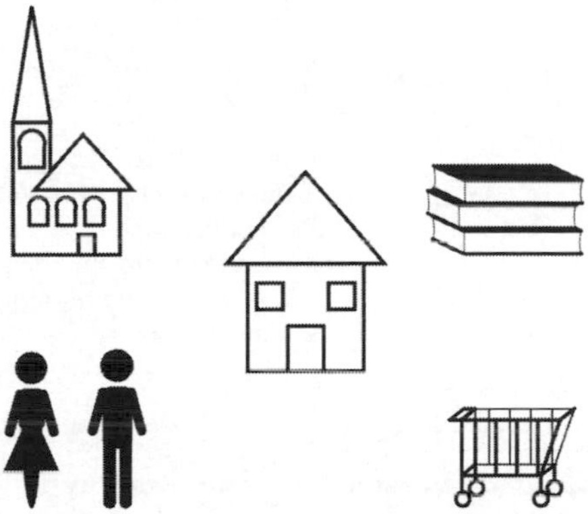

To be treated as an individual

To be able to have as much control as possible of care programmes

Hopes for the future Doing 'being human'

My friends to be close by

Make new friends

Be listened to

Recognise my feelings and where I am emotionally/culturally

Get a job and/or do something I enjoy during the day

To have choices

To be able to move on if I become more independent

Acknowledge my history

- There was a lack of choice in the services offered. Almost half felt they had no choice at all *'in the services they use'*.
- One of the most significant findings, and a very disturbing one, was that service users 'were not routinely provided with sufficient opportunities to discuss what was happening to them, nor were they always given information about their legal rights', during compulsory admission to hospital. This will be discussed further in Chapter 8.

Strategies for living

One of the most influential studies has been the Mental Health Foundation's *Strategies for Living* report of user-led research into people's strategies for living with mental distress and mental illness.

As the first service user quoted puts it:

> We are all *primary experts on our own mental health and about what works for us . . . We can and should value the coping strategies we have developed for ourselves . . .*
> Mental Health Foundation, November 1999

And the main findings demonstrate:

1. *A demand to be seen as fellow citizens and treated with humanity and dignity.*
   Something that is often said by users, carers and frontline staff is 'nobody listens to me!' The concept of citizenship, dating back to the foundations of Western democracy, and in

many other non-Euro-centric cultures, is that of the citizen partaking, speaking and being listened to in a public forum. Discussion and debate in the political arena or around the family/community hearth required well-honed listening skills. In modern society, we seem to have lost, in many instances, the art of narrative, of telling a story and giving it and the teller space to be valued.

2. *A need to be in as much control as possible of one's diagnosis, treatment and care.*
   Linda Hart recalls her psychiatrist changing his mind about her diagnosis 'What peeves me most, is that on the first or second interview I ever had with Graham (the Psychiatrist) I said I was suffering from depression with psychosis and he said, "no, you're straight down the line, schizophrenic". Pity these doctors don't listen to their patients' (Hart, 1997: 232).

   Of course, being offered a diagnosis and an opportunity to discuss symptoms and causes is usually very helpful: 'Yes, it made sense of all the symptoms, but I hadn't thought of it myself . . . It just made sense, not sleeping, waking up early and not being able to get to sleep and not being able to eat, being constantly worried about what was going to happen, that sort of thing'.

   A woman on being given a diagnosis of endogenous depression, quoted in Mental Health Foundation, 1999

Table 3: What was helpful about relationships.

Good relationships gave people:

Emotional support
- acceptance
- self-acceptance
- understanding

Meaning
- sense of belonging
- sense of purpose
- someone to live for

Companionship and friendship
- shared experiences
- shared interests
- someone to live for

Practical support
- dealing with professionals
- domestic tasks
- personal care
- help managing mental health problems
- financial help

Mental Health Foundation, 1999, p21.

3. ***The importance of relationships and informal support.***

    Strategies for Living found that about two thirds of their respondents rated the relationships they formed with others as the most important factor in helping them to cope with mental distress.

The study groups the aspects of relationships which people found helpful into four categories:

    From my own experience of depression, stemming from work-related stress, I found a combination of both professional and personal relationships helpful in enabling me to steer through what seemed like treacherous rapids (see Chapter 1 in this book and Basset and Stickley, forthcoming). One without the other would not have worked for me.

4. ***Being able to give as well as to receive.***

    Very few of us feel comfortable in a purely receiving mode once we leave childhood. Being a constant recipient feeds into a feeling of powerlessness and losing our rights and responsibilities as citizens.

    Some of the most powerful testimonies on this is listening to members of the medical profession who have themselves been recipients of health services (e.g. Wield, 2006 and Miller in O'Hara, 2009).

    The following case example demonstrates the upward spiral which can result when people are engaged in activities to help others while also receiving support themselves.

Case Example 4

Julie was a recently separated mother of four. She suffered with anxiety, clinical depression and a history of self-harm. The

---

two children living at home, both in their mid teens, had been identified as the main carers and involved in all aspects of domestic care. Julie was often incapacitated by her depression and stayed in bed. The community team worked with her to identify a care plan which worked on self-confidence issues, enhancing social opportunities, identifying support for the two young carers and exploring alternative ways of managing her anxiety.

    The community support worker identified voluntary work as an area of interest for Julie, and together they spent time approaching suitable agencies. Julie was successful; in her application as a volunteer and began working in the community. The young people in the family were offered support from a young carers support service, which they accepted. Because of the growing confidence between Julie and her community support worker (CSW) the former admitted her problems with debt, which she hadn't mentioned to other members of the team. The CSW assisted with negotiating issues around the Court summons and repayment. Citizens' Advice was contacted and a meeting with a debt counsellor arranged. The CSW assisted Julie in contacting all the companies to whom she owed money (while waiting for the CAB appointment) and supported her in visits to the Benefits Agency and the County Court.

    With the input of the CSW, Julie felt confident enough to liaise with the District

Council (Housing issues) and the Water/Gas/Electricity suppliers (arrears).

After some months, Julie negotiated her own increase to her voluntary hours and applied for a placement relating to vocational training. Julie now feels confident enough to fully engage with all aspects of self-management in the home and in the community. Further self-harming and hospital admissions have so far been avoided.

5. *Therapeutic supports.*

One of the most frequent everyday sayings is: 'there must be a cure for this'. One of the myths of modern life is that there must be some form of 'magic bullet' to deal with every health situation. So on one side there is a pull towards medication as a supposedly quick cure, and on the other there is a push against from publicised examples of medical interventions going wrong.

The power of the drugs companies is also an issue and recently Support Coalition International, the United States survivor rights organisation, has accused the makers of '*A Beautiful Mind*', the film about the Nobel prize winning mathematician, John Nash, and his struggle with a schizophrenic illness, of deliberately subverting Nash's message that he controlled his symptoms and rebuilt his life without medication, to an end line where he is stating that he is taking the newer form of antipsychotics. In 2009 concerns were raised about the prescribing of some anti-depressants for pregnant women.

The Sainsbury Centre's User Perspectives report (Rose, 2001: 53) demonstrates that 'Users do not show a blanket rejection, or a blanket acceptance of their medication. In a user-focused interview, they discriminate between different questions and show that they balance the cost and the benefits of being on psychotropic medication'. Laura Lea (2008: 172) argues for an approach which is centred in the individual's 'daily experience of life'. Lea argues for the usefulness of the Wellness Recovery Action Plan (WRAP) and for a shared way of working which encapsulates a person's 'dreams, ambitions and hopes'. Speaking with a service user partaking in a partnership programme, in the summer of 2009, he spoke of the importance of anti-psychotic

medication in keeping him safe, but also its depressant effects, and the disappointment that every time he hit a crisis he seemed to climb out of a chasm and have to begin his journey from a different point, losing much that he had gained before the crisis.

The Mental Health Foundation's study shows a very similar finding:

One of the key things to emerge from a reading of interviews on the subject of medication is that of ambivalence. Many people have very mixed feelings about taking medication whether or not they found it helpful. It carried with it associations of long-term illness, concerns about physical health and potential long-term damage, particularly where side-effects were found distressing.
Mental Health Foundation, November 1999: 37

Diana Rose, for the Sainsbury Centre, points out that there is a huge significance in the way that general practitioners and psychiatrists are prepared to negotiate medication levels with their patients. Those who felt they still had some control over what they were prescribed had a greater sense of overall control of their lives. As we have seen from the Westminster Study, medication itself is very much only part of a strategy within a wider perspective of environmental and social supports strategies and services.

When I experienced my own bout of depressive illness, two of the things that impressed me most about my GP were firstly her very human reaction to the condition I was in, and her anger at the state in which I arrived in her surgery and her view of the circumstances which had led to my illness. Also the clear descriptions she gave me of the medication she felt would be most appropriate, and giving me a great deal of control as to when to start it. To be honest, my advice as a professional and as a friend to someone in my situation would have been something along the lines of that it was very much their choice, but that medication could be a very helpful aid in becoming strong enough to bring other strategies into play to recover one's health. In practice, however, I was very wary about taking medication for all the reasons outlined in the user surveys: I didn't want to lose control, I was worried about side effects, I wanted to do it all myself, and even relatively small things troubled me, for instance I was running the London Marathon for my local MIND as part of my recovery strategy, and feared that anti-depressants would cause me a dry mouth – very difficult for marathon running! In hindsight,

Figure 16: The seven principles in relationship (Biestek, 1976).

First Direction: The *need* of the client	Second Direction: The *response* of the caseworker	Third Direction: The *awareness* of the client	The name of the *principle*
1 To be treated as an individual			1 Individualisation
2 To express feelings			2 Purposeful expression of feelings
3 To get sympathetic responses to problems	The caseworker is *sensitive* to, *understands*, and appropriately *responds* to these needs	The client is somehow *aware* of the caseworker's sensitivity, understanding, and response	3 Controlled emotional involvement
4 To be recognised as a person of worth			4 Acceptance
5 Not to be judged			5 Nonjudgemental attitude
6 To make his own choices and decisions			6 Client self-determination
7 To keep secrets about self			7 Confidentiality

I should have taken my GP's advice to start the anti-depressants earlier than I did, but her willingness to allow me maximum control, while keeping an eye on my condition, was very helpful for my sense of autonomy.

6. *Professional support.*

Fundamental to the relations with professionals was a person-centred approach which accorded people a sense of respect, dignity, value, equality and being heard. As described above, I found a human reaction, rather than professional detachment, to be extremely helpful, and this is one of the major challenges for professionals in being warm and genuine, yet keeping that emotional involvement detached enough not to disempower the person one is working with, and to ensure that professional knowledge is brought into play. These values were well defined in the classic work of Felix Biestek in the 1960s and 1970s in his classic text: *The Casework Relationship*, Biestek, 1976.

Work on values in social and health care have understandably developed since the 1970s, especially around issues of empowerment, but the kind of values and attitudes desired by users in the various studies (Rose, 2001; Mental Health Foundation, 1999; Macdonald and Sheldon, 1997; Fulford and Woodbridge in Coyte et al., 2007) demonstrate the same concerns around:

- being valued
- genuineness
- accessibility
- continuity
- help to maintain and regain independence

Strategies for Living states that 'The most helpful professional interventions combined both emotional and practical support; people tended to experience such workers as genuinely interested and caring' (p44). These were precisely the kinds of values and behaviour found useful by users and carers in the Leeds Survey (Leeds, 1997) 'I find my social worker excellent, reliable, reassuring, punctual, helpful and genuine' (service user). 'It's good to be able to talk to a person who understands my son's problems' (carer).

As society becomes considerably more complicated, supporting existing networks, where appropriate, and reinforcing individuals' and groups' coping strategies, becomes even more vital. This is particularly important in issues around culture and race where it's all too easy to cut across existing mechanisms for support (see Sewell, 2009; Keating, 2009).

. . . (the social workers) help me fill out all the forms and go to the right people to speak to about getting a place of my own . . . and how to deal with it and learning how to pay my rent and how to manage my money, and how to buy clothes and shopping and stuff like that. They teach you all those kinds of things, of basically how to live independently, they teach you, and it's been a great help. Because without that support, I wouldn't have been able to have made it.

service user quoted in *Mental Health Foundation*, November 1999

Case Example 5

Give me my life back

How a man diagnosed with schizophrenia can be helped out of his apathy.

Case study

The names of all service users mentioned have been changed.

Situation: Roger Castlemaine is a 48-year-old white male who has been a diagnosed schizophrenic since he was 18-years-old. He receives depot injections for his condition. Castlemaine, whose son is likewise on medication, also looks after his 82-year-old mother.

Problem: Castlemaine feels that his life has been wasted, although he has been grateful to hold down the occasional low-paid job. He believes very strongly that his injections have made him 'a pathetic man'. He feels so 'un-alive' while on medication (he uses Largactil, an anti-psychotic drug) that music, once a passionate love, now does nothing to lift him. He feels he has no emotions – he can't get happy, sad or angry. He has been told that this is his schizophrenia but he rejects that. He believes he is suffering from drug-induced apathy. He says he would rather be ill than be on medication. Feeling so numb and 'out of it' has depressed him, to such an extent that he has even considered suicide. During these low points, Castlemaine has embraced Christianity, finding a comfort and understanding, he says, that has not been on offer to him from his doctors. His son takes Olanzapine which, says Castlemaine, helps him to cope 'without turning him into a zombie'. His 30 years of medication have, for Castlemaine, quite simply 'ruined my life'.

Mark Trewin, approved social worker, Bradford District Care Trust:

'Roger Castlemaine's situation is a reminder to mental health professionals that service users have to consider the effects of the medication that they take against the possible benefits. While medication can help, the side-effects mean that there are also major risks involved. Mental health professionals are increasingly discussing these issues with service users and supporting them to find a balance. An attitude of 'compliance at any cost' can be damaging.

In this situation, Castlemaine would probably benefit from a fresh assessment of his health and social needs. The needs of people with a stable but long-term mental health problem can often be overlooked. It appears that there are many issues that are important to Castlemaine in addition to medication, such as his role as carer, his physical health, his spiritual needs, his access to employment and leisure activities. This assessment should be undertaken from his point of view and with his full involvement and should lead to a care plan that identifies the changes he feels are important and how these would be achieved. Castlemaine is likely to gain a great deal from feeling much more involved with the way his care is planned and carried out.

The mental health team could support Castlemaine to change or reduce his medication in an attempt to reduce the side-effects. There may be alternative ways of supporting his positive mental health. It could be time to review the relevance of his diagnosis. It is important that he feels that he is being listened to and this may be a vital part of that process.

His role as a carer, both for his mother and son, should be tackled, as he may need support in this area that is separate to his own mental health needs. Castlemaine is depressed and has expressed suicidal thoughts. Giving him the opportunity to express how he feels, while attempting to resolve some of the issues could reduce the risk of increased depression.

The important principle in this case is that people with a mental health problem have a right to live full and satisfying lives. If our treatment of mental health problems compromises this basic right then we need to reconsider the way that we support people.'

Gill Rowe-Aslam, team leader, Bradford home treatment service, Bradford District Care Trust:

'Roger Castlemaine's aspirations have not been fulfilled. He gives a clear impression that, despite his achievements, he wishes for more. He does not feel motivated enough to actively pursue his interests. In addition to this he describes his emotions as very flat, which appears to be a source of further frustration to him.

This hinders his ability to care for himself, has a negative impact on his self-esteem and prevents him from feeling able to offer any practical or emotional support to his son or mother.

Through the care programme approach the issue of a medication review could be addressed in a structured and focused way. Castlemaine may wish to explore alternative types of medication or treatment. The benefits of complementary medicine and alternative approaches could also be considered. For example, the Hearing Voices Network – a self-help organisation for people, many of whom have been diagnosed as schizophrenic – or the Hearing Voices workbook[1] (a way of understanding and managing voices). He may also wish to be involved in a local user or self-help organisation, which he may use for support of his own needs, or prefer to be more actively involved in supporting others. It may be helpful for an advocate to accompany him to a meeting to assist him in representing his views.

Assuming the outcome of this was successful, Castlemaine would hopefully feel more in control and motivated. This would then give him and his care co-ordinator room to address the further issues of his daily activities and pursuing interests. He could be supported in taking up job-related training with a view to re-entering employment.

If Castlemaine has found Christianity a source of comfort and understanding for him, it is important for this to be acknowledged and any wishes to work within a spiritual framework should also be explored.

It appears that Castlemaine actually holds two roles in all this, in that he is both the cared for and the carer. Therefore, not only is he entitled to an assessment of his own needs, but also of any additional needs he may have as a carer of both his son and 82-year-old mother.'

[1]J Downs (ed), *Coping with Voices and Visions*, Hearing Voices Network. Available from 91 Oldham Street, Manchester M4 1LW. Tel/fax: 0161 834 5768.

User view

'I find this man's situation tragic', writes Kay Sheldon. 'There are many people with long-standing mental health problems who have been overlooked by current mental health practice and policy. It is often easier to 'maintain' us, carrying on with the same regime, year after year, without considering the impact this has on quality of life.

Roger's mental health needs should be completely reviewed by his community mental health team in a user-centred and holistic way, including a review of his medication. In addition, his social set-up and his occupational status should be discussed in depth with him. The team should establish a mutually respectful partnership with Roger, encouraging and supporting him to make decisions himself.

I have little doubt that, having been there myself, Roger's apathy is due to his medication. It may be that Roger would like to come off medication altogether – this should be supported and facilitated by the team, including developing a contingency plan with Roger, should he start to become unwell. A different anti-psychotic, maybe one of the newer ones, or an anti-depressant or both may be preferable alternatives to Roger. He could find it quite difficult to come off his current medication because of withdrawal reactions, especially from the Largactil, which, contrary to popular belief does cause such effects. Also, psychologically it can be daunting to let go of something that has been part of your life for so long. Whatever is decided, it is important that Roger feels both in control of his mental health and supported enough to take this responsibility.

At 48, Roger obviously feels that he has missed out on a large slice of life. Counselling may be helpful in coming to terms with his loss and to help him think more positively about his future. Counselling may also be beneficial when, or if, Roger recovers his emotions, which can be difficult to cope with after such a long time of numbness.

On a practical level, Roger could be helped to make changes to his life and to rekindle some of his former passions. Help with caring for his mother might be useful, if he is tied to the home. Efforts could be made to reignite his musical interests.

Voluntary work or doing a course could help him put some meaning back into his life. Roger deserves all the help the services can offer him to move on from just existing to actually living once again.'

Kay Sheldon is a mental health service user.

Reprinted by kind permission of *Community Care*, 9–15 May, 2002.

7. **Talking therapies and complementary therapies.**

There is a danger that we see talking therapies and complementary therapies as a middle class occupation. In fact, both of these go back to primary needs to talk, to be listened to, to have thoughts and feelings reflected back to one, to retain control of one's coping and healing strategies, to seek for a reduction in stress and a better harmony between mind and body.

I am concerned that some people I meet in long-term therapy have gained a form of personalised insight but at the expense of a tendency to become self-absorbed.

There is some evidence that these therapies are less available to people from black and ethnic minorities and those from more deprived socio-economic groups. Again, the issue of race and culture is most important:

> *... You tend to feel more at home with a black person ... it is just a general feeling, you feel more relaxed and you can talk, you can be more open with yourself talking with a black person rather than talking with a white person ...*
>
> Afro-Caribbean man

> *... When I came I wanted to talk to somebody of my own culture and my own age with similar children and problems, and who should understand what I'm going through.*
>
> Asian woman

Assumptions are, however, extremely dangerous. Increasingly, people do not feel themselves to be in one culture, but perhaps moving from one culture to another, or part of inter-cultural, multi-cultural groupings, so in all other aspects of mental health, the key worker needs to explore carefully with the user how they see their needs (see Fernando, 1995; Bennett, 2009).

8. **Personal and self-help strategies.**

As Thompson writes in *Existentialism and Social Work*:

> *Discovering that one is responsible for one's own actions can be a very disturbing and destabilising realisation, but it is also a moment of liberation – a liberation for the illusions which deny freedom. As such, it is a significant source of potential empowerment.*
>
> Thompson, 1992

In the end, however helpful our family, friends and professionals are, we are as a service user, a carer, a professional, or an amalgam of all of these, essentially alone with our own history, strengths and weaknesses, belief systems etc.

Some of the self-help strategies described in the literature are:

- positive self-help approaches
- managing distress and negotiating peace
- sport and physical exercise
- approaches to physical health
- relaxation and stress relief
- motivational approaches
- creativity
- spiritual and religious beliefs
- support of others

Fundamentally, there is another major connection between users, carers and professionals in that we all need to feel that there is a meaning and purpose to life in general and our life in particular. Without that, it is very difficult to face the daily grind.

A recognition of the spiritual dimension of everybody is essential (see Copsey, 1997; Copsey, 2001; Mental Health Foundation, 1997; Coyte, Gilbert and Nicholls, 2007; Cook et al., 2009; and see Chapter 9 of this book).

- Spirituality is all about making sense of our lives and discovering meaning and purpose.
- A belief in a personal god or gods or a specific belief system may be individual or based within a faith community.
- Faith communities may have very different approaches to mental distress and mental illness – either supportive and nurturing or negative and excluding.

John Swinton's work on *Spirituality and Mental Health Care* states that: 'Systematic reviews of the literature have consistently reported that aspects of religious and spiritual involvement are associated with desirable mental health outcomes' (Swinton, 2001: 68) though clearly there can be negative aspects as well. The long-standing faith communities need to be less defensive about the broader aspects of spirituality, while mental health professional need to listen to what users are saying about the spiritual aspects of their lives (see Lea, 2008 and Chapter 9 in this book).

9. **Making sense.**

When I was Director of Operations for Staffordshire Social Services, I worked closely with partners on developing a mental health strategy for the North of the county. Some very participatory workshops elicited a strategic direction which made sense to all partners, and had some very vivid and powerful depictions of the sort of services that users and carers would find helpful – one I recall was described as 'asylum in the community'. 18 months on, the vivid imagery had been 'professionalised' out of the strategy, and I couldn't recognise any of the issues that users had raised in the ways that they had described them!

In work on a one-to-one basis, with groups and communities, the language and the concepts have to be such that they make sense to everybody and are owned by everybody. In terms of the National Service Framework, and its successor, *New Horizons* (DoH, 2009) an approach that many other parts of health and social care and many other countries are wanting to copy, it is worth looking at this also from a user's point of view. The following diagram by Alison Faulkner and Thurstine Basset brings a user perspective and language to the process:

10. *Making connections.*
    Frameworks such as the NSF aim to bring together what users and carers want from services and how national policy envisages the delivery of Mental Health Services.

Effective social work has to be about bridging the overarching strategy with the individual aspirations of people

I was struck the other day by a mental health manager with over 20 years experience in social services relating to me 'what got her out of bed' every morning even when the pressures of work were intolerable:

When I joined the social work staff at XXXXXXX hospital, early on I met 'Glynis' who had been compulsorily admitted to XXXXXXXX in her early twenties as a 'moral defective' because she'd had an illegitimate child. 'Glynis' certainly wasn't suffering from a mental illness, and wouldn't have gone within a million miles of the hospital in today's climate. My greatest satisfaction was being able to place Glynis, now in her early seventies, in a community setting of her choice, with other friends; and the spur to my continued commitment to social work is helping people to try and take control of their lives and supporting people who without help would be denied the life experiences which we all wish for ourselves.
Senior manager, Mental Health Services (social work background, but managing health and social care services)

Professionals and managers have a tendency to overlay user and carer issues – usually expressed in powerful and compelling images – with a coating of jargon. Faulkner and Basset's diagram (Figure 17) is extremely useful because it translates the language of strategy into the lived and living experience of people who use (and may in the future require) services.

We use the words 'modernise' in the health and social care world, and so we should, but we also work in a post-modern world where the 'grand narratives' of the past have lost some of their force, and we need to listen to 'the view from below and within, individual narratives, different viewpoints, the personal experience' (Professor Anthony Clare, in the foreword to Priebe and Slade, 2002, *Evidence in Mental Health Care*).

At the end of the day, services are for those who use them, not for those who provide them.

Figure 17: Do it with us, not to us . . . (Faulkner and Basset, 2002).

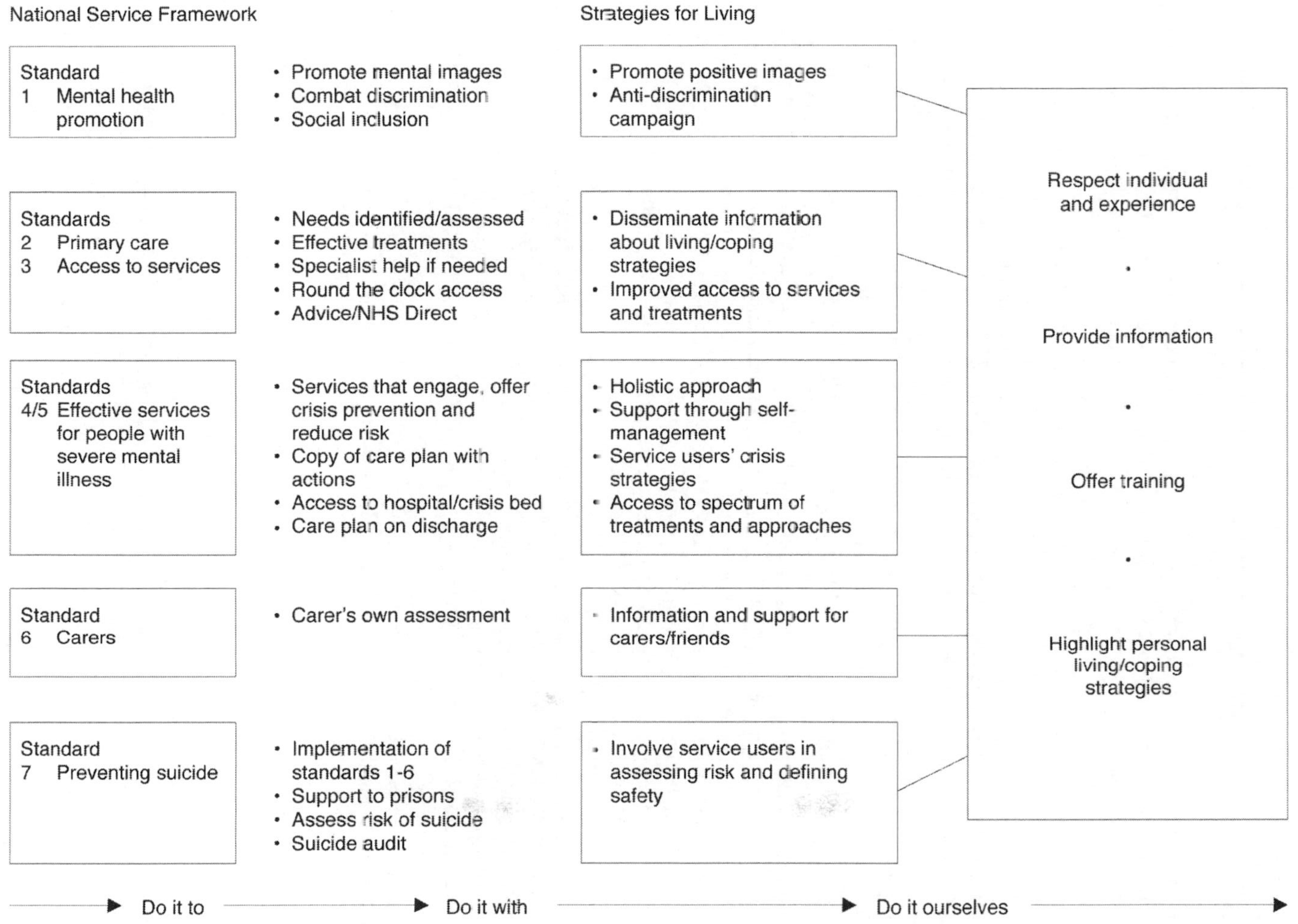

National Service Framework

Standard		
1	Mental health promotion	• Promote mental images • Combat discrimination • Social inclusion

Standards		
2	Primary care	• Needs identified/assessed • Effective treatments • Specialist help if needed • Round the clock access • Advice/NHS Direct
3	Access to services	

Standards		
4/5	Effective services for people with severe mental illness	• Services that engage, offer crisis prevention and reduce risk • Copy of care plan with actions • Access to hospital/crisis bed • Care plan on discharge

Standard		
6	Carers	• Carer's own assessment

Standard		
7	Preventing suicide	• Implementation of standards 1-6 • Support to prisons • Assess risk of suicide • Suicide audit

Strategies for Living

• Promote positive images
• Anti-discrimination campaign

• Disseminate information about living/coping strategies
• Improved access to services and treatments

• Holistic approach
• Support through self-management
• Service users' crisis strategies
• Access to spectrum of treatments and approaches

• Information and support for carers/friends

• Involve service users in assessing risk and defining safety

Respect individual and experience

Provide information

Offer training

Highlight personal living/coping strategies

Do it to ——→ Do it with ——→ Do it ourselves

CHAPTER 6

Personalisation – Choice and Control: The Issues

Sarah Carr

At a fundamental level, the concept of personalisation is nothing new in social work. In most conceptions of social work, there is a core philosophy that the purpose is to support people to maximise their independence and life chances in whatever ways fit their unique circumstances. The personalisation agenda in social care re-connects the wishes of people who use services with the values of professionals who work with them.

Personalisation is a way of expressing a value-based concept that is driving much of current public sector development, including that in social care and mental health. It means thinking about care and support services in an entirely different way, starting with the person as an individual with strengths, preferences and aspirations and putting them at the centre of the process of identifying their needs and making choices about the support they need to live their lives. In short it means 'putting people first' and the social care policies and reforms were set out in the Putting People First Concordat in December 2007 (HM Government, 2007).

The traditional service-led approach has often meant that people have had to fit around services rather than the services being responsive to their individual needs and preferences. For example, many disabled or older people have had their bedtime determined by having to fit in with the time slots of home care and support providers – they have had no choice about what time they go to bed – a level of control so many take for granted. So, personalisation is about giving people much more choice and control over their lives in all social care settings. It is also far wider than just giving direct payments or personal budgets to people eligible for council funding, although this is an important element. It also means addressing the needs and aspirations of whole communities to ensure everyone has access to the right information, advice and advocacy to make good decisions about the support they need. It means ensuring that people have wider choice in how their needs are met and are able to access universal services such as transport, leisure and education, housing, health and opportunities for employment regardless of mental health status, age or disability (Carr, 2008).

Although the term personalisation is relatively recent, it has grown from a number of different ideas and influences from social work values. Good social work practice has always involved putting the individual first and values such as respect for the individual and self-determination have long been at the heart of social work. Personalisation can be associated with existing practice approaches such as strengths-based perspectives, self-determination, person-centred planning, empowerment, mental health recovery, independent living and self-directed support. It is also informing developments in health and the NHS, including the idea of having personal health budgets for people with long-term conditions (DoH, 2008).

Personalisation, choice and control: how far we've come

To fully understand personalisation for 21st century social work practice, it is helpful to know how the approach fits in with the history of social care in the 19th and 20th centuries. Such an overview can give a picture of how society is moving towards accepting people with mental health problems, disabled people, people with learning disabilities and older people as equal citizens and important members of the community, with much more choice and control over their care and support. Where people were once incarcerated in hospitals and institutions, they are now being supported to live independent lives in the community.

During the 19th century, people regarded as having mental health problems or learning disabilities and disabled people were classified by a medical condition and kept in large institutional or hospital settings where they were rarely treated as individual human beings. After a series of 'Lunacy Acts' in the 19th century asylums and institutions for people with mental health problems, people with learning disabilities and people with conditions like epilepsy expanded rapidly. By 1914 there were over 120 asylums in England, the largest of which housed up to 4,000 people. Often 50 people shared a single open dormitory ward (Rutherford, 2008). The staff in these large institutions were in complete control and people had no choice about food and clothes or control over their activities and relationships. The institutionalisation of people with mental health problems, people with learning disabilities and disabled people was standard health and social care practice for the majority of the 20th century.

In 1961 Enoch Powell made his famous 'water tower' speech to the National Association for Mental Health (which is now MIND) calling for the closure of huge psychiatric institutions (Gould, 2008). This proposal became more urgent in 1967 when the News of the World exposed abusive treatment and inhumane conditions at Ely Hospital in Cardiff. Government inquiries into this and other cases of abuse and patient deaths were to change policies concerning long-stay institutions, inspection and the rights of people living in hospitals (Butler and Drakeford, 2005). Gradually, popular, political and professional opinion turned against the old institutions and people began to explore other ways of developing mental health and social care services. In 1990 the NHS and Community Care Act introduced a 'needs led approach' for people using social care services and new arrangements for assessment and care management. The government stated that this would lead to individuals receiving 'individually tailored packages of care'. With further deinstitutionalisation and more people going to live in the community as long-stay hospitals were closed, the emphasis was on providing flexible care and support so that people can live 'as normal a life as possible in their own homes'.

The influence of the service user and survivor movements

Service users, survivors and their allies have been pivotal players in the development of personalisation. Out of the civil rights movement of the1960s and 1970s, which questioned the way power is used and distributed in society, came the disability movement and anti-psychiatry/mental health user and survivor activity (Glasby

and Littlechild, 2009). Campaigning, support and research groups of psychiatric survivors emerged out of the anti-psychiatry movement in the late 1960s. The psychiatric survivor and mental health service user movement became very critical of the medical model in mental health and campaigned for the closure of long-stay psychiatric hospitals and for people with mental health problems to have a greater say in decisions about their lives (Campbell, 1996). In 1972 the Union of Physically Impaired Against Segregation (UPIAS) became the first disability liberation group in the UK. In 1975 they published *Fundamental Principles of Disability* which developed the 'social model of disability' to gain insight into their situation and to recognise how they were oppressed: 'It is society which disables physically impaired people. Disability is something imposed on top of our impairments' (UPIAS, 1975). The group highlighted the fundamental lack of control disabled people have over their lives and the power relationship with social care staff and they started to campaign for independent living and rights for disabled people (Campbell and Oliver, 1996). In 1973 a group of disabled students at Berkeley University in California pioneered the use of personal assistants (PAs) and go on to found the first Centre for Independent Living.

So, personalisation has roots in the disability, mental health survivor and service user movements, where individuals and groups undertook direct action and lobbied for change. Independent living, self-determination, participation, control, choice and empowerment are key concepts for personalisation and they have their origins in the independent living movement, the social model of disability and the survivor movement in mental health (Glasby and Littlechild, 2009). Independent living is one of the goals of personalisation. It does not mean living on your own or doing things alone, but rather it means 'having choice and control over the assistance and/or equipment needed to go about your daily life; having equal access to housing, transport and mobility, health, employment and education and training opportunities' (Office for Disability Issues, 2008: 11). Self-directed support is a term that relates to a variety of approaches to creating personalised social care, and the influential In Control programme (Poll and Duffy, 2006) sees self-directed support as the route to achieving independent living. It says that the defining characteristics of self-directed support are:

- The support is controlled by the individual.
- The level of support is agreed in a fair, open and flexible way.
- Any additional help needed to plan, specify and find support should be provided by people who are as close to the individual as possible.
- The individual should control the financial resources for their support in a way they choose.
- All of the practices should be carried out in accordance with an agreed set of ethical principles.

Direct payments and personal budgets

Personalisation is taking place within the practice context of individual care management and person-centred planning in adult social care services. Some approaches to personalisation and achieving independent living, such as direct payments and personal budgets, are already being tried or are in place in some local social services. In practical terms, a major impetus behind the development of the personal budget option has been the experience of direct payments that became available, initially to disabled adults of working age in England, as a result of the Community Care (Direct Payments) Act 1996, and have since been extended to other groups, including people with mental health problems (Glasby and Littlechild, 2009; Leece and Bornat, 2006). Significantly, direct payments were championed by disabled people themselves and have allowed people the option of having a cash sum in lieu of social care services so they can purchase their own support (SCIE, 2005). Personal budgets can be taken in a variety of ways, such as a notional allocation of funding to be managed and spent as the individual wishes. People have several personal budget management options to choose from: they can be managed by the individual as a direct payment, or by the care manager, by a trust, as an indirect payment to an approved third party or held by a service provider (Carr, 2008; see also Dowson and Greig, 2009). The key to the personal budget approach is giving a clear idea of the amount available to someone so they can influence or control the spend in ways that best meet their support needs. It is a deliberate attempt to shift control away from the provider (which often offers a fixed range of services and little choice) to

allow the individual to design the services (frequently non-traditional) to achieve the agreed outcomes in their care plan.

The popularity and success of direct payments has stimulated much of the thinking around personal budgets, and research clearly shows that people with mental health problems can benefit from having their own budget to make choices about their own support. When personal budgets were piloted, the study found that mental health service users reported a higher quality of life and a possible tendency towards better psychological well-being (Glendinning et al., 2008). People with mental health problems have found innovative ways of using direct payments and personal budgets to manage their mental health and to take part in social and community life (MIND 2009; Coldham and Spandler 2005; Spandler and Vick, 2006). However, research has also shown that there are barriers to the uptake of direct payments and personal budgets by people with mental health problems because of perceptions of risk, decision making capacity and the fact that people with mental health problems are exploring non-traditional support (Glendinning et al., 2008; Newbiggin and Lowe, 2005; Spandler and Vick, 2005; Carr and Robbins, 2009). What mental health social workers need to remember is that 'whilst a person's social care needs have to be assessed by a mental health professional, the *way* they decide to meet these needs should (in theory) be up to them (Spandler, 2007: 21).

Mental health recovery and personalisation

The development of the recovery model in mental health is a key example of the way that a service-user led, person-centred approach provides a framework for improving services. The recovery model is being used as a core principle in mental health service reform in the US, Australia and New Zealand. It is now being promoted as an approach to the development of more holistic, personalised mental health services across the UK (New Horizons). The US Department of Health and Human Services Administration and the Interagency Committee on Disability Research issued a *National Consensus Statement on Mental Health Recovery* which stated that 'mental health is a journey of healing and transformation enabling a person with a mental health problem to live a meaningful life in a community of his or her choice while striving to achieve his or her potential' (US Department of Health and Human Services, 2005). This work drew on the long history of the recovery movement in the United States (Hennessey, 2004).

The *Journey to Recovery* (DoH, 2001) stated that the UK mental health system 'should support people in settings of their own choosing and enable access to community resources including housing and work or whatever they felt was crucial to their recovery' (Lester and Gask, 2006). This type of recovery approach reflects the principles and aims of personalisation.

The central tenet of recovery is that 'it does not necessarily mean cure (clinical recovery). Instead it emphasises the unique journey of an individual living with mental health problems to build a life beyond illness (social recovery). Thus a person can recover their life, without necessarily recovering from their illness' (Shepherd et al., 2008). In the UK the challenge of system-level change has been identified for the implementation of the recovery approach in mental health service modernisation: 'If we want to develop recovery-oriented services for people with serious mental illness, we need to offer systematically organised and personally tailored collaborative help, treatment and care in an atmosphere of hope and optimism' (Lester and Gask, 2006). This is clearly one of the aims of the personalisation agenda and there are already specialist recovery staff working in mental health teams to offer person-centred support. Current discussion on the development of UK mental health services based on a principle of self-determination asserts that this means moving towards a system of support built by the person and their advocates to help them achieve their ambitions and goals (The Future Vision Coalition, 2008).

The role of the social worker

Although the term personalisation is relatively recent, it has grown from a number of different ideas and influences from social work values. Good social work practice has always involved putting the individual first; values such as respect for the individual and self-determination have long been at the heart of social work (International Federation of Social Workers, 2004). As an example of the ways the professional

bodies might integrate this thinking into training and education policy, the English General Social Care Council (GSCC) concluded that social work skills were critical to achieving the ambitions of the personalisation agenda, precisely because of the profession's core values and principles.

There has been some concern about the professional role of the social worker being undermined by the implications of creating more personalised services, but people have also argued that social work could have the opportunity to reaffirm and clarify its role. There is now the potential for social workers to move away from gatekeeping and resource management to advocacy and support tasks. But people who use social care services and their carers are clear about the qualities they value in social workers:

> *People value a social work approach based on challenging the broader barriers they face. They place a particular value on a social approach, the social work relationship, and the positive personal qualities they associate with their social worker. These include warmth, respect, being non-judgmental, listening, treating people with equality, being trustworthy, open, honest and reliable and communicating well. People value the support that social workers offer as well as their ability to help them access and deal with other services and agencies.*
>
> General Social Care Council, 2008

As the last point suggests, social workers can also draw on their skills in counselling and community development to take forward personalisation. Here it is important to remember that personalisation is not only about personal budgets.

Social workers will need to be empowered by their organisations to in turn empower the people who are using the services, so organisational issues need to be considered. People who use social care services have recognised the limitations social workers can face when working within the constrained rules and resources of organisations (Beresford, 2007) but these do not always appear to be recognised in the various official documents. One of the current roles for social workers is to ration resources and identify priorities.

So people have indicated that although having greater choice of services may be a good thing, there also needs to be an improvement in how current services are provided, including addressing issues concerning budgets and rationing, along with the impact this has on the quality of social work.

Co-production

Co-production is a term increasingly used as a way of talking about participation and community involvement in social care services in the UK in the context of personalisation, but it is sometimes difficult to define (Needham, 2006; Needham and Carr, 2009). In proposals for new ways of organising and delivering social care services, people who use services have suggested that 'service user controlled organisations can be a site where social workers are employed working alongside service users in a hands on way' (Shaping Our Lives et al., 2007: 13). This would seem to encapsulate the essence of co-production in adult social care and user led organisations have a particular role to play in the development of personalisation and the provision of care and support services (HM Government 2007; HM Government, 2009).

Co-production has been going on in communities and in public services for more than 20 years. In America the term began as 'a general description of the process whereby clients work alongside professionals as partners in the delivery of services' (Boyle et al., 2006). It has also been described as 'the involvement of citizens, clients, consumers, volunteers and/or community organisations in *producing* public services as well as consuming or otherwise benefiting from them' (Alford, 1998). Organisations like the New Economics Foundation (NEF) have thought about how public services in the UK could be made better through co-production (Cummins and Miller, 2007; NEF, 2008) seeing it as going much further than consulting people or getting them to get involved in meetings (Boviard 2007). The idea is to recognise that the people that use the services are also the people that can help produce the services and change them for the better – they are not burdens but assets.

Research on co-production has demonstrated the value of frontline workers focusing on people's abilities rather than seeing them as problems (Boyle et al., 2006) and highlighted the need for the right skills to do this. It has also identified the importance of developing staff confidence and improving how they feel about themselves and their jobs. Co-production should mean system reform and more power and resources being shared with people on the front line – service users, carers and frontline workers – so they are empowered to co-produce their own solutions to the difficulties they are best placed to know about (Gannon and Lawson, 2008; Needham and Carr, 2009).

Conclusion: social work, 'choice and voice'

It is hoped that as a result of personalisation, people who use services will become more confident and assertive when it comes to choice and control over their own individual support packages and will become co-producers in the new services designed to meet their needs on a local level. This is a very powerful ambition with radical implications. However, the people most likely to be marginalised or underserved in social care services (people known as 'seldom heard' such as some black and minority ethnic people, lesbian and gay people, homeless people, people living in poverty, people living in residential or secure settings, frail older people, refugees and people with cognitive and communications difficulties) are often the least likely to be involved with service development and strategic decision making (Carr, 2004). There is concern about some of the current policy assumptions about the opportunity and capacity people have to exercise power on both an individual ('choice') and collective level ('voice') in social care (Manthorpe et al., 2008).

Implementing the 'choice and voice' aspect of personalisation will need to take account of varying levels of equality, advantage, aspiration, esteem and social inclusion among the different people who use social care services. Some people are already able to be active citizens and take advantage of the opportunities reformed public services will offer, but some people who use social care services are very disadvantaged, both socially and personally. Recent research into designing citizen-centred governance showed that 'citizens and service users in disadvantaged areas receive considerable demands to become involved in governance of their communities. They face a double disadvantage, as they have to negotiate the complexities of public service delivery to meet their immediate needs and also respond to the many consultation initiatives set up by the various institutions of community governance' (Barnes et al., 2008: 2). In the process of transformation, public services should not lose sight of their role in promoting social justice and should 'aim to achieve a fair distribution of outcomes, paying particular attention to the narrowing of unjust inequalities (such as between people from different social class backgrounds, or of different gender, ethnicity or sexuality)' (Brooks, 2007: 6). Many people with mental health problems experience great social and economic disadvantage as well as social exclusion and discrimination and 'ultimately, ideas about 'choice and control' which are so central to individualised funding, do not operate in a vacuum but in a wider social context of constraints, conflicts and competing ideologies' about mental health (Spandler, 2007: 23).

The conceptual person who uses services in the current dominant policy model is educated, articulate, assertive, informed and confident. This has been challenged as having limitations for understanding some people who use social care services:

> The failure to engage with the effects of structural inequalities also vitiates [the] conception of people who use services ... we know that the most common shared characteristic of those who use social work services is that they are poor ... they are also likely to experience a range of other difficulties, including mental health problems ... The combination of poverty, multiple discrimination, a lack of resources in every sense and (frequently) physical or mental impairment means that the typical user of social work services will not often match Ulrich Beck's description of the 'choosing, deciding, shaping human being who aspires to be the author of their life'... most social work clients have more modest ambitions.
>
> Ferguson 2007: 395–6

In the light of their own similar observations, the UK National Consumer Council have warned that: 'choice can compound inequalities as take-up of choice varies across the social divide' (National Consumer Council, 2004: 9). Social workers in mental health and in adult social care in general have a particular role to play in ensuring that issues of social inequality are accounted for because 'in addition to seeking individual solutions, it is essential to address root causes that create social exclusion' (Lyons, 2005: 250).

CHAPTER 7

The Skilled Helper – The Role of the Social Worker

Peter Gilbert

I had help from some wonderful social workers who supported me and helped me achieve my goals in life.

Actor, Samantha Morton, speaking at a social work recruitment campaign, *The Guardian*, 1 September 2009

I am very satisfied with my social worker; she is very helpful and always treats me with the utmost respect.

Quoted in an Inspection report, September 2001

Social work can make a particularly valuable contribution to improving the quality and delivery of services, given that the causes and consequences of poor mental health are significantly influenced by the environment of which we are all a part. Social work is by nature holistic in approach and views the individual within a wider context of their personal, familial, cultural and socio-economic circumstances. Its ethos is on empowerment and promoting independence through a focus on 'working with' rather than 'doing to' which helps to increase personal achievement, self-fulfilment and create a much stronger sense of citizenship.

David Joannides, former lead Director and chair of the ADSS Mental Health Strategy Group

The social worker is the point of contact at a time of crisis or focused need. They have a professionalism that offers a useful distance from the problem in hand and allows them to deal dispassionately with the situation . . . The person who becomes a social worker wants to make a difference to the lives of people and communities, and their commitment is often clear to see in their practice. The practice of social work can be frustrating due to lack of suitable resources. Social workers should be closely involved in planning services for people and communities as they are best placed to provide advice and ideas on the needs, gaps and processes of communities and disadvantaged groups.

co-ordinator of a voluntary sector service

A lot has been written recently about the extent to which social workers are undervalued. But in Mental Health work their value is beyond doubt.

Margaret Clayton, former Chairperson of the Mental Health Act Commission, *Community Care*, 23 May 2002: 38–9

Placing yourself where the user is

At a particularly hectic time as a director of social services, I contracted a bad sinus infection. Wanting to get back to full health as soon as possible, I queued up for evening surgery and

was seen by a GP in his 50s who, when I said what work I was in, launched into a eulogy about the practice-based social worker (and yes, I did contact the social worker and her manager the next day to give them the positive feedback). What were the most important factors in her work, I asked the GP?

She seems to be able to put herself where the patient [sic] is and, as somebody who has been in general practice many years, the life we live now seems to me to be a lot more complicated than it used to be; the social worker can find her way through the maze which is society today in a way that makes things easier for the patient and for us.

It has always struck me from the time I was a social work trainee on attachment to a GP surgery in the mid 1970s that there is, or should be, a natural affinity between social workers and general practitioners. Both have to pull off the conjuring trick of working with individuals, with their unique natures and circumstances, and help them cope with and develop in an increasingly complex world, where people cannot depend on the certainties they once put their trust in.

As a generic (general) social worker in the late 1970s/early 1980s, I worked with an older, single mother, with a very poor self image, who had married late in life, given birth to a daughter, and then faced the tragedy of her husband dying suddenly. Mrs T found herself not only grieving but **extremely** angry with life for snatching happiness away from her, and angry with her daughter, that it was her daughter who was still alive and not her husband.

This was a very middle class family and although it soon became clear to the GP and her neighbours that Sally, the daughter, was at risk, and that Mrs T was in acute mental distress, nobody had felt it appropriate to contact social services, because middle class families in middle class neighbourhoods coped – didn't they? As Mrs T's mental health deteriorated, however, her expressions of pain became more extreme, and her attitude towards 'Sally' declined. Neighbours ran out of capacity to cope with the demands and the anxiety.

When social services were eventually involved,

Mrs T was very frank about her feelings of extreme anger to her daughter, and the occasional desire, especially when washing her hair in the bath, to actually drown her. A psychiatrist and clinical psychologist were involved, but the day-to-day work was through a social worker and a family support worker. The social history was especially vital to the psychiatrist and GP, as it was through this that Mrs T's deep-rooted sense of worthlessness and that life had 'cheated' her became starkly evident. The intensive work by the social worker and family support worker was required to ensure both the safety of Sally in the short term, and also the viability of the family unit in the long run. If the professionals had completely taken control of the situation, then Mrs T's feelings of worthlessness would have been reinforced: 'I'm a worthless wife who couldn't save her husband from the heart attack that killed him; I'm a worthless mother because you've taken my child away'.

Some excellent work was done by the psychologist, but as Mrs T's self-awareness and recognition of the issues troubling her surfaced, the danger to Sally actually increased as the mother became more volatile. The psychologist, though excellent in one-to-one work, was not aware of this, but the social worker and family support worker were. It became clear that therapeutic work to heal Mrs T's wounds could not be carried any further until Sally was more comprehensively safeguarded. Mrs T was persuaded to request Sally's reception into care in a partnership arrangement with the Local Authority, and she was informally admitted to the local psychiatric hospital under the 1959 Mental Health Act. She was treated for depression and therapeutic work undertaken to address her feelings of low self-worth. The social worker continued to work with Mrs T and supported Sally in the foster home. Sally was a very intelligent and strong-minded nine year old who was quite aware of the danger she had been in while in her mother's care and the ambivalent feelings her mother had for her. Despite this, she was very clear that she wished to return to her mother as soon as possible, and this was expressed with some hostility towards the social worker.

In the end, Mrs T came out of hospital with her depression lifted, and a number of feelings about herself and her circumstances ameliorated if not fully resolved. Sally was considered to be no longer at immediate risk, and she was very clear that she wished to return home. Intensive work continued from the social worker, and even more especially by the family support worker who worked with Mrs T on the care tasks with Sally which Mrs T found particularly difficult. The social worker co-ordinated input with health staff and rebuilt the capacity for support within the local community, through the church that Mrs T and Sally belonged to. In the end, the family and the community learned to cope again.

For the social worker, there was the challenge of assisting a parent and child to rebuild a relationship both in the present and for the future; high risk elements around childcare and mental health; the need to balance the safety of the child which was paramount with the fact that any increasing feeling of powerlessness and worthlessness on Mrs T's part would have made the mother-child relationship non-viable in the future; there was complex networking to take place both with health professionals, with communication between the GP and the consultant psychiatrist, not always of the first order, and competing agendas between a concentration by the Mental Health professionals on the mother, and the social worker and GP balancing need to concentrate on the safety of the child as well; there was the imperative for the social worker to supervise the family support worker, without whose character and skills the child would have been at risk and the relationship might not have been viable in the long run.

Without social work intervention, the child would not have been protected adequately and the mother-child relationship would almost certainly have broken down permanently. The social worker's balancing of risk around the paramount safety of the child but also her long-term need for a stable relationship with her mother; the need to network with professional bodies and the wider community; knowledge of child care and mental health law; an understanding of psychological processes for both the child and the mother; and holding both the short-term and the long-term issues together creates a pressure on the social worker which not many professionals would wish to have.

As a debate is current in 2009, following the Baby 'Peter' tragedy in Haringey, as to whether the education of student social workers should be split between children and adults, this case study demonstrates the need to keep the whole family in focus.

Professor Andrew Cooper, of the Tavistock, in a recent article, quotes a friend and colleague as saying: 'I don't think they really understand in Health what we mean when we call ourselves a therapeutic service. It is not about individual treatment programmes, it is about all the things that you and I have talked about over the years – a total response to the complex dynamics of family plus professional system that you get presented with' (Cooper, 2002: 7).

As we have seen from the preceding chapters, users value:

- Somebody to work alongside them as they make sense of themselves and themselves within the world around them.
- Being valued as individuals and as citizens.
- Help with both the emotional and the practical side of life.
- Assistance in working through the maze of agencies.
- Mediation in both family, group and community relationships.
- Balancing personal liberty with care.

Carers value:

- Appreciation of their individuality and citizenship.
- Help in preserving their essential relationship with the person cared for as husband/wife, mother/father, son/daughter, rather than being viewed primarily as a 'carer'.
- Accurate and accessible information.
- Assistance in finding their way through the maze of agencies, benefits etc.
- Contact with other carers with similar circumstances.
- Time to talk with an empathetic listener about the particular pressures on them as carers, and their aspirations for the future.

Both users and carers wish to be able to influence service policy, systems and education in a dynamic way, and with a clear commitment from providers that this isn't simply lip service (see Beresford, 2002; Moss, Boath et al., 2009). Societies and governments have expectations as well. Whether we define government in the highly optimistic tones of Charles James Fox:

> *What is the end of all government? Certainly the happiness of the governed.*
>
> Charles James Fox, MP, House of Commons, 1 December 1783

Or, in the words of the French proponent of minimal government:

> *To be governed is to be inspected, spied upon, directed, law-driven, regulated, preached at, controlled, censored . . .*
>
> Pierre-Joseph Proudhon

Or again, the pragmatic, utilitarian approach which informs much of modern governance:

> *That action is best which procures the greatest happiness for the greatest numbers.*
>
> The words of Francis Hutcheson, developed by Bentham and John Stuart Mill

As Banks, Davies and others point out:

> *Social workers are not autonomous professionals whose guiding ethical principles are solely about respecting and promoting the self-determination of service users. They are employed by agencies, work within the constraints of legal and procedural rules and must also work to promote the public good or the well-being of society in general.*
>
> Banks, 1995: 31

And Davies:

> *The practice of social work takes place almost wholly as a result of **either** statutory legislation or policy decisions taken by politicians in central or local government. The functions of the social worker and the focus of her work are not self-selected but are politically sanctioned and authorised by the agent which employed her. The point that makes as many questions as it answers, but it does at least indicate the source of social work legitimacy, and emphasises that social workers are not, and can never be, a law unto themselves.*
>
> Davies, 1994. (See also Smale, et al., 2000: Ch. 1)

Governments therefore desire:

- The fulfilment of social objectives through the carrying out of legislation and agency practice.
- The promotion of citizenship and the healthy functioning of individuals, families and communities.
- The maintenance of equilibrium between the liberty of the subject and the safety of the subject and other people.

Of course, as we can see from the case description given above of Mrs T and Sally, there are numerous tensions inherent in the effective delivery of social work. Users and carers are often lumped together in policy documents and statements, and yet their needs are often different and may well be conflicting. The state and its legislation may be beneficent, but can also be oppressive. Britain's uneasy compromise between American libertarianism and European communitarianism is under pressure from both sides. We tend to regard 'the Law' as neutral, but legislation is a reflection of society especially as

Mental Health law has oscillated between care, legalism, treatment, rights and safety over the centuries (see Chapter 8 in this book).

It is into this complex and conflictual environment that social work has to operate. Not only are there obvious dichotomies between different individuals and groups but also within the world of the person one is working with. In such a world, the utilisation of precise science, the application of the scalpel and laser are not appropriate. In essence, the social worker is a skilful mariner, navigating a fragile bark among the shoals and reefs and currents of life together with those they are working with. As my social work tutor Hugh England asserts:

> *The source of social work's potential strength, and the conviction of its proponents, is the very fact that it does not separate the world experienced by those in need of help into component elements. Such experience is always a complex, composite experience, it is always a unique synthesis; yet it cannot be impossible to construct such a synthesis, because the client – and everyone – does so all the time. The strength of the able worker lies in his [sic] ability accurately to join the client in a construction and experience this synthesis. It is only through such sharing that people sometimes say to others . . . 'you seem to understand' – and we know that to be understood by others is a necessary and a therapeutic experience.*
>
> England, 1986

It is worth noting that the 'Ten Essential Capabilities' set out by NIMHE's workforce programme, link closely with the values of Social Work. The ten are: working in partnership, respecting diversity, practicing ethically, challenging inequality, promoting recovery, identifying people's need and strengths, providing service user-centred care, making a difference, promoting safety and positive risk taking, personal development and learning (see McGonagle et al., 2008).

Historical roots and routes

> *. . . there seems something else in life besides time, something which may conveniently be called 'value', something which is measured not by minutes or hours, but by intensity, so that when we look at our past, it does not stretch back evenly but piles up into a few notable pinnacles, and when we look at the future it seems sometimes a wall, sometimes a cloud, sometimes a sun, but never a chronological chart.*
>
> Forster, *Aspects of the Novel*,
> The Clark Lecturers, 1927

> *The unifying element . . . is the professional skill of the social worker whether deployed in field work, in primary care, in residential or day care, or in hospital.*
>
> *Better Services for the Mentally Ill*, 1975: 23

As Jordan states:

> *In societies which are relatively simple in construction, there are no social workers. 'Vulnerable people' are looked after within the extended family or the tribe. Unconventional behaviour is either tolerated, venerated or punished by retributive methods.*
>
> Jordan, 1984: 31

Younghusband makes a similar point about social care being regarded 'as something private or as an attitude, a concern for welfare, rather than as a practice based upon knowledge and skill' (Younghusband, 1978: 24). This is not so different from how nursing was regarded in the mid 19th century, because, after all, it was thought that anyone can nurse, and the portrayal of the professional nurse, such as Mrs Gamp in Dickens's *Martin Chuzzlewit* (1843) is hardly flattering. The professionalism of the doctor also is not something which has been fixed for all time. The doctor in Flaubert's *Madame Bovary* or Mr Perry in Jane Austen's *Emma* have an ambiguous professional persona and before that the English radicals used to refer to the doctors' limited skills in 'purging and bleeding' (see Hill, 1972) in the same way that some users now refer to 'chemical straightjackets'.

As Midwinter points out (Midwinter, 1994) the mediaeval monasteries were the first welfare state, and the almshouses were the forerunners of both the hospitals and care homes. When they were abolished at the Reformation, the state had to find other means to alleviate the direct effects of poverty and ill-health while ensuring that social unrest was averted.

The 1601 Elizabethan Poor Law set out a system of outdoor relief, reversed in 1834 by the new Poor Law and its emphasis on institutions.

Andrew Scull, Professor of Sociology at the University of California, highlights 'the transformations underlying the move towards institutionalisation' being tied 'to the growth of the capitalist market system and to its impact on economic and social relationships' (Scull, 1984: 24). Increasing geographical mobility (echoed in the 20th and 21st centuries) the alienation and anonymity of the urban slums; the destruction of the old paternal relationships; the breakdown of rural patterns as described in Hardy's *Far from the*

Madding Crowd; and rapid technological progress (again an echo in our own day) meant that 'the situation of the poor and dependent classes became simultaneously more visible and more desperate' (Scull, 1984: 22).

Scull identifies a number of connected features to distinguish deviance and its control in modern society:

- The substantial involvement of the state, and the emergence of a highly rationalised and generally centrally administered and directed social control apparatus.
- The treatment of many types of deviance in institutions providing a large measure of segregation from the surrounding community.
- The careful differentiation of different sources of deviance, and the subsequent confinement of each variety to the ministration of 'experts' (Scull, 1984: 15).

This drive towards greater organisation would have been recognised by Edwin Chadwick as he pushed forward the social reforms of the mid Victorian era (see Midwinter, 1994: Chapter 3.) Though we are indebted to Chadwick in many ways for his social environmental reforms – in fact had Chadwick been able to enlist wider support among the governing classes, we might be living today in a country with a markedly cleaner environment and a health service less concentrated on individual pathology (see Small, 1998) – the Earl of Shaftesbury's concern for people in mental distress was much more based on principles of care, than Chadwick's preoccupation with social order.

The historical pendulum described in Chapters 3 and 4 is in full flow in mental health services from the mid 19th century.

For those at the receiving end of care, treatment, control etc., the picture could be very stark and there is nobody like Charles Dickens to describe the social environment and our need to work towards a common good so as to avoid it 'raining social retributions' (*Dombey and Son*, 1846) and the reaction of those who were deprived to the power of the state on the one hand and the machinations of an unregulated private sector, e.g. Dotheboys Hall (*Nicholas Nickleby*, 1838) on the other.

Dickens's description of Betty Higden in *Our Mutual Friend* (1864), she of 'indomitable purpose and a strong constitution', is demonstrative of the poor's attitude to the state:

God help me and the like of me! – how the worn-out people that do come down to that, get driven from post to pillar and pillar to post, a-purpose to tire them out! Do I never read how they are put off, put off – how they are grudged, grudged, grudged, the shelter, or the doctor, or the drop of physic, or the drop of bread . . . then I say, I hope I can die as well as another, and I'll die without that disgrace (of entering the workhouse) . . . sooner than fall into the hands of those cruel jacks we read of, that dodge and drive, and worry and weary, and scorn and shame the decent poor.
Dickens, 1864, 1988 edition: 248

It is Mrs Pardiggle, the visitor of the poor, with her certainties (*Bleak House*, 1853) who might be seen as the negative caricature of the social worker, whereas Esther Summerson , with her greater self-awareness could be speaking as a social work student when she says:

That I was inexperienced in the art of adapting my mind to minds very differently situated, and addressing them from suitable points of view. That I had not that delicate knowledge of the heart that must be essential to such a work. That I had much to learn, myself, before I could teach others and that I could not confide in my good intentions alone . . .
Bleak House, 1852, 1911 edition: 127

As Bill Jordan points out in his admirable *Invitation to Social Work* (Jordan, 1984) it was the social reformer, Octavia Hill, who talked about the defining quality of relationship between her and her helpers and the tenants as 'respectfulness', a phrase which chimes very much with modern social work values (see below). Hill added that 'each man [*sic*] has had his own view of life and must be freed to fulfil it . . . In many ways he is a far better judge of it than we, as he has lived through himself what we have only seen' (Jordan, 1984: 37–41). The social reform tradition; the growth of therapeutic approaches stemming mainly from the USA and a local government strand began to come together, with some aspects of collision as well as cohesion in the 1950s.

Submission to the Department of Health from the Northamptonshire Approved Social Workers Standards Group on Proposed Reforms of the Mental Health Act, 1983.

Historical Context
The first documented appointment of a trained mental health social worker in Britain was in 1928. From this inception,

there were new opportunities in ways of working with people with mental distress both within institutional and community settings. The role of the social worker was new and different from the profession of psychiatry which dominated hospitals at the time, and one of the tasks of the social worker encompassed recording service users' social history as part of their treatment plan.

In addition, social workers arranged after-care services for patients being discharged. The underlying belief was that some did not need to be detained in hospital provided that adequate support services were available on discharge. Social workers at the time were the only mental health professionals to work across the hospital/community boundary.

In 1939, the Association of Psychiatric Social Workers turned down the BMA proposal that social workers should be registered as medical auxiliaries. At the time it was clear that the value base and theoretical orientation of social workers differed significantly from a medical model.

Despite this, the disciplines, at least locally, worked well together. The Social Work Department at St. Crispin's Hospital, Northampton, in 1950, was described as being of 'great value in the total treatment effort', and in 1958, 'special attention was paid to outpatients and long-stay patients who wished to return to life outside the hospital'.

Mental health social workers were the first discipline to move out of psychiatric hospitals and base their practice within a community setting. They were also keen advocates of the closure of psychiatric hospitals, believing that, where possible, community resources should be mobilised to enable service users to have the opportunity to receive care and treatment outside institutions.

Social workers, therefore, have traditionally been, and continue to be concerned, with enabling people to have control over their lives, promoting people's right of citizenship and protecting those who are at risk in the least restricted way.

21st March 2000

Table 4: Routes towards the social worker in mental health

- 19th century social philanthropists:
  - social action
  - community approach
  - insistence on independence and self-help.
- American psychotherapy:
  - therapeutic approaches
  - understanding of history to unlock the present
  - advent of psychiatric social workers
- Local Government (Poor Law and afterwards):
  - social control
  - alleviation of extreme poverty
  - work with individuals and families
  - duly authorised officers and mental welfare officers

(See Timms, 1964; Jones, 1972, 1988; Younghusband, 1978; Butler and Pritchard, 1983; Olson, 1984; Ulas and Connor, 1999; Heimler, 1967; Golightley, 2008; Gould, 2009.)

Mental health social work encapsulates some of the tensions which exist in social work as a whole, and came to a head in the *Barclay Report*, 1982: 199, which argued that: 'The personal social services must develop a close working partnership with citizens focusing more closely on the community and its strengths' while the minority report by Robert Pinker stressed a more professional and casework approach (see Jordan, 1985: 139). The more highly qualified psychiatric social workers tended to be more readily found in the main psychiatric hospitals, while the mental welfare officers came from the administrative and supervisory tradition within local authorities stemming from the Mental Health and Mental Treatment Acts of the early part of the 20th century. When Goldberg's studies in the early 1960s concluded that: 'Some understanding of the whole family constellation is essential before any plan for treatment can be formulated' (quoted in Younghusband, 1978: 167), clearly much of the social work resource was in the wrong area to effect change.

Gradually, PSWs and mental welfare officers moved closer together. The Macintosh Report (1951) and the Younghusband Report (1959) both recommended extensive initiatives on training for social workers in mental health, and the 1968 Seebohm Report reinforced the value of social work for people experiencing mental ill-health:

The families of mentally disordered people tend to suffer from inter-related social disabilities which are often caused or aggravated by the mental disorder, *which may precipitate breakdown or incapacitate the family for caring for the chronically sick member. The social worker should be concerned with the **whole family**, learning how to make a family diagnosis, and be able to take wide responsibility and mobilise a wide range of services.*

Seebohm, 1968: para. 353, my emphasis

Seebohm, of course, saw the creation of social services departments in 1971, bringing together the old children's, welfare and mental health departments, with children moving across from the Home Office, and mental health from the Health Service. This had the effect in some areas of simultaneously creating increased understanding of common issues across generations; effecting more 'clout' for social and community aspects of care; diluting some elements of specialist knowledge; dislocating some of the old relationships with other professionals and organisations in the mental health and learning disability fields.

The reintroduction of specialist social work, with a reasonable amount of permeability of experience and training between childcare, adult mental health and the mental health of old age, coupled with an acceptance, as Cooper points out, that one can have, and indeed should have, a foot in the two camps of social action and individual casework (Cooper, 2002: 8), has led to a strengthening of professional practice, coupled with a strong focus on the needs and rights of individual users and their families.

There is a danger that unless the values, knowledge and skills of social workers are not appreciated and nurtured, then the move into specialist mental health trusts, which occurred from 2002 onwards, could have the effect of emasculating the social and environmental perspectives, which are essential to counter the profound disadvantages in which many users with mental health needs find themselves (see ADSS/NIMHE, 2003; Bogg, 2008).

Defining social work

Because social work performs so many different functions with such a range of individuals and groups, and interacts with a wide range of statutory and voluntary agencies, it is often difficult to define what it is in essence. As Hanvey and Philpot point out:

The problems social workers face are not so neatly dealt with as are problems faced by professionals who have to handle the arrest, the fire hose or the scalpel. The material

clues, the heartbeat and the pulse are, whatever the problems faced by others, more specific and scientific than what is often available to social workers.

Hanvey and Philpot, 1994: 3

As Professor Thompson opines in his admirably clear *Understanding Social Work*, one can define social work in terms of theoretical constructs; through a descriptive approach and list of what social workers do; constructing it through an historical process; placing it in the broader context of social welfare; placing it in the tension between social stability and social change etc. (Thompson, 2000.)

Calling on his earlier work (Thompson, 1992) Thompson then considers an existential approach concentrating on:

- Ontology – concerning questions of human existence and meaning, and how existence presents us with a number of challenges that we have to meet and face in a variety of ways.
  – Life event challenges – those we face as we move from the cradle to the grave.
  – Challenges of circumstance and/or trauma facing traumatic events and the issues we face as we try to reach our goals.
  – Socio-political challenges – stemming from our position in society, including poverty, racism, ageism, sexism, sexual orientation and other forms of exploitation.
- Uncertainty and flux, as we can see from all the case examples, appeal to a corpus of knowledge and personal experience is important, but 'a basic task for the social worker in very many situations is the management of uncertainty' (Thompson, 2000: 21) and one might add as well, the management of paradox.
- In these situations, social work practice needs to be:
  – Systematic – having a clear focus on what we are trying to achieve and why.
  – Reflective – reflecting on practice with an openness to change and develop (see also Brechin et al., 2000; White and Taylor, 2000).
- Moral commitment – taking account of and attempting to ameliorate existing inequalities so that social work needs to be explicit about its value base and committed to demonstrating those values through 'supporting people in their struggles to break free from the disadvantage, discrimination and oppression they experience as a result of their social location' (Thompson, 2000: 23).

The social work profession's own description of *The Social Work Task* is:

> *Social work is the purposeful and ethical application of personal skills in interpersonal relationships directed towards enhancing the personal and social functioning of an individual, family, group or neighbourhood.*
>
> BASW, 1977

Most professions' descriptions of themselves have a certain pomposity about them, and some critics of social work rounded on this description of its task but, in effect, it's a pretty accurate summary of what social work does, though demographic, budgetary and policy pressures have tended to push social work away from having any impact on neighbourhoods in the way that it attempted to do in the 1970s and 1980s.

Social workers don't have the Benefit Agency's cash or the surgeon's scalpel (or laser); for them the instrument is the use of the self in situations where gauging where an individual is in the light of their mental and physical state, culture, past, beliefs, values, current circumstances etc., is immensely complex.

Individual social workers and the profession as a whole have to engage with the issues of care and control, especially in the context of the Approved Mental Health Professional (APMH) role (see Chapter 8) where the worker is accountable for the actions as an individual professional, rather than as a member of an agency.

Social workers derive their role from:

- The legislative framework.
- A policy framework.
- A professional body (BASW).
- A regulatory body (GSCC).
- The agencies in which the workers operate, either statutory or voluntary.
- What users and carers need.

There are arguments as to the looseness or tightness of the task:

> *Those who commit themselves to social work contribute, in my view, to the sensitisation of our society. In doing so, they will not be popular; they must seek to hold, and to mediate in, the multiplicity of conflict in interpersonal relationships. They deal in shades of grey where the public looks for black and white. And they are bitterly resented for it. They are brokers in lesser evils, frequently faced with the need for choice followed by action whose outcome is unpredictable.*
>
> Professor Olive Stevenson, 1974, quoted in Hanvey and Philpot, 1994: 2

'The truth is that social workers are employed to do a wide-ranging but quite specific job, which necessarily involves them in risk-taking, decision-making and the exercise of judgement' (Davies, *The Essential Social Worker*, quoted in Hanvey and Philpot, 1994: 3). There is also the argument as to how much social workers are agents of stability or change. Inevitably, if they are going to behave with integrity to the people they work with to serve, their colleagues, the agency they work for and their professional body (see Smale et al., 2000; Thompson, 2000) they will look to reinforce those aspects of society which promote individual and social welfare (social stability) and seek to change negative and destructive aspects of society, such as discrimination (social change). Hugh England, in *Social Work as Art: Making Sense for Good Practice* (England, 1986: 8) quotes Noel and Rita Timms as saying 'Boundaries are loosely drawn and often permeable . . . this looseness constitutes one of the major challenges, if not one of the glories'. As England comments, 'There is no doubt about the size of the challenge; I hope there will be no doubt that it is also a matter for glory'.

Case Example 6

T is a 44 year old woman who has lived with severe mental illness for most of her adult life. Her first admission to hospital was at age 32, although she had been treated as an outpatient for the previous ten years. Her original diagnosis of depression began to move towards the more accurate diagnosis of schizophrenia over the years. By 1999, she had had 15 hospital admissions and had become a 'revolving door patient', with little hope, apparently destined to become a continuing care patient on a long stay ward.

Her husband, whom she met during her second hospital admission, was an alcoholic and was usually in a very intoxicated state. Medical staff would not visit the home and would not listen to the couple's views. The home was in a severe squalid state; the carpets were soiled with faeces, most of the floor was covered in rubbish piled several feet in the room, cigarette butts were everywhere and opened tins of dog food were on every surface. The bed was soaked in urine and the smell permeated down to the ground floor of the block of flats, even though the flat was on the third floor and there were several doors between. T was incontinent, had congestive obstructive airway disease and mild cardiac failure. She smoked and drank (anything) constantly and had made numerous serious suicide attempts.

The medical staff was at a loss and requested help from social work staff who had only been invited to become involved at the point of compulsory detention. The nature of the request was more to do with keeping the alcoholic husband from visiting the ward and making demands on staff for his wife to go home. It was at this point that the social worker became involved and began the slow process of trying to gain the couple's trust to see what could be done.

It soon became very clear that the couple were very much in love and that despite their numerous difficulties, wanted to live together. It was from this premise that the social worker began the slow task of getting the couple to feel that they did have some power over the 'mighty medical system'. Through gentle encouragement, the couple were empowered, for the first time in their lives, to make some decisions about how they wanted to live and after a great deal of hard work, we were able to fund the fumigation, gutting and sterilisation of the flat, followed by re-decorating and furnishing it to a reasonable standard. The couple were involved throughout the entire process and although things did not run smoothly, we did not give up and the task was eventually completed. 'It would be fair to say that I experienced huge levels of resistance from medical staff, to the point where I almost gave up because of the pressure.' (SW)

A massive care package was organised to enable the couple to live in the flat. This included daily medication administration, cleaning, attention to personal hygiene, cooking, day-care and regular respite in a rehabilitation ward and becoming appointee for their financial benefits and organising payment of everything. The couple were again involved at each stage and slowly clear progress could be seen.

We are now 18 months on and the couple's lifestyle is unrecognisable. T has gained insight into her illness and is now able to talk about her own relapse symptoms. The flat is bright and clean. The care package has been reduced to only two hours each week and transport to attend a day centre. The couple shop and cook for themselves, keep themselves clean and tidy and have, this week, taken back the total responsibility of their finances. Her husband's alcoholism is greatly improved and the couple have a quality of life that could never have been envisaged only a few years before.

The most difficulty was experienced in attempting to provide care on a flexible basis, with the local medical services being very rigid and unimaginative in their approach. Indeed, it is ironic that various medical establishments still complain, despite the exceptional progress that T has made.

Without social work intervention, T would be in a long stay ward, probably still very unwell, unhappy and unsafe and the couple would be apart. It is only the clear social work values that enabled this couple to have their current lifestyle and for T to be mentally stable and happy.

The values of social work

They (the social workers) treat me with dignity and respect.
> service user from the Westminster Study
> (McDonald and Sheldon, 1997)

The love of liberty is the love of other people; the love of power is the love of ourselves.
> William Hazlitt, 18th century essayist

Only one thing prevailed – strength of character. Cleverness, creativeness, learning, all went down; only real goodness survived.
> Pierre d'Harcourt (Nazi concentration camp
> survivor) *The Real Enemy*, Longman, 1967

As Zofia Butrym states in her *The Nature of Social Work*:

Implicit in the discussion of the nature of social work . . . is the fundamental importance of moral issues. This importance is derived from both the objectives of social work and the means by which it attempts to reach these objectives.

Concern with the quality of human living which ... is what social work is basically about, cannot operate in a moral vacuum but on the contrary must be based on certain beliefs. Regarding what constitutes 'a good life' and also on ethical considerations in relation to the ways by which such a good life can be sought and promoted.

Butrym, 1976: 40

As Sarah Banks has flagged up in a book entirely devoted to ethics and values in social work (Banks, 1995: 4) 'values' is one of those words that tends to be used rather vaguely and has a variety of different meanings.

Dictionary definitions state that values are one's judgement of what is important in life, stemming from the Latin *valere*: to be strong, well, worth, and leading to the French *valoir*: to be worth, and related to the old Slavic *vlasti*: to govern. And indeed, it is essential to realise that as Professor Preston-Shoot so pertinently remarks 'Values are only as good as the actions they prompt' (Preston-Shoot, 1996: 31).

Ethics stems from the Greek *ethikos*: moral philosophy, and is the science of morals in human conduct; moral principles; rules of conduct. (See Thompson, 2000; Banks, 1995; Philpot, 1986; Butrym, 1976; Smale et al., 2000; Hanvey and Philpot, 1994; England, 1986; Davies, 1994; Braye and Preston-Shoot, 1995; British Association of Social Workers, 1986 and 2002).

Values have a vital role to play in organisations as long as they are 'real'. They:

- Provide the bedrock for the organisation – how people should behave to patients/clients/users/customers/partners, and towards each other.
- Create a benchmark against which the prevailing culture and actions/responses of the organisation can be measured.
- Offer a framework for making sense of practice.
- Provide motivation and give a sense to staff that they are valued and are adding value to the lives of others.

If values do not lead to appropriate actions, however, then they are, in that lovely North Midlands phrase: 'neither use nor ornament'! When I was Director of Operations for Staffordshire Social Services, two deaths of residents at the hospital for people with learning disabilities resulted in a team from Central Government being sent up, and led eventually to a county-wide partnership to close the hospital, re-provide the service and improve the lives of people with learning disabilities in the county. One of the deaths involved ward staff leaving a woman tied to a lavatory by her clothing while they went for lunch. The woman strangled herself in her efforts to get free. One of the Trade Union officials justified the event as the staff being under pressure and needing a break! The loss of dignity and freedom leading to the loss of the life of this woman happened not in Dickens 19th century, not even in the 1970s where a number of scandals led to a real drive to improve services and the values underpinning services, but in the mid 1990s!

I was recently concerned to hear of a consultant psychiatrist who questioned the use of 'citizens' as a description of users in the Statement of Principles and Practice produced by his trust. It seems to me that the tragedies where human beings are cruel to other human beings occur when we fail to recognise the shared humanity in the person facing us. That distancing, of course, comes so often from humankind's innate sense of separateness, disease and anxiety, leading to a need to distance ourselves and see ourselves as superior.

Raymond Plant, summarising Immanuel Kant's philosophy in his book, *Social and Moral Theory in Casework*, says:

> *A man [sic] deserves respect as a potential moral agent in terms of his [sic] transcendental characteristic, not because of a particular conjunction of empirical qualities which he might possess. Traits of character might command admiration and other such responses, but respect is owed to a man, irrespective of what he does, because he is a man [sic].*

see Plant, 1970, quoted in Philpot, 1986: 143 and Kant, *The Fundamental Principles of the Metaphysics of Ethics*, 1785

Anti-oppressive practice is not an area which has a great deal of impact in Health Service thinking. It is imperative that social workers continue to strive to achieve this, and challenge when it is not happening.

mental health social worker

Of course, it is important that social work is not precious about the issue of the values. A whole range of professions who are concerned about the health, well-being and care of vulnerable people in the community e.g. youth workers, counsellors, clergy, chaplains, nurses, occupational therapists, housing officers etc., will subscribe to a broad set of values and professional identities, and some of the common themes will be commitment to:

- humanitarianism
- a value base
- a professional knowledge base
- a set of skills
- professional discretion and accountability

Thompson, 2000: Ch. 1

Social workers will be familiar with the seven principles developed by Felix Biestek of Loyola University (Biestek, 1976: 17). These are still of great merit today, but as Banks makes clear, they were developed primarily within the context of voluntary, one-to-one casework relationship. Banks, Thompson and Braye and Preston-Shoot consider:

- The Kantian approach – with its accent on human beings as free individuals.
- Utilitarian approaches – where human beings are seen as free individuals, but participation in society involves a compromise of freedom in order to promote the public good as well as the welfare of individual users.
- Radical approaches – where human beings are social beings whose freedom is realised in society, and where there needs to be individual and collective empowerment and a challenging of inequalities in the working for social change.

These writers perceive a development of **traditional values**:

- Respect for persons – recognising each person as a unique individual. Acting: 'so act as to treat humanity, whether in your own person or that of any other, never solely as a means but always also as an end' (Kant quoted in Banks 1995, 28).
- Protection – protecting the vulnerable when they are under threat from others or themselves.
- The purposeful expression of feelings – providing a safe environment for user or carer to express their negative as well as positive feelings in a safe environment; upholding those emotions so that, perhaps for the first time, the individual can consider and evaluate those emotions without the fear of condemnation or being overwhelmed by them.
- Acceptance – 'Acceptance is a principle of action wherein the caseworker perceives and deals with the client as he [*sic*] really is, including his strengths and weaknesses, with congenial and uncongenial qualities, his positive and negative feelings, his constructive and destructive attitudes and behaviour,

maintaining all the while a sense of the client's innate dignity and personal worth' (Biestek, 1976: 82).

A good example of this would be from the Macdonald and Sheldon Study (1997: 42) where one of the people interviewed comments 'He (the social worker) doesn't always agree about my voices, and says "no, it's your sickness". I can talk to him about it. I feel quite comfortable discussing differences of opinion with him.'

Here, the social worker accepts the reality of the voices to the user, but also allows the individual to stand back from the voices and evaluate their reality and significance.

- Controlled emotional involvement – as the voluntary sector co-ordinator commented at the beginning of this chapter, social workers 'have a professionalism that offers a useful distance from the problem in hand and allows them to deal dispassionately with the situation'.

At the same time, as we've seen from the *Strategies for Living* research, users and carers need to feel that social workers are both genuine, and genuinely committed to working with them and in tune with their experience of their world.

- Non-judgmental attitude – clearly this does not mean shying away from making professional judgments. Also the worker needs to be clear with the people they are working with as to the consequences of their actions or proposed actions in relation to the effect on other people, society, the law etc.
- Client self-determination – as we've seen from the case example at the beginning of this chapter, an over-protective approach can in fact mean that individuals can become passive or conversely rebellious.
- Confidentiality – again, the issues around confidentiality will be subtly different for a worker in an agency setting, rather than working within a pure counselling model. This is especially so when issues of risk have to be addressed. The worker needs to be clear with the user as to what the limits of confidentiality are.
- Normalisation – a term which is often misunderstood and misused. It is based on assisting individuals to lead a valued, ordinary life. The founder of this approach, Wolfensberger, updated his approach and re-termed it 'social role valorisation' – seeking

to enhance the perceived status of people with disabilities through their performance of socially desired and valued roles (For a short summary, see Braye and Preston-Shoot, 1995: 39).

- Congruence – as we have seen before, it is most important that the worker is seen as 'genuine'. The relationship between the worker and the user or carer is inevitably a power relationship. This power can be used to dominate or manipulate. Carl Rogers, the doyen of client-centred approaches, makes the powerful statement that:

> *It has been found that personal change is facilitated when the psychotherapist is what he [sic] is, when in the relationship with his client he is genuine and without 'front' or façade, openly being the feelings and attitudes which at the moment are flowing in him. We have coined the term 'congruence' to try to describe this condition.*
>
> Rogers, 1961: 61

I once had the enlightening experience of buying a drink from a bar in an area where I had once practised as a social worker. The person serving had been a young person looked after by the local authority, and I had been one of her social workers. She gave me a succinct pen portrait of all her social workers, and the core of what she was saying was as to whether she had found the workers genuine, or as she described it, 'real' or not! Linda Hart's book (Hart, 1996) is an excellent example of power relationships in a Mental Health setting. For a fictional exploration of power, I would recommend Ursula LeGuin's *The Dispossessed* (1974). Shevek, the hero, a philosopher scientist, finds himself in many ways in similar situations to a social worker, operating on the margins of complex individual social and political situations and with no instruments except the purposeful use of himself. LeGuin's final words in the book are: 'But he had not brought anything. His hands were empty, as they had always been' (p319).

Thompson, then, outlines a number of what he calls **'emancipatory values'** (or **radical values**) which in a sense move the more traditional values forward in a world where it is increasingly recognised that individuals are part of a wider social and political milieu.

- De-individualisation – while recognising the uniqueness of the individual, there are merits in looking at connections and commonalities. Users can be seen in a wider context,

particularly within the perspective of membership of oppressed groups. Thompson uses the example of working with a woman with depression, where the significance of gender can clearly be an issue with her concomitant expectations of female roles in current society (p117).

- Equality – a recognition and a willingness to confront inequalities.
- Social justice – although those social workers who advocated a greater voice for people in the institutions, and subsequently the closure and re-provision of the institutions, may not have recognised such actions as a pursuit of social justice, but that's what it was.
- Partnership – an increasing value put on this in government policies, in respect of engaging with users and carers and a range of agencies as equal partners in a shared enterprise.
- Citizenship – an idea we still seem to struggle with some 1,000s of years after the Greek city states developed the concept!

There were plenty of exceptions to citizenship in Greece, but we should have been able to move beyond that. Arguments for the extension of the franchise in Britain in the 19th and early 20th century now seem so self-evident. There is quite rightly an accent on rights and parallel responsibilities within the value of citizenship. But this should not be used as an excuse to deny care when that is required.

- Empowerment – this is both on an individual basis but also collectively. Both recognising the significance and recognising the severe disadvantages that pervade the everyday lives of people with mental health needs.
- Authenticity – recognising the boundary between those aspects of our lives that we can control and those that we cannot. In this, both the worker and the user or carers acknowledge the role they play and the responsibility they carry for their actions.

In 2002, the British Association of Social Workers reformulated the Statement of Values and Principles of Practice which it had issued first in 1986. The booklet describes five basic values, and then outlines a number of principles attached to each value.

These are:

- human dignity and worth
- social justice

Figure 18: Values, relationships and constraints in the worker–user relationship.

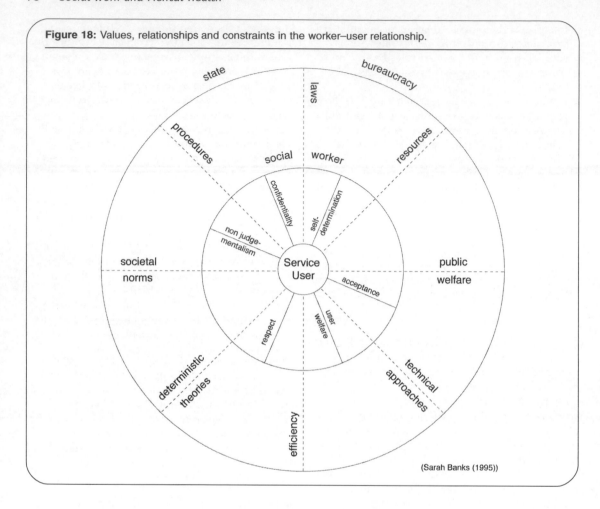

(Sarah Banks (1995))

- service to humanity
- integrity
- competence

There is then a section on ethical practice setting out guidance in particular situations:

- Responsibilities to service users:
  - priority of service user's interest
  - conflicts of interest
  - self-determination by service users
  - informed consent
  - services provided under compulsion
  - cultural awareness
  - privacy, confidentiality and records
- Responsibilities to the profession.
- Responsibilities in the workplace.
- Responses in particular roles:
  - management
  - education, training, supervision and evaluation

- independent practice
- research

A sound value-base is essential for a profession, for individual workers, for organisations and for the protection of vulnerable individuals who use services. Some, such as a commitment to recognising the humanity of each individual, must, I believe, be written in stone, others may ebb and flow in proportion to the type of agency and the state of society.

My voluntary sector contact, who is so positive about social work, also articulates the warning that when workers lose touch with their values and their own sense of self, then that hardness will be very hurtful to the user. Richard Titmuss, the social philosopher, spoke movingly that:

There cannot be one unambiguous goal for social work: human needs and desires are complex, interdependent,

simultaneously rational and irrational and often in conflict. Nor is there one unambiguous objective for the social
services. It would be terrifying if there were and if we
thought there could be. All one is left with (or I am left
with) is the philosopher's thought that increasing sensi-
tiveness to the claims of others (and claims which cannot
be wholly satisfied on the material criteria of the market)
is one important element in the definition of moral
progress in society.

Knowledge, skills and tasks

*Integrity without knowledge is weak and useless, and
knowledge without integrity is dangerous and dreadful.*
Dr Johnson

*Social work as a profession has often been divided between
a focus on individuals (casework) on the one hand, and on
groups and communities (group work and community
work) on the other. It also tended to suffer from a schism
between social work educators and researchers, representing 'theory' on the one hand and the practitioners,
representing 'practice' on the other hand.*
Professor Shulamit Ramon, Conference Paper,
27 April 2001

*It is one thing to show a man he is in error and another to
put him in possession of the truth.*
John Locke, *Essay Concerning Human
Understanding*, 1689

The National Institute for Mental Health in
England was launched in 2001 with a remit to
'Reshape services and practice in line with the
evidence base bringing together the research,
development and dissemination functions of
Mental Health Services' (DoH, 2001).

Social work, as Butrym points out, is an
'applied discipline' 'in the sense that relevant
knowledge acquired is for direct use in the
pursuit of its objectives'. It has often had an
inferiority complex where knowledge is
concerned (see Chapter 10 in this book) partly
because, as we can see in this text, the range of
user needs, government imperatives and social
work tasks is such that a broad spread of
knowledge is required, and social workers'
qualification training, set at two years, is clearly
only long enough to skim the surface of the
theoretical base required. Doctors, for example,
not only have longer qualifying training, but have
a greater investment in post qualifying training as
well.

Not all of the self-abnegation is justified,
however. In an applied discipline, experience
reflected upon in an appropriate way is valued
enormously by users and colleagues. As Taylor

and White comment in their searching text:
*Practising Reflexivity in Health and Welfare: Making
Knowledge* (Taylor and White, 2000) they point to
'professional practice in health and welfare' being
'characterised by a greater degree of anxiety
about its goals and outcomes. As we have seen,
social workers have to deal with uncertainties
much more than certainties, and too often the
dominant answer to this uncertainty has been a
technical, procedural, and often bureaucratic one'
(Taylor and White, 2000: 4).

Progress is based on exploration; often the
major improvements in human welfare (the
discovery of penicillin, for example) are founded
in accident rather than design. Human beings
crave certainty, and modern society believes that
there is always a magic pill for every ailment. In
some senses, we feel happier with the
pronouncements of 'science': from the Latin
scientia – knowledge, and from Latin and French
root words meaning to know, but also to
separate, and divide into separate parts. This is
connected but different again from 'knowing',
from Greek, Latin and old English roots: to come
to know, to recognise. Knowledge, as Thomas
Kuhn (Kuhn, 1962) asserts, is a series of
paradigms which are developed and then
challenged and replaced. The Greek philosopher,
Socrates, asserted that wisdom is: 'knowledge of
what it is one does not know', echoed in modern
times by Popper's assertion that 'our ignorance
grows with our knowledge' (see Butrym, 1976: 63;
Popper, *The Logic of Scientific Discovery*, 1934). For
man science is not enough on its own because
human beings do not simply come as one-size fits
all. In the context of international management,
Geert Hofstede has demonstrated that if a
business person with considerable expertise fails
to shape their knowledge to the culture of the
country they are operating in, they are doomed to
failure (Hofstede, 1980).

It is very clear that the general practitioner and
psychiatrist most appreciated by service users
and carers is someone who combines both the
scientist and the artist. As Magee has expressed it
in his writings on Karl Popper: 'the scientist and
the artist, far from being engaged in opposed or
incompatible activities, are both trying to extend
the range of understanding and of experience by
the use of creative imagination, subjected to
critical control. They both use irrational as well as
rational faculties in the pursuit of this objective;
they are both exploring the unknown and trying
to articulate the search and its findings; both are

seekers after truth who make indispensable use of intuition' (Magee, 1973: 72).

Thompson indicates the danger, which is too often evident, of social workers remarking: 'I prefer to stick to practice' (Thompson, 2000: 72–3, see also Thompson, 2009) and the problems which follow from this dichotomy between theory and practice.

In 2001, the government set up the Social Care Institute for Excellence (SCIE) with its three main functions:

• To review current knowledge about social care.
• To develop best practice guides based on that knowledge.
• To ensure that those guides contribute to positive practice and policy change.

SCIE recognises that knowledge comes from diverse sources, including from research, service reviews and from the experience of people who use and who provide social care services. As Mike Fisher, Director of Analysis and Reviews, emphasises: 'it's not "what works" but "what works for whom and under what circumstances"' (quoted in *Community Care*, 25 April 2002: 35).

As Professor Olive Stevenson once wryly commented: 'to try and build a social work house on the shifting sands of social science theory is asking for trouble. Social work should probably concentrate on erecting strong, portable, flexible tents rather than houses' (Stevenson, 1971: 226).

Incidentally, when I did my CQSW course at Sussex University in the mid 1970s, one seminar running right the way through the course was one integrating theory and practice so that the student placements always related back to theoretical concepts and vice versa.

As the poet T.S. Eliot saw it: 'perceptions do not, in a really appreciative mind, accumulate as a mass, but form themselves as a structure' (quoted in Kermode, 1975) and of course in a pilgrim profession, this may well be Stevenson's 'tents' rather than houses. Hugh England, in *Social Work as Art*, quotes Bowers in saying that:

> The subject matter of social casework is the individual human being as he [sic] exists in reality, that is, in a total situation ... casework does not deal with some particular segment of the individual, but with the individual as a **whole person** (my emphasis).
>
> England, 1986: 105

Knowledge is one thing, how we use it is another; and I know that the times when I felt I have 'got it wrong' is when I have inappropriately used knowledge from one setting and imposed it on another, e.g. having worked in a community, multi-disciplinary team, and feeling I knew the issues well, I made presumptions about the operation and issues of another community team in another place, and was told firmly by team members that I was out of context! We therefore need to use knowledge through:

• Selection – what we need at any one time.
• Integration – interlinking different forms of knowledge and theory with practice.
• Reflection – thinking through our actions and their consequences.
• Reflexion – interrogating our previously taken-for-granted assumptions (Taylor and White, 2000).

Case Example 7

This case example looks at the issues for the mental health of an elderly couple. The social worker requires considerable knowledge about human development, the psychology and physiology of ageing; the cultural issues for a couple coming from the Ukraine, and the issues around oppression and its effects impacting on people both in the present and in the future.

The social worker, Alison Kilbride, demonstrates an ability to listen, to empathise, to assess, to liaise with a range of other staff, and co-ordinate complex care packages, to assess risk and have the courage to stick with a risky situation including the experience of aggression from the user.

Reprinted with kind permission from Community Care, 17–23 May 2001

Knowledge and skills

Truth lies in the quality of the user's experience of the service.

Baroness Jane Campbell, former Chair, SCIE

There is still an insufficient commitment to applied social science in NHS Psychiatry. At the level of the frontline practitioner that is exactly what the social worker can provide ... but social science has yet to realise its full potential as a contributor to the study and management of illness and disability because it lags a long way behind the more dominant biochemical framework as far as the strength of its theoretical underpinnings are concerned.

Case Example 7

Rights and wrongs

An older couple with deteriorating physical and mental health and poor command of English provided social worker Alison Kilbride with the tough task of co-ordinating different agencies to ensure the couple's health and well-being while respecting their human rights.

Case notes

Social worker: Alison Kilbride

Field: Senior practitioner in a mental health specialist team for older people Location: Oxfordshire social services

Client: Jak Navard (not his real name) is in his 80s and has progressive dementia. He lives with his wife, who has had a stroke, which resulted in physical and cognitive deterioration. Both were anti-fascist activists in eastern Europe during the war, and have English as a second language.

Case history: They were referred to the team when Mrs Navard was in hospital because of a stroke. A few days later her husband's mental confusion became evident to professionals. She was then sent to a rehabilitation unit for intensive physiotherapist and occupational therapist inputs. Mr Navard joined her because both became hostile when separated. She was discharged with a substantial community care package, and Kilbride's team arranged for a psychiatric assessment of Mr Navard, which confirmed progressive dementia. He began to exhibit paranoid behaviour towards care assistants and Kilbride, often refusing them access to his wife. They also stopped speaking and understanding English, as a result of which Ukrainian interpreters were employed.

Then Kilbride and her colleagues were assaulted, which led to the care assistants being withdrawn. A subsequent psychiatric assessment confirmed the earlier diagnosis, changes were made in work practices to protect staff, and a mental health assertive outreach team employed to assist. They were admitted to a community hospital, and subsequently referred to a psychiatric assessment centre – the department of psychiatry and old age at a local mental health trust.

Dilemma: Their health and cognitive functioning is deteriorating, but they want to return home, and their wishes must be respected.

Risk factor: Even with an intensive care package, their health and safety is at risk.

Outcome: The centre wishes to discharge them back home.

The government's social care agenda with its emphasis on evidence-based practice and effective outcomes seems to have been broadly welcomed, despite continuing concerns about the future role of social services. But of course social workers are often faced with the difficult job of trying to sort what an effective outcome is. In many situations this is far from clear.

Alison Kilbride, a senior mental health practitioner in a specialist team for older people, is still grappling with this question in her work with Mr and Mrs Navard (not their real names). The couple, who are now in their 80s, suffered political persecution in the Ukraine prior to and during the Second World War, and came here as refugees many years ago. They were not known to statutory services until Mrs Navard had a stroke and was treated in hospital. At that time it became clear that she was malnourished and showed other signs of self-neglect, and two days later when their GP visited the husband, he admitted that he was becoming confused.

They were referred to the hospital social work department, and subsequently agreed to enter a rehabilitation unit, where she received intensive physiotherapy and where an occupational therapy assessment was made. It was noticed that the couple became hostile when separated.

The hospital social work department decided to refer the couple to Kilbride.

She says that it was clear to everyone that Mr Navard had progressive dementia, and that as a result of this and his wife's condition, they were at significant risk. Consequently, a substantial care package was put in place, and Kilbride and her colleagues arranged a psychiatric assessment for the Navards. The assessment confirmed that they were suffering from progressive dementia. Meanwhile, their home had been thoroughly cleaned, and adaptations made to assist Mrs Navard, who had significant physical impairments.

The couple had expressed a wish to remain in their own home, and at first the care package, which included many personal care services for Mrs Navard, appeared to be working. But then her husband started to exhibit paranoid symptoms. He began to make it difficult for the care assistants to attend to his wife, and at times refused entry to them, to Kilbride and to the community psychiatric nurse, all of whom had been visiting very regularly. Also, at about this time he began to be unable to understand or speak English, and she subsequently arranged for Ukrainian interpreters to visit alongside the care staff in an effort to persuade him to allow them to attend to her. Kilbride had offered the couple the option of residential care, but this had been rejected. Malnourishment was now becoming a major concern.

Meanwhile, the state of their home was deteriorating to such an extent that rats were often seen, and on more than one occasion the Navards' deteriorating cognitive functioning caused safety problems, for example the microwave oven had burst into flames.

Consequently, a case conference was called, and a decision was made to intensify the care package, basically to ensure that one carer could distract Mr Navard while the other attended to his wife. Additional attention was given to ways in which the daily visitors, namely Kilbride, the community practice nurse and the care assistants, could act to ameliorate his 'very excitable' state. She had also engaged an assertive outreach team from the local NHS department of old age and psychiatry to help.

Shortly after this, and despite these efforts, Kilbride and her colleagues were assaulted by one or other of the couple, as a result of which the care agency withdrew their staff. 'This happened to me despite the presence of a Ukrainian-speaking interpreter, because by now Mr Navard was unable to recognise me. Thankfully, my manager and others in the authority supported me a great deal after the assault, but we had obviously reached another crisis,' she says. Consequently, the couple did not have the support of care assistants for a few weeks. In the meantime, Kilbride had contacted the GP, who the couple still trusted, in the hope that he would arrange another psychiatric assessment, she also asked the same of the assertive outreach service.

'By this time the various agencies had already decided that compulsory admission under the Mental Health Act 1983 was inappropriate, even though it was clear that their health was deteriorating and the risks to their safety were increasing,' she says.

The GP persuaded the Navards to enter a community hospital so that their physical health could be attended to, but while they were there their behaviour deteriorated rapidly and a decision was made to transfer them to a psychiatric assessment centre. The centre has now decided that they should be discharged back to their home.

'I'm now faced with them returning home, with only a minimal amount of care assistance, which I've managed to secure from another care agency. There are enormous health and safety risks, which are also recognised by the community practice nurse and the psychiatrist, but there are no legal means to avoid this situation. I am investigating the use of an electronic keypad on their front door, so that access can be assured, although I'm concerned about the human rights implications of taking this step. I'm keeping all the agencies informed about what's happening, and exploring residential and nursing home options,' she says.

'I'm terribly concerned about both of them, and particularly about Mrs Navard's health and her very low quality of life,' Kilbride concludes.

Arguments for risk

- Mr and Mrs Navard have always stated that they wish to remain together in their own home.
- Suitable residential or nursing home care facilities are hard to identify, given the couple's loss of English, and his paranoid behaviour.
- A co-ordinated approach by care staff, members of the assertive outreach service, and their GP, could help to secure and operate a new care package.
- It may be possible under Mental Health Act 1983 provisions to put Mr Navard on a medication regime, which would ameliorate his paranoid behaviour, although the department of psychiatry and old age would need to be in full agreement.
- Social services, with the Navards' agreement, administers their finances.

Arguments against risk

- Mrs Navard's health is at serious risk unless she receives regular assistance in washing, feeding and other personal care.

- Both of them are living in squalid conditions, and their behaviour creates serious risks to their personal safety.
- The state of their home is beginning to impact on neighbours, and there is a likelihood that the environmental health service will be called in, which would undoubtedly create further distress.
- Their increasingly aggressive behaviour could lead to care staff being injured.
- They are socially isolated, and now unable to use English, which effectively precludes the option of organising any wider support, befriending or other care network to underpin statutory services.
- Their progressive dementia, allied to their personal histories, make it ever more likely that they will view the intrusion into their lives of care services as a threat.

Independent comment

The challenges here are enormous. Kilbride has done an admirable job in trying to maintain an isolated older couple in the community who have both physical and mental difficulties and specific cultural needs, *write Alisoun Milne and Jayne Lingard.* The key risks are around the safety of Mr and Mrs Navard and also the safety of the care staff. Despite the best efforts of Kilbride, the couple remain very vulnerable and have retreated into a world that isolates them from help and support.

Although use of the Mental Health Act 1983 has been considered, a formal risk assessment that takes account of Mr Navard's dementia has not been conducted. This may help decision making by locating risk in a coherent framework that respects user rights and applies the principles of person-centred care. A jointly administered risk assessment, which takes account of the needs of both Mr and Mrs Navard, may be helpful.

Although an interpreter has been employed, we do not know if this person has any understanding of the nature of dementia. An advocate trained in communicating with people with dementia may help the Navards to make informed decisions about their future care.

The Navards and Kilbride have been failed by the separate delivery of health and social care services, and the even wider gap between the care of people's physical health and their mental health. The couple were assessed in a number of settings and by a range of social and health care teams. Neither the Audit Commission's report on mental health services for older people with mental health needs[1] nor standard seven of the National Service Framework for Older People[2] directly confront the current pattern of services failing to meet the needs of the whole person.

Alisoun Milne and **Jayne Lingard** are consultants to the Mental Health Foundation's programme of work on Mental Health in Later Life and are both qualified social workers.

[1]Audit Commission, *Forget-Me-Not: Mental Health Services for Older People*, Audit Commission, 2000
[2]DoH, National Service Framework for Older People, March 2001

Reprinted by kind permission of *Community Care*, 17–23 May, 2001.

With acknowledgements of the need to re-humanise our patients, and of the shortcomings of our current treatments, mental health services are faced with the challenge of embracing social science in a way that they haven't to date.

consultant psychiatrist

The body of knowledge that social workers need to become proficient in consists of:

- Human development – the increasing accent on specialising and sub-specialties, means that sound knowledge on human development is more than ever important for helping to understand the individual and the individual's family.
- Social processes and power dynamics – as we have seen in previous chapters, the construction of society, power dynamics within or outside institutions, and the issues of race and culture, bear heavily on the individual and their relationship with the world around them (see Thompson, 1998; Fernando, 2007; Sewell, 2009).

In a case example, Suki Desai and Aasra Garib (1998) demonstrate how in inter-cultural situations in mental health the worker has a complex role of 'social interpreter' from the individual to the family, and vice versa, and from the individual and family to the other professionals involved so as to get round the cultural incomprehensibility that pertains.

- Social policy – not only what it is but why and how it has developed.
- Law and constitution.
- Interpersonal and group dynamics.
- How organisations function.
- The value base – and how it works in practice.
- Theoretical paradigms:
  - psychodynamics
  - psychosocial casework
  - humanistic psychology
  - behavioural
  - systems theory
  - radical approaches
  - participatory approaches
  - emancipatory practice

Methods of intervention

Methods of intervention are likely to follow closely on from theoretical perspectives and may include:

- Client-centred approaches – based on the work of Carl Rogers and Gerard Egan, starting where the person is, and moving from exploration to understanding, and then to action followed by evaluation.
- Task-centred practice where Reid and Shyne's work pointed to the benefits of short-term goals to boost self-esteem rather than an open ended therapeutic relationship.
- Crisis intervention – rather like judo, using the energy inherent in a crisis to move forward.
- Behavioural work – based on the work of behaviourists such as Skinner, and developed by social learning theorists, e.g. Albert Bandura, who 'emphasised that learning behaviour is a social act, acquired through modelling, imitation and observation' (Pierson in Hanvey and Philpot, 1994: 83).
- Radical emancipatory intervention – based on confronting oppressive social structures.
- Care management – the procurement, delivery, monitoring and evaluation of care packages (see below).
- Advocacy – but professional workers need to be very aware that there are a number of times when it is inappropriate for the professional to act as advocate, and an independent advocate needs to be brought in. As a service user once remarked to me: 'I have an excellent social worker, she battles on my behalf, but she and I are both aware that she works for social services, and sometimes I need somebody who works just for me.'

For greater detail and more exploration of the issues see Thompson, 2000; Coulshed and Orme, 1998; Hanvey and Philpot, 1994.

Skills and tasks

The former Central Council for the Education and Training of Social Workers (CCETSW) published a set of competencies for social work students in respect of the Diploma in Social Work (which replaced the Certification of Qualification in Social Work and the Certificate in Social Services). The 1996 version sets out the competencies under six headings:

1. Communicate and engage – with users and carers, colleagues and partner organisations.
2. Promote and enable – 'promote opportunities for people to use their own strengths and expertise to enable them to meet their

responsibilities, secure rights and achieve change' (CCETSW, 1996: 11).

3. Assess and plan.
4. Intervene and provide services.
5. Work in organisations.
6. Develop professional competence.

Social workers have retreated from the social model, as they experience difficulties in finding a voice.
consultant psychiatrist with a strong emphasis on social perspectives

Anti-oppressive practice is not an area which has a great deal of impact in Health Service thinking. It is imperative that social workers continue to strive to achieve this and challenge when it is not happening.
social worker in a multi-disciplinary team

Skills are intrinsically linked with the values, the humanity and human construct of the individual, and the knowledge base. It clearly helps if the worker has innate human skills of being integrated (in terms both of personal integrity, integrity and self-belief) sensitivity, open-mindedness, patience and being well organised. In fact, recent research by the Sainsbury Centre (Murray et al., 1997) demonstrates that the innate qualities of the support workers, their trust-worthiness, caring attitudes and availability were more important to users than professional qualifications e.g.

I can talk to her, she's normal – there's no professional fence, no prying and less making me do things. I do things for her because of the way she approaches it. If things are hard for me to do, then I know she will be there to help. It's not just, 'do this because I say so and maybe I'll help', which you get from professionals. They give less pressure and far less criticism.
Murray et al., 1997: 44

The skills I describe below, however, are not theoretical, but ones I have seen demonstrated by social workers I have worked for, worked with and managed. Social work education, if it's effective, should be able to build on, consolidate, enhance and sharpen existing skills, and develop new skills (Thompson, 2009):

Self-awareness

Awareness of the user's history, hopes, fears, abilities, needs, aspirations etc.

Awareness of our own formative influences, preconceptions etc.

How we come across to users and carers.

How external factors affect us, e.g. I once managed a heroic and very skilled unqualified

social worker, who had been placed, in my view quite irresponsibly, within an organisational minefield of an institution, with no adequate support. Her supervisor, social work trained, had never overcome his fear of and distaste for institutions, and therefore rarely set foot in the hospital to support her and to battle for the rights of the individuals within the institution.

Self-management

'Good people skills' writes Neil Thompson, 'have their root in personal effectiveness' (Thompson, 1996: 7). The ideal helper for Gerard Egan 'realises that he [sic] must model the behaviour he hopes to help others achieve. He knows that he can help only if, in the root sense of the term, he is a 'potent' human being, a person with the will and the resources to act' (Egan, 1975: 22). The workers must be able to manage themselves, their time and their record keeping. Resilience is also important and workers must strive to ensure that they do not become over-stressed and that they preserve a work-life balance (see Gilbert and Thompson: 97–107).

With the realisation of one's own potential and self-confidence in one's ability, one can build a better world.
The Dalai Lama

Communication skills

One of the earliest management texts in the post Roman western world has the line: 'listen with the ear of the heart' (Benedict of Nursia, AD 540) and the skill of listening, hearing, responding and then acting is a fundamental social work facility. Too passive a listening or jumping in too quickly with proposed actions undermines the user or carer. Communication skills (see Moss, 2008) need to be both verbal and non-verbal (attempting to listen while seated behind a desk with your arms folded does not normally denote receptivity!). Written skills in reports for courts, tribunals, communication with other agencies etc. is a vital function when representing a user, as is also technical facility with phones, emails etc.

Analytical skills

Identifying key issues, and sifting the important items from the accumulation of facts which often cloud rather than clarify the issue. Identifying patterns and acting to check these out and connect them. As Noel and Rita Timms urged in an early social work text '. . . acceptance should describe the active search to discover *the point*' (Timms and Timms, 1997: 88). Analytical skills, then, need to be brought forward in all elements of the helping process from working with the user to explore their world, helping to create patterns which assist, planning actions and reviewing them.

Sensitivity and observational skills

Empathy with the individual. Identifying issues of culture, gender, race, position and role, and other power-related factors and acting to address these.

Reflection

A constant reflection on practice and challenge to our existing presumptions and practices (see Taylor and White, 2000).

Handling feelings

Acquaintances sometimes say 'Well social work is just about listening to people, isn't it? We all do that', but when they see the strength, sometimes violence, of the emotional interplay, they usually change their mind. As Donald Winnicott pointed out in his influential 1963 work, *Casework and Mental Illness*, part of the social work role is one of 'holding', staying with the individual through many trials and tribulations. It is this 'stickability' which Macdonald and Sheldon point to as one of the most helpful factors in the Westminster Study.

Planning and co-ordination

This aspect of work has been sharpened by care management (although not all social workers would agree with this!) and one can see a change in emphasis in Gerard Egan's work as he moves from his 1975 version of *The Skilled Helper*, to the 7th edition in 2002. Timms and Timms pointed out that in the 1970s, workers sometimes seem to have been 'so preoccupied with understanding a situation that they have not been free enough to do much to change it' (Timms and Timms, 1977: 1000) but Winnicott in 1963 was quite clear that 'integration is vitally important in this connection, and your (social workers) work is quite largely counteracting disintegrating forces in individuals and in families and in localised social groups' (Winnicott, 1963: 227).

Partnership skills

'What service users value', writes Professor Peter Beresford, Professor of Social Policy, and Director of the UK Centre for Citizen Partnership at Brunel University, and a long-term user, 'are participatory ways of working, whether in the production of services, support or knowledge. It is not a question of reducing the role of other stakeholders, but of ensuring service users are routinely included among them and have opportunities to speak for themselves and offer their own discussions on equal terms. Service users must be involved and included in *everything* from the start and at every stage' (Beresford, 2002: 16).

George Bernard Shaw once remarked that 'all professions are a conspiracy against the laity' and this can be as true of social work as any other profession. The voluntary sector service co-ordinator who was so positive about social work in a earlier part of the text also remarked:

> *There is a real need to meet each client with an open mind and listen hard to what they are saying – the solution is probably very deep within their words. There is a tendency to go with the history of the client when they might have changed, or the history might have been written by someone who wasn't listening properly.*
>
> voluntary sector, service co-ordinator in conversation with the author, May 2002

Creativity

Some people are naturally creative, but creativity in the helping professions will develop from active listening to individuals and reflection on practice, either individually or in groups. One of the main benefits of multi-disciplinary working should be increased creativity – if it isn't, we should be asking why not!

Presentation skills

Social work inevitably means assisting a user in presenting their case for resources, benefits, or in a legal/para-legal situation, or presenting on their behalf. Presentational skills are not only important in formal situations but discussions with influential others. The approved social worker not only has to have knowledge and skills but has to argue their case influentially with those who have more overt organisational power than they do. In conclusion, as we can see, these are skills which are in some sense technical, but by no means *just* technical. If they are simply a mechanical working out of techniques, then the individual being worked with will readily spot that. As Bill Jordan puts it:

In suggesting that to be helpful the helper must be a real person, I am making it clear that I think helping is not simply a skill or expertise or technique. Helping is a test for helper as a person. It involves the disciplined use of the **whole** *of the personality . . . he has also to retain his own values and standards, his own strengths and virtues. He has to recognise that the other person's feelings and fantasies are real to him, and to share in the discomfort of them, yet also to stay in touch with his own reality.*

Jordan, 1979: 26 (my emphasis)

Or as Winnicott colourfully puts it:

They (the users) take a risk, and first they must test you to see if you may be able to prove sensitive and reliable or whether you have it in you to repeat the traumatic experiences of their past. In a sense, you are a frying pan, with the frying process played backwards, so that you really do unscramble the scrambled eggs.

Winnicott, 1963: 227

Perhaps the main fault is that social workers feel they have to resolve things. They are needed by the client to listen, respond effectively and sensitively and then to come up with some practical measures to alleviate some aspects of the problem. The punter knows that social workers are not miracle workers, but they need a professional person to help them through the mire and to access useful support in order to move forward.

voluntary sector service co-ordinator

Case Example 8

Brief history

John H is in his mid thirties and has experienced schizophrenic illness since his teenage years. Six years ago he was admitted to hospital under Section following an episode of self-mutilation. He expressed a strong wish to live in his own flat on discharge and has spent the last six years living independently with a support package co-ordinated through the care programme approach, with a multi-disciplinary team providing ongoing professional support.

Current situation

John rents his own council flat with daily visits from a home care agency to provide practical support around budgeting, meal preparation, medication and maintaining the flat. Members of the multi-disciplinary team meet with John every six weeks to review the support package and work

---

with any arising difficulties. For example, harassment from a neighbour or falling out with a support worker. The high level of support has been felt appropriate because John's levels of motivation, concentration and self-worth mean that self-neglect is a significant risk.

John is offered some structured day activities. In the past, he used a day centre but with growing independence, it became increasingly clear that this provision was inappropriate and John could receive a better day service from mainstream services. John now attends one group session with a day service for people with disabilities because he particularly likes the session, has someone to work with him on a one-to-one basis for recreational community activities and is beginning to engage with sessional groups with a mental health day service.

John is someone with a dual diagnosis of mental health needs and a mild learning disability. There is always the risk that he may fall between services and not receive proper support around his mental distress from either learning disability or mental health services. The support package that John has recognises this dilemma by providing day care which he feels is appropriate, while ensuring that he has ongoing support to develop his daily living skills.

Social work support

The key contributions made by the social worker to the support package are: care planning skills to co-ordinate a multi-agency and cross-service package. The stability to provide ongoing professional support over a number of years, enabling good relationships to be built and engagement with long-term aims. A person-centred focus to ensure that the client's needs are met when they do not fit established service provision. Local knowledge is used to provide practical support, e.g. pay as you go leisure facilities. Professional support has overcome stressful crises, e.g. burglaries and moving flats.

The tasks for social workers are:

● *Assessment* – this is an assessment looking at the whole person in the context of their close relationships, family, community, neighbourhood, culture and faith, past experiences, future aspirations, strengths and needs (see Figure 18 above).

As the 1959 Younghusband Report stated:

We regard the essential functions of social workers in the Health and Welfare Services as being to assess the disturbance of equilibrium in a given 'individual' and his [sic] family and social relationships so as to give appropriate help. The aim will be to offer a supporting relationship in which his and their fears, frustrations and anxieties are understood, and measures used to meet or lessen them.

Younghusband, 1959

Malcolm Firth, 2000 (From the Manchester Care Assessment Schedule). (See also Firth, 1999, for a description of a generic approach to mental health needs assessment.)

The user is essentially the 'owner' of their own 'story'. Butler and Pritchard are clear that the 'social worker should be conscious of the potential strengths that exist within client and family, as well as apparent weaknesses and areas of dysfunction (Butler and Pritchard, 1983: 43) and the report into the care and treatment of Christopher Clunis, remarked on the fact that the strengths that the family had had to offer were never properly brought into play (Ritchie et al., 1994).

Smale, Tuson and Statham describe a number of types of assessment process, and look closely at what they call the 'questioning model' and the 'exchange model'.

The questioning model

Assumes the worker:

- Is expert in people, and their needs.
- Exercises knowledge and skill to form their own assessment to identify people's needs.
- Identifies resources required.
- Takes responsibility for making an accurate assessment of need and taking appropriate action.

The exchange model

Assumes that people are expert in themselves. Assumes that the worker:

- Has expertise in the process of problem-solving with others.
- Understands and shares perceptions of problems and their management.

- Gets agreement about who will do what to support whom.
- Takes responsibility for arriving at the optimum resolution of problems within the constraints of available resources and the willingness of participants to contribute.

Smale et al., 2000: 140

Working towards positive change

As we have seen already, social work operates at the margins of society, and is often in the position of interpreting the user's world to members of his/her family, groups and professionals, and conversely, interpreting the outside world and various groups and cultures to the user.

Egan's development of the skilled helper model has three stages:

1. What's going on? Telling the story, looking at 'blind spots' and considering leverage.
2. What solutions make sense for the user? Possibilities – change agendas and commitment to change.
3. How does the user get what they need or want? Possible strategies – best fit plan.

The social worker will arrive on the scene at a time of crisis, as can be seen by most of the case examples in this text, and therefore 'no change' is very rarely an option, while change without consent, participation, empowerment and self-direction will cause problems with self-determination later on.

Every day social workers help people from all walks of life, connecting thousands of people to appropriate resources. Social workers help people understand their own personal power to overcome life's adversities.

Elizabeth Clarke, Executive Director, National Association of Social Workers, USA quoted in Snell, What About the Social Workers? *ADSS Inform*, April 2002

Ongoing support

Martin Davies sees one of social work's prime tasks as: 'contributing to the maintenance and growth of those citizens seen to be deprived and underprivileged, and trying to enrich the lives of those on the margins of society' (Davies, 1981). It is one of the features of social work that many workers' fear has been neglected following the introduction of care management. In 1993, which had a greater emphasis on short-term interventions and co-ordinating practical care packages with a lesser emotional component. The

Figure 19: Assessing the individual's needs in their historical context.

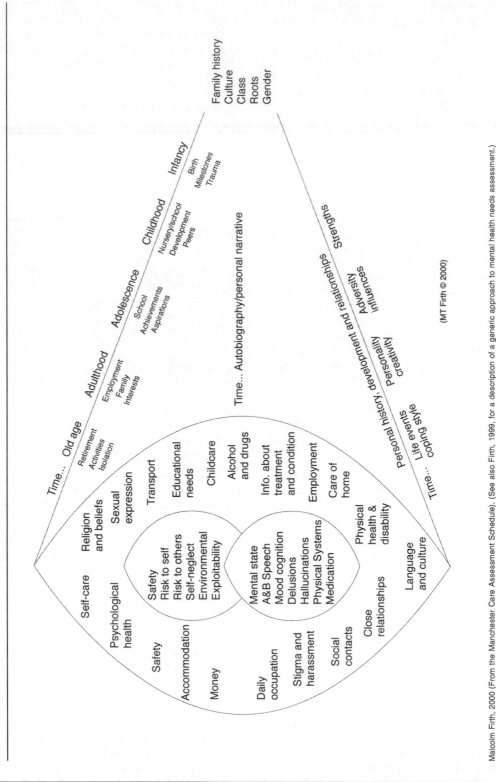

(MT Firth © 2000)

Malcolm Firth, 2000 (From the Manchester Care Assessment Schedule). (See also Firth, 1999, for a description of a generic approach to mental health needs assessment.)

Westminster Study is essential reading to understand how vital the ongoing support is for people with multiple social and environmental needs and environmental as well as personal needs, and as one colleague in the voluntary sector said to me recently 'Who else is going to deal with the nitty gritty of life?'

Planning, monitoring and review

This can be a cycle of interventions, on a partnership basis, around behaviours and interactions, and/or the bringing into play of packages of care (see also Care Management below) which is a feature of a number of the case examples in this text where users are particularly vulnerable and there are major elements of risk.

Co-ordinating

The world doesn't get any simpler! One of the prime tasks of the social worker is to co-ordinate work across a number of professional disciplines and agencies so as to ensure that the user is in as much control of the situation as is possible, they are not subject to multi, individual consultations or subject to the oppressive posse of professionals; while at the same time ensuring that all the professionals and agencies deliver.

Information gathering

One of the universal rules of information is that one is always overwhelmed with a plethora when one doesn't need it, but accurate and understandable information is not around when you do.

Because of their social perspective and links with a wide range of social agencies, social workers are in a good position to gather information or signpost.

When I was researching the needs of carers with disabled offspring in West Sussex in the early 1980s, one of the major pleas was for better information. We produced an information handbook, which one parent described as 'A real hand of friendship' (conversation with the author).

Nowadays, information changes so rapidly that a careful judgement has to be made as to whether information is printed or produced for electronic distribution. Issues of race, culture and language are, of course, crucial as has already been mentioned earlier in the text (see Fernando, 2002; Bennett, 2009).

Empowerment

The social work task is to empower the people we work with, and to ensure that issues of citizenship, rights and empowerment are at the forefront for other professionals working with users and carers.

Linda Hart's autobiographical work, *Phone at Nine Just to Say You're Alive* (Hart, 1997) is a powerful description of the issues around power relationships between users and professionals. See also works such as Harding and Beresford, 1996 and Wield, 2006.

Education

All professions should be a source of education for colleagues and other agencies in the values, strengths, knowledge and skills which they have. While social workers sometimes have a lack of confidence in this, the emphasis on a social and community agenda in the United Kingdom at present should give them confidence if espousing and propounding the social perspective.

In all of this, it should never be forgotten that the social worker is working alongside the most vulnerable people in our society at the margins of identity, recognition and tolerance, and in situations of conflict, distress and paradox. There is often an underlying assumption in public life that another structural change, procedure or initiative will reduce 'the complexity, ambiguity and uncertainty inherent in the workers' pivotal position':

> *A more realistic position is to recognise this lack of certainty as an inevitable and integral dimension of the role of the social change agent. The task is to balance these different perceptions and reconcile conflicting behaviours. Ambiguity, confusion and complexity are not problems to be solved before the job can be done: working towards their resolution is the work.*
>
> Smale et al., 2000: 94

When the draft statement on the roles and task of children's social workers was released in the summer of 2009, it came under criticism from Professor Eileen Munro of the LSE, among others, because 'The words 'poverty', 'social exclusion' and 'racism' do not appear anywhere in the document, although they apply to so many of the families who need social work services . . . it downplays structural factors that create adverse conditions for families' (quoted in *Community Care*, 27th August, 2009: 5).

Table 5: The social work contribution to mental health services.

Knowledge	Skills	Ethics
Mental health, Social welfare, family and human rights law. Sociology. Social administration. Social and individual psychology. Social philosophy and the ethics of social welfare. Social work methods. Models of social intervention and empowerment. Research. Race, gender, and disability studies.	Individual and family casework. Group work. Social brokerage, mediation, and advocacy skills. Advocacy. Use of relationship as an enabling process. The assessment of a person's social circumstances and needs, and communication of the conclusions. The compilation of assessment reports for specific purposes. Assessments regarding the potential need for compulsory detention and treatment under the Mental Health Act. The co-ordination and implementation of community care packages. The evaluation of complex needs on a more general level to assist planning and development. Advising fellow professionals on the relevance of social factors. Reflective analysis.	All that is included in the BASW Code of Ethics including the following commitments: • To a distinct set of professional principles and values based on the worth and the social and civil rights of each individual and groups as an integral part of the work. • To anti-discriminatory and anti-oppressive practice. • Commitment to promoting and upholding self determination and social inclusion. • To the least restrictive alternative. • Commitment to ongoing learning and professional development.

Table compiled by the Mental Health Special Interest Group, a National Forum representing Social Work in Mental Health. From the BASW Website, May 2002.

If I were to summarise my reflections, it would be to encourage you to be bold, and emphasise not only the statutory and supportive contributions social work can make to Mental Health Services, but to come out of the shadows, so to speak, and emphasise the intellectual contribution as well.

consultant psychiatrist

Social work and care management

There isn't time here to go into the whys and wherefores of the NHS and Community Care Act, 1990 (implemented 1 April 1993). The tensions between the increasing numbers of vulnerable people requiring care and an escalating social security bill; between the Treasury and 10 Downing Street; the ambitions and fears of both the NHS and local authorities; and the challenge to simultaneously promote choice while keeping a lid on the pot of available resources is a complex seesaw well set out in Lewis and Glennerster's *Implementing the New Community Care* (1996: 8). Lewis and Glennerster's conclusion is that:

They (the reforms) were not primarily driven by a desire to improve the relations between the various statutory authorities, or to improve services for elderly people, or to help those emerging from mental hospital. They were driven by the need to stop the haemorrhage in the social security budget and to do so in a way that would minimise political outcry and not give additional resources to the local authorities themselves.

The new care managers, or those social workers re-designated care managers, were the people who had the creative role of assessing individual needs and creating care packages out of the former social security money transferred to social services under the Special Transitional Grant, and simultaneously balancing those individual needs with the amount of money available.

'Choice' was a word on everybody's lips, yet as Lewis and Glennerster point out:

The new policy was precisely designed to ration that choice in order to save public money. The right to be assessed and sensitive care management that would take account of everyone's preferences, including carers, seemed a way of squaring the circle. The difficulty was that circles have the rather irritating property of not being squares!

Lewis and Glennerster, 1996: 14

Figure 20: The process of care management.

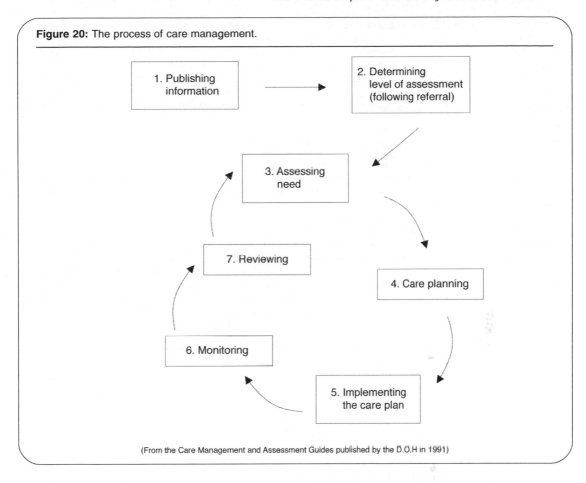

(From the Care Management and Assessment Guides published by the D.O.H in 1991)

This is worth recalling as the new wave of 'personalisation' (see Chapter 6 in this book) gathers momentum (see Leadbeater, 2009) at a time of severe budget restrictions and tight eligibility criteria.

There is no doubt that care managers did in fact make far better use of the social security money, in retaining people's independence, and re-abling those who had been admitted to institutions of various kinds. At the same time, finances were never adequate, some authorities running out within the first year, and therefore, to quote one Director of Social Services: 'social workers have become the public face of denial'.

Lewis and Glennerster's studies of a number of different kinds of authorities found some people feeling that 'it would erode much valued aspects of social work practice' (p141) 'turn them into administrators and financial processors' (p140) but there were also numerous occasions when social workers/care managers found that they could produce positive outcomes for the users

and carers they were working with, through the budgets delegated to them or their team managers, rather than scraping together resources from a whole range of different agencies. The process of care management, as set down by the Department of Health Care Management and Assessment Guides in 1991 show a great deal of congruence with the social work task described above.

Social workers feared, however, that the therapeutic aspects of their role would be eroded, and in fact some social services departments did appear to see the advent of community care as a way of moving away from that particular aspect of the work; while others integrated the process with traditional social work; and others again split social work and care management. The parallel issue of whether nurses wished to take on the care management role in addition to their therapeutic one has been mirrored in the debate over the 'Approved Mental Health Practitioner' role in the reform of the 1983 Mental Health Act (see Chapter 8). Many other professions have found the complexity of the role too challenging.

In many cases, there seems to have been a misunderstanding as to what people like Challis at the PSSRU envisaged care management to be. Challis and his colleagues in fact made a distinction between 'administrative' and 'complete' care management (or case management). They wrote:

> It is possible to define a rather limited form of case management – described here as 'administrative' case management – where service arrangements and co-ordination are seen as the central tasks. The other tasks of case management such as counselling, dealing with psychological stresses and tensions arising from caring or providing advice to families would be undertaken by persons other than the case manager . . . An underlying weakness in the 'administrative' model of case management is the failure to recognise the nature of the responsibilities and decisions which have to be made by the case manager.
> Challis et al., 1990: 15 (see also Smale et al., 1994)

My belief is that it simply isn't sensible to separate care management and social work. My own experience as a social worker and as a manager, added to the research, leads me to the conclusion that users and carers need and want attention to *both* their emotional/psychological needs and their practical concerns, in a way which values them as unique individuals. Social work and care management are two sides of the same coin. Social workers who veer too much towards a counselling perspective, and do not address the practical needs of users or combat oppression, are in danger of pathologising the individual. Those who only address practical concerns are in danger of dehumanising the individual so that the whole process becomes caricatured as a package, whereby the user is processed and 'boxed' in a way that denies them their dignity and uniqueness.

The Westminster Study, conducted three years after the implementation of Community Care demonstrates again what some American commentators had already warned their English counterparts of, namely that a purchaser/divider split within the main professionals delivering care (i.e. social workers/care managers) 'is an artificial macro construct which has nothing to do with micro practice in the human services and which is being imposed on a natural helping process' (Phyllis Sturgess, San Jose State University, in Clark and Lapsley, 1996).

Macdonald and Sheldon demonstrate clearly that:

> Clients value the opportunity to discuss and clarify their worries and fears, and examine ways of overcoming them ('emotional support and reassurance'). This important aspect of service provision has been shown to be one that needs protecting within current organisation changes towards a purchaser/provider split and privatisation. The growing pressure here is to purchase what is easy to define and to monitor what it is easy to count, whether or not those inputs have a close 'logical fit' with the qualitative nature of clients' problems.
> Macdonald and Sheldon, 1997: 43

The Sainsbury Centre Study on Care Management in Mental Health quoted a range of reactions, but several positive ones are worth quoting:

> I think the advantage of care management is that it brings a structure to the social work process.
>
> I wish assessment and care . . . management had come in twenty-five years ago, because it would have made me a better social worker . . . the creative professional can mould together different traditions and approaches so as to improve their practice.

As one experienced senior manager put it in Staffordshire 'We're still doing social work but we are doing it in a more organised, systematic and effective way'. Some of the same difficulties in melding together two strands of work, reappeared in the requirements and difficulties in merging care management and the care programme approach. I will leave the last word to Macdonald and Sheldon:

> The role of specialist social workers was obviously pivotal in the system of care. They both arranged for services, and were a service themselves (an awkward principle for those who speak and write about 'services', as if these were always 'things'). In this study, the social services staff emerged as individuals to be relied upon, to promote emotional support and counselling, for a range of practical services, and for their well-respected 'advocacy' function. This appears to have been carried out with a distinctive friendliness, openness and professionalism which, for the majority of respondents, was thought to be the best thing about the help they received.
> p51

The social worker in the community mental health team

> Mental health issues have predominantly been within the domain of psychiatry, concentrating on mental ill-health rather than mental health. This approach is in the process of being cemented further in the 'ill-health' camp with the movement of social work to the NHS. The NHS has traditionally spent many millions on reacting to ill-health

and relatively little on maintaining health and social well-being. I am of the opinion that psychiatry should be an adjunct to social inclusion and social support for those suffering from mental health problems, rather than the lead profession. The role, training and model of social care within psychiatry needs to be enhanced greatly if the traditional view of mental ill-health being a lifetime problem is going to be challenged. Social workers are in a great position to influence this challenge but the overall philosophy needs to be addressed by the policy makers and traditional psychiatric services.

Director of Integrated Mental Health Services,
from a nursing background

I am profoundly disappointed when I come across community mental health teams where there seems to be more of a focus on inter-disciplinary rivalry than inter-disciplinary working. Clearly, forming a team (though sometimes the teams seem more like groups) – as Malcolm Payne's work demonstrates is a complex process and the effective team needs to operate more like a creative football team, rather than like an athletics team concentrating on their own individual pursuits (see Payne, 1982). When teams are not functioning properly, the following problems are mentioned frequently by staff:

- Poor leadership, either providing no structure or control, or imposing an authoritarian style.
- Lack of clarity about roles and responsibilities within the team.
- Absence of or infrequent meetings.
- Poor communication about team functions, and between members of the team.
- Time not managed to enable members to meet.
- Opinions not sought and talents not recognised and used.
- Lack of training.
- Poor working conditions.

Gilbert and Scragg, 1992: 158

My disappointment stems partly from being part of a very positive community team for people with learning disabilities in the mid 1980s (see Gilbert and Spooner, 1982). The senior community nurse had been appointed to lead a community nursing team only, but he was quite clear that a multi-disciplinary approach would be better for the people we served, both users and carers, and would have a long-term positive effect for the working together of the two major statutory agencies; also creating better links with the voluntary sector. Some of the features of the team were as follows:

- A very clear focus, at the outset, on producing positive outcomes for users and carers.
- A shared operational policy for the team with an explicit value-base.
- Right from the beginning, recognising and celebrating the strength and skills that each profession had to bring to the team.
- A lack of defensiveness about professional roles, but within the operational policy, being clear with ourselves and our clientele what the core roles of each profession were, and also what the positive overlaps were.
- An open referral system with an initial team discussion of each case referred, and an agreement over which worker/workers would work with the user and their family at any one time; who the key worker was, and when key workers changed.
- A sharing of skills and a celebration of people's work, which saw people developing skills which they almost certainly would not have done if they had remained in a uni-professional setting.

The chairing of the team was done on a rotational basis, and this was very useful in addressing some of the power issues between professions, and presenting a changed and more radical focus to the agencies concerned.

Professional supervision was undertaken through the professionals' lines of accountability.

We are taking relatively senior people in Health and Social Services and asking them to do something different. People have risen to the challenge and developed and enhanced their transferable skills.

Director of Mental Health Services, from
a background in clinical psychology

In team working across disciplines, people sometimes forget the basics. John Adair's description of effective leadership as paying attention to three interlocking circles of mission or task, the team and individual needs, is sometimes lost sight of within the complexity of organisational concerns (Adair, 1987).

Cormack describes the needs that should be met for the team to achieve success as follows:

- Mission or task.
- To set clear targets for the task.
- To set standards of performance.
- To make full use of resources.
- To clarify responsibilities.
- To ensure members' contributions are complementary.

- To achieve the set targets and standards.

Team needs:

- To know and respond to the leader's style and vision.
- To feel a common sense of purpose with members.
- To have a supportive climate.
- To grow and develop as a unit.
- To have a corporate sense of achievement.
- To have a common identity.

Individual needs (your own and others):

- To be accepted by the leader.
- To be valued by the leader.
- To be able to contribute to the task.
- To know what is expected in relation to the task.
- To be part of the team.
- To know what is expected of you by the team.

Cormack, 1988

To provide positive outcomes for people with mental health needs you have to connect primary care, secondary care and health and social care in a way so as they enhance each other.

Director of Social Services and former
Chief Executive of a Mental Health Trust

The Sainsbury Centre's study of Community Mental Health Teams (Onyett, Pillinger and Muijen, 1995) shows a changing picture of CMHTs increasingly working as 'teams' in Payne's sense of the term, with team managers or co-ordinators, an organised and consistent referral system, shared record keeping etc. But at the time of the study, a large number were still operating as groups, for example, 53 per cent of the teams taking referrals via individual members rather than by a referral route which ensured that the team considered each referral with a team perspective.

The authors pay considerable 'attention to role ambiguity', because that 'is often cited as a source of stress and job dissatisfaction'. Putting:

Practitioners into teams places them in a special dilemma. They become members of two groups: their discipline and the team. As a result, they may find themselves torn between the aims of the Community Mental Health Movement that explicitly values egalitarianism, role blurring and a surrender of power to lower-status workers and service users on the one hand, and a desire to hold on to tradition, socially-valued role definitions and practices on the other.

The authors go on to say that:

It might, therefore, be predicted that the ideal conditions for team membership would be where a positive sense of belonging to the team can exist alongside continued professional identification. This is most likely to occur when the discipline has a clear and valued role within the team, which in turn requires that the team itself has a clear role.

Onyett et al., 1995: 21–2 (my emphasis)

Who is going to keep my professional feet on the ground as I try and support people against the system?!
social worker in a multi-disciplinary team

The Sainsbury Study looks at the pressure on all the members of CMHT, and a great deal of those pressures do seem to be around role ambiguity and role changes, where individuals and groups have not been able to, or been allowed to, develop new ways of seeing themselves as valued. Psychiatrists, for example, appear to be 'vulnerable to burn out because they see themselves as having 'a lot of responsibility but not the corresponding authority' (quoted in Onyett et al., 1995: 35).

The study shows that 54 per cent of the social workers are:

Highly exhausted emotionally. Compared with other disciplines, they also have a comparatively low sense of personal accomplishment and a high degree of de-personalisation. They also have the least satisfaction with work relationships and least overall job satisfaction.

Onyett et al., 1995: 34

The authors believe that this dissatisfaction may stem from:

- Confusion about their roles and their place in the team.
- Comparatively unclear about the role of the team and their focus within it.
- Low identification with their team and profession.
- Least positive sense of belonging to their profession.
- Confusion in regard to their roles as purchasers or providers of services (at the time of the study, community care and the care management role was relatively new. See also Macdonald and Sheldon's comments on the dichotomies of purchasing and providing).

The relationship between psychiatrist and social worker as both contribute to the care of people with mental health problems has shifted in various directions over the years, but it has always been an intimate one. In many ways, future Mental Health Services can be expected to be less dominated by a biomedical model as has been the case in recent years. All of the major

Case Example 9

Gambling on independence

A former social care manager is diagnosed with a disease that affects people with HIV and which severely impairs his cognitive ability. He develops mental health problems and is sectioned. A return to independence seems far off until social worker Paul Hatchman intervenes.

Case notes

Practitioner: Paul Hatchman
Field: Social worker, health team (specialist HIV)
Location: London
Client: Richard Fraser (not his real name)
Case history: Just over two years ago, Fraser's health was deteriorating so badly that he was persuaded by friends to go to hospital. He was subsequently admitted and tests showed that he was HIV positive. Further tests showed that he had suspected progressive multifocal leukoencephalopathy (see Fact File, page 43), a disease associated with HIV that severely impairs cognitive ability. For example, Fraser became unable to wash himself, dress himself and so on. Survival is very rare, with death occurring usually between one and four months after contracting PML. He spent three months in an HIV specialist ward at a general hospital and was then admitted to a north London respite hospice. He was discharged home with an intensive 24-hour care package, but within a month began to display mental health difficulties that resulted in him being sectioned. He returned home only to be sectioned once again.
Dilemma: Fraser, an ex-social care manager, had difficulties in coming to terms with his illnesses, believing he could return to his usual way of life.
Risk factor: By increasing Fraser's independence, there is a danger that he might not manage his medication resulting in him being sectioned again.
Outcome: Fraser continues to improve and it is possible that future assessments might reduce his level of care further.

No longer considered newsworthy, you might be forgiven for thinking that HIV was no longer with us. But by the end of 2001 some 48,226 people in the UK had been diagnosed HIV positive, of which 3,342 were newly diagnosed that year. Since the introduction of combination therapy in 1996, death rates have dropped dramatically. More people (currently estimated at 33,000) are finding themselves able to live with HIV.

Life, however, was not something that Richard Fraser (not his real name)was thought to have much of left. Encouraged by his friends, who were alarmed at the deterioration of his health, he went to hospital and was subsequently diagnosed with HIV. Worse followed: he was also diagnosed with progressive multifocal leukoencephalopathy, a terminal and incurable illness that affects the nervous system.

PML usually takes between one and four months to claim its victims. It is very rare to survive this disease, but somehow Fraser did so. He was eventually discharged home, but with an intensive 24-hour care package.

Fraser, now 46, also developed mental health problems that resulted in him being sectioned twice. It was at this point that Paul Hatchman, social worker with the health (specialist HIV) team, became involved.

He immediately set about sorting out 'the nuts and bolts stuff', such as Fraser's housing benefit, disabled living allowance and professional pensions. It was clear that Fraser, an ex-social care manager, was in denial over his illness – possibly stemming from the shock of the dual diagnosis. 'He had come to terms with the HIV but not the PML. He wanted to go back to work. But I explained that wasn't realistic and he'd get angry and agitated. The pointers were all there, towards him getting violent and being sectioned again,' says Hatchman.

Hatchman supported Fraser through this traumatic period. 'I tried to understand where he was coming from,' he says. He was increasingly isolated, his circle of friends having faded away. 'We tried to address his aggression and convince him that we only wanted what was best for him. But he went through a stage when he wouldn't return calls or left rude messages.'

The other big challenge for Fraser was the loss of privacy that inevitably accompanies 24-hour care. 'There's only so much a carer can do and they'd sit with him and he'd just feel watched,' Hatchman says. He had four carers (all trainee doctors) who worked a rota. On occasion one would fail to turn up. What could have been a problem actually became an opportunity, as Fraser would manage to cope without a carer. 'After this had happened a few times we started to think about reducing the care hours,' says Hatchman. 'We agreed to take away the night care and that worked out fine.'

Further opportunities presented themselves: 'He'd call up and say that the carer hadn't turned up and he needed to go to the bank. So I'd say "well, just go then". And he would. So, slowly but surely he took on more independence.'

There have been times when Hatchman has 'sailed close to the wind' in his work with Fraser. Occasionally Fraser hasn't taken his anti-psychotic medication. 'He had worked in the drugs field and knows what these drugs can do to your head, so he wouldn't take them. But he'd become aggressive.' His carers had informally monitored his medication, but with their reduced hours this was no longer possible.

However, Fraser has managed his medication well. The community psychiatric nurse visits fortnightly now rather than daily. He even attends courses at the London Lighthouse, studying for a teaching qualification. Although he is aware that he may never teach, the personal esteem and confidence this promotes is immeasurable.

Fraser's continual improvement, mentally and physically, has meant that he now has just two care hours in the morning and three in the evening. And this may even be reduced further. Hatchman says that Fraser recently facilitated a group at the Lighthouse on HIV and drugs awareness: 'I went along and there were about five other professionals there as well. And apart from me, no one knew about his status. I was very impressed and the feedback was very positive.'

Hatchman's work with Fraser highlights the positive support that can help bring some normality back to a life shattered by HIV and, most impressively, PML. 'I compare him now with those times when he has been very low, depressed, confused and disorientated. And he is such a different man.' And quite a remarkable one, too.

Arguments for risk

- Fraser's physical health was improving and it was reasonable to build on this and encourage more independence. The more that he was able to do things for himself the more his confidence and self-esteem would improve, thereby positively affecting his mental health.
- Clearly the more independent Fraser is, the better his quality of life. By moving, however gradually, to developing his independence, it would go some way to combating the trauma of the double diagnosis of HIV and PML and restore some normality back to his life.
- The isolation suffered through his condition and loss of work and friends needed to be tackled, or else there would be a real danger that Fraser might deteriorate further. Attempts to introduce social contacts may help to reduce Fraser's helplessness and, in turn, his frustration and aggression.
- Fraser had demonstrated that on occasion he could manage with reduced care, and he was willing to try and do more for himself.

Arguments against risk

- Fraser had not always managed his medication well – either forgetting or deliberately refusing to take it (on one occasion his carers found a small number of tablets tucked away in his pockets).

The removal of full-time care meant that the informal monitoring of his medication by his carers would be lost – adding to the risk.
- Should he not take his anti-psychotic medication, his subsequent aggressive behaviour may be misinterpreted, resulting in him being possibly sectioned.
- Should he not take his HIV medication there would be a strong possibility that he would build up a resistance to it. This may lead to the further possibility that he may run out of effective medicines to stabilise his health. The side-effects can also be quite harmful.
- There is always the possibility that if things were not working out and he believed he would never have his old life back, he might at best deteriorate further, or worse take his own life.

Independent comment

Fraser faced the complexity of an HIV positive diagnosis and possible deteriorating cognitive impairment at a time when his physical health was severely affected, writes Grainne Morby. Any diagnosis of a potentially life threatening condition, particularly HIV with its associated stigma, has a damaging effect on self-esteem.

Fraser was provided a 24-hour medical care package by four different people, which also helped combat perceived risks such as self-harm and non-adherence to treatments. He, however, believed it was over-controlling and did not welcome it.

Breakdowns in the care package led to an increased emphasis on supporting Fraser's independence which, with the peer support and personal development opportunities, suggests that he is learning to live independently with HIV. It is very likely though that, without Paul's encouragement and practical support on diagnosis, the positive outcome would have been less certain.

A person is better equipped to deal with the consequences both of their HIV diagnosis and the knock-on effect it will have on the rest of their life if health and social care are combined early enough after diagnoses of HIV.

Terrence Higgins Trust and Lighthouse are in the process of establishing a social care centre. This will enable people living with HIV to receive both medical and social care support, and reflects the growing need for a more holistic approach to the delivery of care packages.

Grainne Morby is director of London services at the Terrence Higgins Trust.

Reprinted by kind permission of *Community Care*, 7–13 March, 2002.

developments: assertive outreach, home treatment, early intervention, etc. are around the development of different forms of psychosocial intervention.

consultant psychiatrist

The social worker in primary care

Social workers have a specific contribution to make to the government's modernising agenda, with its emphasis on rights and responsibilities, citizenship and participation. Delivery of social care will be best offered in a collaborative approach from a range of professionals and agencies with the emphasis being around meeting the needs of individual consumers, their families and their communities.

GP with a regional and national role on mental health

As we have seen from Chapter 1, the general practitioner is so often the first point of contact for individuals suffering from mental distress and their families. GPs recount a significant psychological component in 70 per cent of consultations, and in 20–25 per cent of patients a mental health problem will be their sole reason for consultation. As we have also noted, the interaction between physical and mental states of health and ill-health are profound, and it is the GP and members of the primary care team who are likely to be crucial in making a real difference for people who use their services.

Many of the issues around roles and team working, that have already been set out in the section on the Community Mental Health Team above, appertain to Primary Care Teams. Inevitably, resources in Social Services Departments are limited, and although some have made significant investments in attaching social workers to Primary Care Teams with great benefits (see Le Mesurier and Cumella's Study of Worcestershire, in Managing Community Care, 9: 1) but these social workers are normally targeted towards older persons and their families – including of course older people with a mental health need (either functional or organic). Studies, such as Le Mesurier and Cumella, demonstrate considerable benefits in preventing hospital admission and effecting speedier and effective discharge back to home or homely settings.

A model of innovative practice described by Firth et al. (2000) looks at five part-time and two full-time mental health workers attached to seven practices delivering services to patients/users referred directly by GPs. Of 200 referrals, only a dozen required assistance from secondary care services.

Social workers in primary care are also in a strategic position to affect partnership working and break down the silo mentality so as to ensure proper partnership in the service of users and carers.

The creation of the large and unified Health and Social Care Mental Health Trusts has produced a powerful and specialist focus for mental health services. One of the dangers is, however, that without clear leadership and an environmental perspective, they could become the children of the 19th century asylums, institutional and inward looking. It is absolutely essential that primary care drives the agenda as much as possible with a strong user, familial and social perspective, though this clearly has a lot of issues about strengthening mental health commissioning within primary care trusts and ensuring that they are really reflecting community needs in the way that Primary Care Groups had begun to do before their demise (see Behan and Loft, 1999).

The really effective primary care team is invaluable in promoting sound mental health. As one general practitioner puts it:

● Most patients present their problems as undifferentiated mixtures of physical, emotional, family and social symptoms. And yet we organise whole systems of health and social care, which separate the biomedical from the psychological and social. The limitation of such a simplistic 'body and mind' approach is challenged by several studies of mental disorders in primary care which consistently report the co-occurrence of physical, emotional and social problems in patients, and furthermore show such patients to be the highest utilisers of these services.

General practitioner with a policy role

Conclusion

With society and family life increasingly fragmented and under a range of pressures, the need for skilled helpers to consider the needs and aspirations of individuals within their family, community and social context, is even more acute now than when social work first began to put down roots in the middle of the 19th century. In times of crisis, or when life becomes a long and bitter struggle for survival, then people in distress turn to someone who is genuine, who listens,

Figure 21: From silo to strategy.

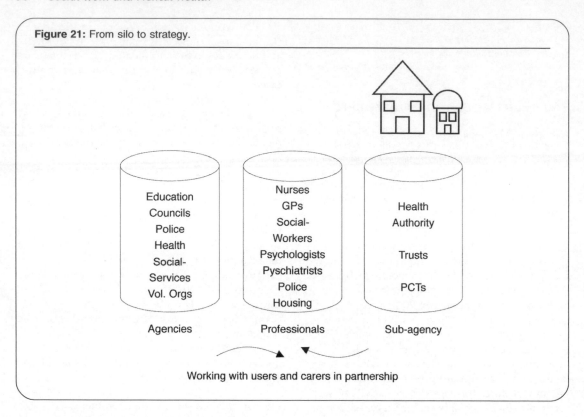

hears, and who produces practical results. As the GSCC puts in its 2008 document on the roles and tasks of social workers:

People value a social work approach based on challenging the broader barriers they face. They place a particular value on Social Work's social approach, the social work relation-

ship, and the positive qualities they associate with social workers. These include warmth, respect, being non-judgmental, listening, treating people with equality, being trustworthy, open, honest and reliable, and communicating well. People value the support social workers offer as well as their ability to help them access and deal with other services and agencies.

GSCC, 2008

CHAPTER 8

The Vital Equilibrium – Social Work and the Law

Greg Slay

What is liberty and how can it best be safeguarded? All societies have these problems. How they answer them depends on what they are and the values they hold.

Jones, 1972: xiii

It is essential for people to move on from being service users to being people with fulfilling lives, with hopes and ambitions, in control of what happens to them. They may well continue to use services, but this should not define them.

Future Vision Coalition, 2008: 17

The causes of mental ill-health are complex but their impact can be reduced by intervening quickly and effectively when people are showing early signs of problems. This can be done by identifying and providing appropriate support to those at higher risk of mental health problems and by the provision of timely and good quality services when people do become unwell.

DoH, 2009b: 11

From the service user's perspective, a crisis is always a frightening experience.

Watkins, 2009: 33

Introduction

Much of the way in which we live our lives today is not merely the result of a recent determination by politicians, of whatever political persuasion, or by academics such as Bunting (2005) and Bauman (2007) who have highlighted the complexities of contemporary identity. Or even by those with an interest in the importance of a spiritual dimension to mental health and well-being (Slay, 2007; Coyte, Gilbert and Nicholls, 2007). Irrespective of the tragedy of the September 2001 terrorist attacks in the USA, the July 2005 bombings in London, and the global economic crises of the end of the first decade of the twenty-first century, much of the way in which British society is ordered actually has its roots in public debate and powerful lobbying over many years.

The need for a synthesis between authority, legislation and the practice of governance is not a new phenomenon and has a long history (Wallace-Hadrill, 2000). But so much of what takes place in terms of political discourse at the

present time is about the nature of Government and authority, and who should wield that authority and in what circumstances.

The importance of countervailing influences, both ethical and pragmatic, in moderating the weighting of the scales of law should not, and cannot, be underestimated. Mental health care and treatment is no stranger to these debates. The way in which mental health care has been viewed and provided over the decades and centuries has long been the result of a search for consensus and equilibrium.

Values-based social care practice

Into this search for public consensus comes the nature of the laws that stem from the development of social policy and practice (Jones, 1972; Olsen, 1984; Jones, 2008). Social work and social care practice are fundamentally moral activities, underpinned by a set of values that centre on the uniqueness and worth of individuals, their right to freedoms and justice, and the importance of community (General Social Care Council, 2002; Golightley, 2008).

The rich perspectives of people in the UK who have themselves experienced mental distress at first hand have only comparatively recently been added to this discourse (Rogers, Pilgrim and Lacey, 1993; Pilgrim, 2005; Survivors History Group, 2008). Many who have experienced at first hand the often apparently negative benefits of a stay – enforced or otherwise – in a psychiatric hospital, have emerged from that experience both chastened and emboldened. But they face a difficult challenge in overturning the powerful forces at play for the maintenance of all that has gone before, particularly those that argue for custodial and/or medicalised approaches to mental health care.

In today's 24-hour news-driven world the role of the media often exacerbates and reinforces negative stereotypes and stigma – irrespective of the evidence otherwise (Taylor and Gunn, 1999; Mental Health Foundation, 2000). And the powerful role of the media in promoting and sustaining what one might, perhaps generously, refer to as 'mental health illiteracy' is also a global phenomenon (Granello, Pauley and Carmichael, 1999; Wilson, Nairn, Coverdale and Panapa, 2000; House of Lords European Union Committee, 2007).

At the centre of this discourse, alongside the voice of the consumers of mental health services, is the key role now being performed in England and Wales by Approved Mental Health Professionals (AMHPs). From 1984–2008 this role was undertaken by Approved Social Workers (ASWs). Values-based practice is the fundamental underpinning of all that is associated with the AMHP role. This is confirmed in the AMHP Regulations (DoH, 2008a); it also formed the basis of the training materials prepared for practitioners in the run-up to implementation of an amended 1983 Mental Health Act in November 2008.

These values are complex and often conflicting – and may often conflict between professionals involved from different mental health service disciplines. The values of the person being assessed must also be taken into consideration. Hence the requirement of practitioners to take proper account of the so-called Guiding Principles set out in the Mental Health Act Code of Practice (DoH, 2008b) as well as the facts, or evidence, available that supports decision-making. And it is for the AMHP to ultimately make sense of any conflicts in the values and evidence inherent in any Mental Health Act assessment, as part of the overall co-ordination of that activity.

The AMHP not only co-ordinates the assessment process but has to be aware of, and manage, the separation of executive and legislative powers, balance issues around liberty and safety, and provide a constitutional 'checks and balance' approach to the assessment outcome.

Independence of the AMHP role

The importance of the independence of the role of the AMHP was initially enshrined in its predecessor ASW role when the Mental Health Act 1983 was first developed. Although ASWs were required to be officers of a local social services authority, and to act on the behalf of their employing local authority, their role under the Mental Health Act was different to the

position of any other employee in that they did not work at the behest of their employers. In other words, their professional judgement in the role was not open to challenge and could not be overridden. The judgements, decisions and actions of ASWs were theirs and theirs alone and ASWs were required to complete their legal responsibilities once they had begun them. It was the ASW's role in the Mental Health Act assessment process that was independent, not they themselves.

In mental health law particularly, where the liberty (both physical and psychological) of the individual is at risk, such liberty has to be balanced against their safety and that of other people. Section 2 (2) of the Mental Health Act 1983 states that an application to compulsorily admit a person to a hospital must be founded on the grounds that:

> *He is suffering from mental disorder of a nature or degree which warrants the detention of the patient in a hospital for assessment (or for assessment followed by medical treatment) for at least a limited period, and he ought to be so detained in the interests of his own health or safety or with a view to the protection of other persons.*
>
> Barber, Brown and Martin, 2009: 142

The history of mental health law, policy and practice shows society as a whole – and practitioners in particular – grappling with the concepts and the practicalities of weighing freedom before the law with a need to protect individuals from the extreme consequences of their own and others' actions. In essence, we still work on the lines laid down by John Stuart Mill in the 1850s that self-protection is the sole end for which society is enabled to interfere in the lives of others, whether individually or collectively.

But these general propositions, whilst being vital foundations and guides, do not provide the whole story for the team of Mental Health Act assessors called to assess a person's mental health needs in the middle of the night in a police station custody centre. Nevertheless, it is philosophy and the development of legislation that provides such a strong impetus to the need for checks and balances to the dominant professional viewpoint. In terms of mental health legislation, the dominant profession is that of medicine and a presumption that in order to access appropriate specialist help it is necessary to become a patient and conform to a number of other powerful cultural norms (Parsons, 1951; Johnstone, 2000). For the past two and a bit decades however it was the ASW, employed by local authorities, who provided the checks and balances to this dominant hegemony. Or, as was described by Professor Peter Jones in 2002, the ASW role provided 'the essential grit in the oyster, helping to produce the pearl of positive outcomes for users' (Jones, 2002).

One only needs to look at the press coverage of causes célèbres in the second half of the 19th century (Jones, 1972) and the similar coverage of a range of Mental Health Inquiries in the 1990s (Sheppard 1996) to understand how vital has been, and remains, the checks and balances role of the mental health social worker in this legislative context.

An historical perspective on current legislative arrangements

The history of the current of mental health legislation can, in the main, be traced back to the 18th century. At that time there was considerable fear both of the mobile poor (described as vagrants) and of people suffering from a mental disorder. The practical tolerance of the mediaeval monasteries had long since vanished under the pressures of social dislocation, agrarian reform and industrialisation (including the emergence of newspapers) and fears amongst the propertied classes.

Public debate therefore began to develop over the wider responsibility of society for people with mental health problems, as a number of academic studies have reported in more detail than space allows for in this chapter (Jones, 1972; Bartlett and Wright, 1999; Bell and Lindley, 2005). Essentially, however, in the 18th century people suffering from a mental illness could be confined as follows:

- In Bethlem – an institution financed by public subscriptions and legacies.
- Under the Poor Laws – and therefore came under the responsibility and jurisdiction of the parish overseer.
- Under criminal law – until 1800 insanity was not an effective defence against a criminal charge.
- Under the vagrancy laws – anyone considered a vagrant was harshly dealt with.
- In a private run-for profit madhouse – where the only defence against confinement was by means of a writ of Habeas Corpus, but the secrecy and restraint used by the owners of

these institutions did actually made it very difficult to issue such a writ.

In addition there were what was referred to as 'single lunatics' who were usually confined out of sight at home unless the family had money or other connections – such as Mrs Rochester in Charlotte Brontë's *Jane Eyre*.

The 1744 Vagrancy Act was the first to identify and emphasise the benefits of detention and restraint in order to provide the curative refuge and tranquillity needed to enable individuals to recover their reason and rationality. It was also the first attempt to see more distinction between vagrants and those suffering from a mental disorder. Several thousand people suffering from mental disorder or mental deficiency already lived alongside ordinary paupers in workhouses and no attempt had previously been made to separate them from other residents.

The 1744 Act also introduced a form of checks and balances in that two or more Justices of the Peace had to be brought into play to confine somebody suffering from a mental illness, whereas a vagrant merited a warrant signed by one Justice of the Peace. However no medical opinion was deemed necessary. The prevailing belief was that mental illness was a distinct state differing markedly from ordinary mental health – and therefore was both easily identifiable and continuous in nature. But this approach also meant that it was very difficult for individuals to prove that they had recovered.

Private madhouses came under scrutiny in the 1760s when instances were discovered of persons being placed there by relatives for sinister reasons. For instance, wives who had become inconvenient and elderly relatives (whose money was coveted) were extremely vulnerable to a stay in a madhouse.

The genesis of regulation can be seen in the passing of the 1774 Act to Licence and Regulate the Private Madhouse. This recognised the many people living in private madhouses in conditions of appalling squalor and deprivation without any form of legal protection. Licensing; the notification of reception of people considered mentally disordered; visits by commissioners; and the introduction of inspection and supervision by the medical profession, were all introduced. In fact these different elements bear remarkable similarity to the regulatory framework with which we have become very familiar in the 21st century.

Although attitudes towards people with a mental illness gradually became more positive during the latter part of the 18th and early 19th centuries, it was still very much a taboo subject in polite society. Public sympathy for King George III in his severe bouts of mental distress helped, as did the passionate championing and legislative muscle of Lord Ashley. Ashley, later the 7th Earl of Shaftesbury, was appointed chairman of the Lunacy Commission in 1834 and served in this role for the next 50 years. His leadership was founded on first-hand observations of the conditions of the poor, deprived, distressed and dispossessed. He was also driven by his own profound religious beliefs and by an awareness of his own tendency to severe bouts of depression.

Predictably, the care provided in madhouses was not based on the use of medicine (which was still in its infancy) but majored on the use of restraint. The Government's select committee set up in 1807 under the chairmanship of Charles William Wynn enquired into the state of pauper lunatics in England. The committee's report probably made depressing reading for the Government – and led to the 1808 County Asylum Act.

The 1808 Act enabled the development of asylums financed by a county rate. For the first time care for people with mental disorder was seen as a responsibility of the state. The legislation was broadly welcomed by enlightened physicians of the time, such as Dr Boyd of the Somerset County Lunatic Asylum (Marshall, 2006) and Dr Ellis of the Yorkshire asylum in Wakefield – who later moved to the Middlesex Asylum in Hanwell (Rutherford, 2008). The Act also introduced new powers aimed at dealing with 'persons dangerous to be at large' who had not previously been covered under legislation. The admission of the latter was however regulated by the need to again secure the support of two Justices of the Peace, who would issue a warrant so that the relevant person could be legally intercepted and removed to the asylum.

Inevitably, though, the development of asylums and madhouses became a minor growth industry with still relatively few checks and balances on what actually happened within the walls of the asylum. Many of the asylums that were built were still largely experimental in the care they offered. The legislation was seen as permissive rather than compulsory and consequently only the most progressive Justices of the Peace used the powers to actually raise county rates in order to build asylums in their midst.

Notwithstanding the early attempts at formal regulation set out in the 1845 Lunatics Act it was not in fact until the 1890 Lunacy Act that the institution came to be viewed as needing to be routinely offering legal safeguards in order to avoid inappropriate confinement. 40 years on again, and as a range of new medical treatments gained prominence (chief amongst which were the emergence of electro-convulsive therapy and the development of brain surgery) the focus shifted back to the asylum being the place to be to get these specialist treatments. Recognising the location of these treatment options, and also that the public might actually want to access them of their own accord, voluntary admission to hospital was also introduced in the 1930 Mental Treatment Act, having been effectively trialled seven years earlier by the Maudsley Hospital in London (Carrier and Kendall, 1997).

The many and various county asylums, run by local government, were effectively nationalised in the 1948 development of the National Health Service. It was not until the mid-1950s however that community-based prevention could start to be developed in any systematic way. It was the development of medications such as chlorpromazine (it was found to significantly reduce the impact of major mood disturbance) that enabled this shift to begin to take hold.

The confidence of the public in the increasing variety of medical treatments for mental disorder – and where those treatments could be best provided – was to some extent anticipated through the 1959 Mental Health Act. This legislation was effectively a 'root and branch' overhaul and replacement of all the legal arrangements that had previously existed. It included the disappearance of the role previously undertaken by Justices of the Peace. The Act was largely drafted on the basis of the recommendations of the 1957 Report of the Royal Commission on the Laws Relating to Mental Illness and Mental Deficiency. The Commission was particularly keen to see the removal of the concept of 'certification' in the hope that the public would no longer stigmatise or label detained people.

The 1959 Act was therefore born out of an optimism in the efficacy of the new drug regimes, and a belief that community alternatives to hospitals would invariably proliferate, whilst recognising that hospital care might be needed for some people as an alternative. The 1959 Act also introduced the new role of Mental Welfare Officer, providing a dedicated specialist assessment and co-ordinating role around the arrangements for hospital admission.

The pendulum swung back again with the 1983 Mental Health Act, crafted at a time of public disillusionment with 'care in the community' as a concept. And not just in the UK, where the rhetoric of the 1959 Act had not really been matched by practical reality. A reduction in the inpatient population was relatively easy to achieve; the development of an equivalent resources base in the community at large had proved a much more difficult aspiration. Again, this was not just the UK phenomenon. Studies in the United States were beginning to report on both the successes and the difficulties with the programme there of deinstitutionalisation. The decline in the public psychiatric hospital population was, as Bachrach (1997) notes, complicated by being accompanied by a series of ideological debates around funding mechanisms and reduced regulation and a series of high profile events associated with what were termed 'landscapes of despair' (homelessness and destitution) and 'the landscape of haunted places' (the re-creation of the Institution) (Dear and Wolch, 1987).

The 1983 Mental Health Act (and its 1984 Scottish equivalent) was for many in the UK a return to the concerns expressed a century earlier and which surfaced in the legally prescriptive 1890 Lunacy Act. Or as Jones (1988: 39) has stated 'In its final form, it represented an uneasy compromise between the civil rights concerns of MIND and what the DHSS lawyers thought it possible to achieve by law.'

Furthermore, many saw the 1983 Mental Health Act as focusing on a very small number of people – and therefore not really touching the issues for the majority of people in hospital and the much greater numbers in community settings. Although policy was becoming increasingly community focused, with the vast majority of people with mental illness living in the community by the late 1970s, the commissioning budget was still very much tied up in hospital buildings, and had not been released to fund any of a broad range of community services (Leff, 1997). This only served to repeat what had been happening in the United States, whose model for community services had so readily found favour with UK politicians and policy-makers from the 1960s onwards. It also made the job of the ASW

more difficult in trying to work out the best outcomes for individual patients following a Mental Health Act assessment. The struggles for many ASWs were encapsulated in a debate they had to have at the time of the assessment itself, and where the ASW had to act as the independent arbiter between hospital or community care-based services, and the use of compulsion versus informal arrangements.

By the late 1990s the Government was beginning to take the view that the legislation was creaking and in urgent need of reform. But it was not as high on the list as some other legislation revision requirements. An interim solution had been found in England and Wales in 1995 by introducing Aftercare Under Supervision Orders. These were seen as a means of placating public anxiety about supposedly high-risk individuals who were at large in local communities. Their introduction followed the Official Inquiry that followed the fatal stabbing of Jonathan Zito on the London Underground network (Ritchie, Dick and Lingham, 1994).

The incoming Labour Government in 1997 established an independent expert review committee under the chairmanship of Professor Genevra Richardson. Her committee reported in November 1999, and the following year the Government published its first attempt at reforming the 1983 Act. Once again the focus returned to emphasise the importance of a whole system approach, although this was hampered by the parallel aspiration that certain people who might develop mental disorder (and who might therefore place people other than themselves at risk of harm) should in effect be removed out of harm's way first. The Government was also well aware that a number of parts of the 1983 Act were at variance with the Human Rights Act 1998 (implemented in England in 2000) and the European Convention of Human Rights, and that increasingly it faced legal challenges about those variances.

With people who use mental health services exercising their right to join in with the public debate – in a manner that had not previously been witnessed – the Government found itself seriously underestimating the strength of opposition to some of the changes it had proposed. It was not until 2007 that an amended version of the 1983 Act was passed into statute. Attempts to revise the 1984 Act in Scotland had also had a rough ride through the Scottish Parliament but eventually the Mental Health

(Care and Treatment)(Scotland) Act passed into statute in 2003.

The revised Act in England and Wales, passed in 2007, implemented in November 2008, and still referred to as the 1983 Act (which continues to be the primary legislation), brought in nine key changes. These included a new, broader, definition of mental disorder; the replacement of specific Aftercare Under Supervision Orders with a strengthened focus on supervised community treatment; new roles for ASWs as Approved Mental Health Professionals (AMHPs); extensively revised arrangements for Mental Health Tribunals; and the introduction, from April 2009, of a new nation-wide Independent Mental Health Act advocacy service (Barber, Brown and Martin, 2009).

The role of the Approved Mental Health Professional (AMHP)

Already it will be plain from our historical survey that one of the main values that the AMHP – and its predecessor roles – brings to the complex process of Mental Health Act assessment is their independence. AMHPs operate:

- As independent professionals accountable for their own professional judgement.
- On behalf of a local social services authority that is not part of the NHS mental health system with which so many specialist resources are still associated.
- Within a context of professional support from an authorising organisation that has responsibilities and connections with a wide variety of social and educational agencies.

To this there are a number of valuable aspects that each AMHP brings to the role, irrespective of their substantive professional discipline (social work, mental health nursing, occupational therapy or psychology):

- Holistic skills in a whole person/whole systems assessment.
- Specific training in social, environmental and legal perspectives.
- The ability to work in partnership with individuals, families and agencies, to mobilise the resources of the NHS and community services, acknowledging and using all as a therapeutic resource.

While the extension of a psychosocial approach has increased health professionals' awareness of

social care issues, social workers who are AMHPs bring a unique perspective that counter-balances the often rather individualistic focus of their medical colleagues in the formal assessment process. To fulfil these complex roles well and to safeguard the interests of the individual while at the same time ensuring proper attention to risk and safety requires enormous skill and confidence.

Moreover, the strength that the AMHP brings to the assessment process is a knowledge of the circumstances, the networks and the resources, which is usually significantly more comprehensive than that provided by any medical input. The knowledge of the AMHP can be a significant factor in the successful use of alternatives to hospital admission.

The AMHP is in charge of the assessment process. The accurate and effective 'stage management' of the assessment is a skilled and time-consuming task that has a major impact on both the outcome, the level of risk, and the service user's perspective of the process. The management of the assessment process also involves the co-ordination of a range of agencies and informal participants, often in the setting of crisis and florid behaviour. It can be a difficult situation to maintain control of – with little in the way of resources in settings such as police station custody centres – that may not be best suited to the purpose of Mental Health Act assessment.

In fulfilling this task, the AMHP will draw upon a range of interpersonal skills. They may be required to use an awareness of group dynamics (as assessments are often in the setting of dynamic group settings). They will be expected to maintain an anti-discriminatory approach. They will need to use their interviewing skills. Most of all, they will need to develop an accurate assessment of all the circumstances surrounding the crisis and to form a clear view upon which to take a decision (Hatfield, 2008). They must then relay their decision to the service user directly. These skills – competences for professional practice – are described in detail in the 2008 AMHP Regulations (DoH, 2008a).

It can be a lonely role, and one that can be seen to exist at the margins of social work practice, given that decision-making does not need to be checked back with the employing organisation, and applications under the Mental Health Act are made by individuals rather than by organisations. But it is a role, if undertaken within a supportive framework of professional supervision and continued practice development and learning, that sits as comfortably within specialist mental health services as it does outside them (Slay, 2002).

Deprivation of liberty safeguards – another role for AMHPs

The Mental Capacity Act 2005 became operational during 2007, following almost the same trajectory of research and a decade's worth of lobbying that characterised the parallel arrangements to reform the 1983 Mental Health Act. Of the statutory principles, set out on the face of the legislation (unlike the Mental Health Act principles that are confined to the Code of Practice) the most important centres on the presumption of capacity unless proven otherwise and consequently this additional legislation can also be seen as both enabling and supportive (Brown and Barber, 2008). But it is what the Mental Capacity Act requires of practitioners in relation to people who lack mental capacity that forms the bulk of the Mental Capacity Act.

The European Court of Human Rights in its October 2004 judgement in the Bournewood case (HL v UK) highlighted that additional safeguards are needed for people who lack capacity and who might be deprived of their liberty in institutional care environments rather than at home or in the community. The Bournewood case concerned an autistic man with severe learning disabilities who was informally admitted to Bournewood Hospital in Surrey under common law. He was not subject to any provisions under the then Mental Health Act and yet the staff at the hospital felt that they were entirely within their rights to be the only people able to make decisions as to his care requirements and also his contact with people outside of the hospital. The European Court of Human Rights found that he had been deprived of his liberty unlawfully, because of a lack of legal procedures that offered sufficient safeguards against arbitrary detention and speedy access to a court.

The Government has closed the 'Bournewood gap' by amending the Mental Capacity Act 2005. The new Deprivation of Liberty Safeguards introduced in England and Wales in April 2009 ensure compliance with the European Convention on Human Rights. The aim is to provide legal protection where deprivations of liberty or restrictions in freedoms for individuals are assessed as necessary. The arrangements only apply to people, aged 18+, in hospital-based care or in establishments covered by the Care Standards Act 2000 and do not cover people detained under the Mental Health Act 1983, who already have the benefit of legal safeguards.

The legislation requires that care homes and hospitals (Managing Authorities) will seek a formal authorisation from the Local Authority or Primary Care Trust (Supervisory Bodies) for that deprivation to continue. The Mental Capacity Act's Deprivation of Liberty Safeguards Code of Practice (DoH, 2008c) refers to deprivation being defined by degree and intensity. Deprivation therefore effectively relates to the exercise by staff of the 'complete and effective control' over the care and movements of residents or patients. From April 2009, deprivation of liberty is unlawful where there is neither a formal deprivation of liberty authorisation nor a relevant decision by the Court of Protection.

AMHPs form the bulk of the workforce who have undertaken additional training in order to work as best interests assessors under the Deprivation of Liberty Safeguards. It is another checks and balances role, in that the task of the AMHP is to co-ordinate an holistic assessment process, covering six separate assessments, and to weigh up what is in the best interests of the person lacking mental capacity. Are the person's best interests served by their needing to be formally restricted in their freedoms or deprived of their liberty, or can changes to the care and treatment practice arrangements be accommodated that are less restrictive? AMHPs, who are already experienced in weighing up the issues when considering the use of the Mental Health Act, are ideally placed to undertake this new role of best interests assessor and to decide on the best outcome that meets the needs of the person being assessed.

There is no reason why, in future, AMHPs acting as best interests assessors need to be directly employed by local social services authorities. However it will be on behalf of a local social services authority that they undertake their duties under the Mental Capacity Act's Deprivation of Liberty Safeguards.

The AMHP – room for a life outside the legislative context?

AMHPS do not just provide a statutory assessment service under either the Mental

Health Act or the Mental Capacity Act's Deprivation of Liberty Safeguards. They are also key players in the ongoing care management and support arrangements for any person in contact with specialist mental health services and/or with wider health and social care services.

The past decade has seen a blizzard of policies and proposals all aimed at improving and modernising mental health service provision in England. There has also been an increasing focus on the need to modernise the workforce and the skills need to work within the new map of service provision. A great deal of attention has been focused on the role of the NHS and in particular the need for practitioners steeped in the biomedical model of care to pay much greater attention to the needs of people with whom the NHS has traditionally struggled to maintain contact. Hence the emphasis on the development of early intervention, assertive outreach, and crisis resolution services that are (primarily) for adults of working age (see also Chapter 4 in this book). The first ever national dementia strategy (DoH, 2009a) broadens this service improvement focus to include the hitherto largely forgotten 570,000 people with dementia and emphasises the development of early intervention and specialist diagnostic services.

To many, the marketing of the non-statutory role of social care within mental health services has been largely invisible over this same period. In the debate as to what roles would best be needed within the revised statutory Mental Health Act framework, there was vigorous (and ultimately largely successful) lobbying for the retention of the ASW role. But beyond this, and within the broader mental health services context, the role of social care has perhaps been less clearly understood. But this belies the true picture. The 'stickability' of the social care approach, with practitioners working quietly and reliably behind the headlines to provide a consistent and recovery-based service for people who use mental health services has in fact been reported and conceptually developed in a number of studies (Slay, 2003; Tew, 2005; General Social Care Council, 2008).

In the late 1990s, a number of local authorities and mental health NHS Trusts started to question the prevailing wisdom that some of their separate but overlapping functions should always remain that way. One of the early pioneering partnerships was that proposed in 1997 between Somerset County Council, Somerset Health

Authority, Bath Mental Health Trust and the Avalon Trust. This led to the creation in April 1999 of Somerset Partnership NHS and Social Care Trust, an organisation that was then critically evaluated over a three year period (Peck, Gulliver and Towell, 2002).

There had already been good examples of inter-agency collaboration around service planning, largely as a result of the drivers associated with the annual Community Care Plan planning framework introduced in 1992. In addition, mental health social workers had been physically based in community mental health services since the early 1990s (Huxley and Kerfoot, 1994). But the Somerset approach set out to take integration to a new level.

During the decade that followed many more partnership arrangements were formally and legally established. They are now the norm, rather than the exception. Into those partnerships went the bulk of the ASW workforce, on a secondment basis, where they remain to this day, albeit now as AMHPs. The legal foundation for these arrangements was the 1999 Health Act that enabled, for the first time, a range of so-called 'flexibilities' including the formal integration of service provision, the pooling of budgets and the nomination of lead commissioners (see Bogg, 2008).

The work on structural integration has been an important development over the past decade. It was assisted by guidance produced jointly by the Association of Directors of Social Services and the National Institute for Mental Health in England (Association of Directors of Social Services, 2003). This guidance highlighted common pitfalls – as well as successes – and was targeted at the many local authorities and NHS Trusts seeking to go down the joint management route.

Structural integration does not of itself change anything and work has also been needed to improve the quality of the interaction between the mental health workforce and its customers. This work was started in 2003 by the National Institute for Mental Health in England and the Royal College of Psychiatrists. After these two organisations provided a ground-breaking report in 2005, the 'New Ways of Working' programme (as this activity had become known) moved on to encompass all the other professional bodies associated with specialist mental health services.

The specific 'New Ways of Working for Social Workers' (NWW4SW) explored the challenges of sustaining an effective social work identity when so much of the role was, at that time, tied up in the distinctive and somewhat isolated (although crucially important) contribution of the ASW. In particular the NWW4SW working group was keen to emphasise and articulate the constellation of values associated with the distinctive contribution of social work within mental health services. The portfolio of evidence collected by the working group clearly demonstrated and supported the raising of the social care contribution based on the following elements:

- Nurturing and maintaining social work identity.
- Promoting the leadership expectations of social workers.
- Encouraging an expectation that research is integrated with, and integral to, social care practice.
- Developing a clear career progression pathway, particularly for social care staff based in NHS Trusts, coupled with strong and ongoing local authority engagement.
- Actively embracing new opportunities and new roles as they emerge.

DoH, 2007, Chap. 10

Subsequently, the Association of Directors of Adult Social Services has taken these elements and interwoven them within a vision document that stresses the importance of mental wellbeing in communities rather than the specific illness management of individuals (Future Vision Coalition, 2008). These policy and practice aspirations need now to be used as the basis for discussions on planning the workforce needed to support a vision of care in the community that focuses on whole-population mental health, the overcoming of the persistent barriers to social inclusion, and most importantly to improve whole-life outcomes for individuals whose own personal experience of mental health is poor.

Concluding remarks

The importance of social care practice within mental health services has been explored in depth. In particular this chapter has emphasised the role played out within the legislative arena, specifically the current 1983 Mental Health Act, as amended in 2007, and its antecedents. That role provides a vital equilibrium between the demands of the biomedical approach that monopolises the provision of specialist mental health services in the UK and the needs expressed by individuals who experience mental distress at a crisis time in their lives.

The prevailing tensions between the needs of the individual and the needs of the wider community are a constantly fluctuating influence on the way in which mental health policy and legislation develop. These tensions continue unabated. The many battles to retain the social care focus and the legal independence of the ASW function within the new AMHP role have however been won.

Buried in amongst the many new policy initiatives has been a determination to secure a role for social work and social care practice within mental health services that is not limited by practice within the Mental Health Act and the Mental Capacity Act. Alongside these vital legislative roles AMHPs, when not carrying out Mental Health Act related functions, are also ideally placed to act as trailblazers in bringing to the fore the contribution of social care to the wider determinants of mental health and well-being.

CHAPTER 9

Spirituality – The 'Forgotten' Dimension?

Peter Gilbert

And would this psychiatrist be able to understand my difficulties in coming to terms with the loss of my religious beliefs, about life seeming empty and meaningless, and those hard to explain 'what am I?' feelings?
Jean Davison, *The Dark Threads*, 2009: 10

... the spiritual perspective reminds us that 'negotiating terms' with pain and suffering is a universal and primarily spiritual task for human beings, which offers evidence of spiritual health, not psychopathology.
Christopher Cook, Andrew Powell and Andrew Sims, *Spirituality and Psychiatry*, 2009: xiii

And so we came forth, and once again beheld the stars.
William Styron, *Darkness Visible*, 1990/2004: 85

Commenting on the New Labour health reforms, the historian of the NHS, Charles Webster states that:

Labour made a serious error of judgement in adopting the hospital inpatient waiting list as the main yardstick of improvement ... put into practice it risked doing more harm than good.
Webster, 2002: 221

Speaking out on both the 'Baby Peter' and the Mid Staffordshire Foundation Trust Acute Hospital scandals, Jo Webber, Deputy Director of Policy at the NHS Confederation speaks of both social care and health organisations placing 'Too much emphasis on targets and too little on well supported, benchmarked professional judgement' (Webber, 2009).

In July 2009 the House of Commons Health Select Committee criticised *disastrously unsafe care* in a handful of NHS trusts where parts of the health sector had become obsessed by government-imposed performance targets (see Parkes and Gilbert, forthcoming).

In both mental health and physical care, all inspection reports point to the fact that people wish to have sound and up-to-date technical care, but also attention to their needs as whole human beings, their dignity, culture and identity; and within the context of their lives outside the confines of the healthcare system. Public health experts stress the need for a whole persons whole systems approach (DoH, forthcoming).

As we have seen in Chapter 1, Bracken and Thomas commented on the reductionist approach in medicine, which has seen human beings as machines to be fixed. In recent years, however, a move towards to a 'medicine of the person' (see Cox et al., 2007) has seen a revival and in the late 1990s, the Royal College of Psychiatrists formed a special interest group on spirituality and psychiatry, which saw the publication of a major text in 2009 (see Cook et al., 2009). In many ways this takes us back to the Greek philosopher, Plato, and his dictum that:

As you ought not cure the eyes without the head, or the head without the body, so neither ought you to attempt to cure the body without the soul ... for the part can never be well unless the whole is well.
Quoted in Linda Ross, 1997: I

As more and more service users and survivors speak out concerning their desire for their spiritual dimension to be recognised and attended to, some of the most persuasive voices come from those with a scientific background. Dr Cathy Wield writes of the problems caused by a reductionist approach in health and social care:

Historically the body had become divided in a completely artificial way as far as the medical world was concerned. The mind, body and spirit are considered separate entities; an attitude which has been highly influential, spilling over into modern society. Consequences are grave for the sufferer. I was entering the world of the 'mentally ill'; no flowers, chocolates and sympathy now ... I felt worthless, useless, a hopeless failure.
Wield, 2006: 17

Embryologist, Lewis Wolpert, uses spiritual/religious language in his description of depression:

If we had a soul – and as a hardline materialist I do not believe we do – a useful metaphor for depression could be 'soul loss' due to extreme sadness. The body and mind emptied of the soul lose interest in almost everything except themselves. The idea of the wandering soul is widely accepted across numerous cultures and the adjective 'empty' is viewed across most cultures as negative. The metaphor captures the way in which we experience our own existence. Our 'soul' is our inner essence, something distinctly different from the hard material world in which we live. Lose it and we are depressed, cut-off, alone.
Wolpert, 2006: 3

In his *Religion and Spirituality*, Bernard Moss (2005) identifies that human beings' drive to identify and own their inner spirit has been profoundly present throughout history as people look for meaning, purpose, connection and a moral framework by which to live (see also Armstrong, 2009). Moss recalls the sociologist Emile Durkheim arguing that one of the main functions of religion 'is to promote the well-being, stability, and integration and social cohesion of society' (p9). Psychotherapist and concentration camp survivor, Viktor Frankl, using his life experience and work, postulated that human beings' primary search was for 'meaning' (Frankl, 1946/1984).

The search for meaning is a striking feature of Jean Davison's moving autobiography. In her conversations with health professionals she is continually saying that she is having problems with the belief system which she grew up with, but in having a struggle with her original belief system she is finding it difficult to find a moral compass. Her struggles with the meaning and purpose of life are constantly redefined for her by professionals as an illness.

When the NIMHE/National Forum Spirituality and Mental Health Project was commenced in September 2001, partly as a response to the tragic events of that year, it was amazing how many people across the country came out to say clearly that they felt that their spiritual dimension had been neglected. When asked why they thought that was, the response invariably was that any discussion of spiritual or religious beliefs would be pathologised and turned into symptoms of mental ill-health. The Oxford English Dictionary defines *spirit* as the *animating or life-giving force*. Clearly, to ignore or neglect this aspect of the human person is to diminish the individual receiving care; the one providing it; and may indeed be delivering a form of treatment and care which is neither effective nor cost effective. Survivor and journalist, Clare Allan in a recent article speaks of the very different perceptions of self which can be gained from listening to one's own memories and those who've provided the care (Allan, 2009) and Jean Davison's autobiography provides references from her case history, as well as her own account. Donn Fraser (see Box 5) a participant in the 2009/2010 Service User Partnership Programme in Jersey, speaks of a strong hope and desire to retain his 'spirit' through a voyage which often proceeds through

many dark tunnels. Service users appreciate staff who treat their beliefs, hopes and aspirations with the seriousness with which they hold them themselves. As a service user interviewed in the Somerset Spirituality Project put it:

The CPN was terrific. Although he was not religious, he asked very pertinent questions about how I could reconcile my faith with what was happening to me, and what God meant to me.

Nicholls, 2002

Box 5: Being Humbled by Mental Illness

I have suffered with schizophrenia for 14 years. The depression which is something I also suffer with is always brought on two weeks after taking anti-psychotic medication. I personally think you can feel worse at times taking medication than you can without it. I know medication is good for some people and for some people some of the time. At times medication has had a beneficial effect on me. I have a more stable life for my family. Their worry is kept to a minimum which makes me feel contented but I feel dead inside and my passion for life has gone.

The meaning of 'soul' in the dictionary is 'that which thinks, feels, desires etc; innermost being or nature; moral and emotional nature, power or sensibility'.

The meaning of 'soulless' in the dictionary is 'lacking in animation or nobleness of mind; empty, lifeless, bleak; extremely monotonous; unrewarding'.

All this I have experienced due to taking atypical medications. It's really the soul which the medication affects. The spirit is the disembodied soul. God if you believe in him is spirit. This is what medication cannot affect.

So, for the sake of peace and society, I will take medication and allow myself to be subdued. But one thing I would say is that medication should be more revered and not something that is given lightly, especially by force.

I am lucky still having such hope for the future. Most believe that their life is over when they develop schizophrenia. Their hopes and dreams are taken away and there is no light at the end of the tunnel. Life becomes futile and pointless.

> The emotion I miss the most is love. After 14 years of struggle that is the worst thing. Not being able to give or feel affection.
>
> **Donn Fraser**

Drivers towards spiritual care

There are a number of strong drivers for embedding an ethos of spiritual care in today's heath and social care service. The first is clearly that coming from services users and carers themselves. As an interviewee for the Mental Health Foundation's *Strategies for Living* put it:

> I often think about how my Gran brought up her children, how she lived her life, and she had a deep spiritual being, not necessarily formatted to a fixed religion – a spirituality within her. In her wisdom she was very wise, very funny and her zest for life, I don't know, that sort of spiritual inner self, that deeper sort of thing.
>
> Quoted in Gilbert and Nicholls, 2003

In the Croydon Mind DVD, *Hard to Believe* (2003) which explores both individual spirituality and a spiritual and pastoral care team in East London working with faith communities, one service user in the group speaks about: 'spirituality is an anchor to my soul'.

Part of the impetus for this comes from a dissatisfaction with the reductionist approach to health and social care; the failure of mere consumption to satisfy human desires, especially in a recession which is decreasing people's ability and propensity to consume (see Bauman, 2007) and a greater complexity of belief systems in the UK. It is often stated that the UK is an increasingly secularised society, and there is some measure of truth in that, but just a drive through a city such as Birmingham, with its prominent mosques, temples, gurdwaras, churches and assembly halls for the growing Pentecostal Christian movement, testifies to a much more complex scenario. In some city wards, there will be far more people who believe in a divine providence than don't believe (see Gilbert and Parkes, forthcoming). The National Census of In-Patients in mental health hospitals, carried out by the Commission for Health Inspection, NIMHE and the Mental Health Act Commission (CHAI, 2005) found a surprisingly high percentage of affiliation, even if this did not equate with specific religious belief. In the Central and North West London Mental Health Trust, 95 per cent of service users in Brent's In-Patient service described themselves as having a religion or faith affiliation.

Professor Kamlesh Patel, as the then Chair of the Mental Health Act Commission, in launching the results of the survey, stated that:

> If you don't know who I am, how are you going to provide a package of care for me to deliver something? When you do not know how important my religion is to me, what language I speak, where I am coming from, how are you going to help me cope with my mental illness? And that is what I am trying to get over to people; the first step is about **identity**. It is absolutely fundamental to the package of care we offer an individual.
>
> Mulholland, 2005: 5, my emphasis

What is spirituality?

For some people from a more traditional religious background, spirituality is too new or too vague a term. But theologian, Ursula King, reminds us that the Greek philosophers used a number of words for spirit, connected with both individual breath and the breath of life. Two words: *psyche* and *pneuma*, King tells us, came to stand for the principle of individual and cosmic life. *Psyche* was the individual soul, whereas *pneuma* related to a transpersonal, cosmic soul, the life of the whole world (King, 2009: 5). Eastern philosophies and religions also talk about the importance of the individual and the cosmic spirit, and this is vital in the Abrahamic faiths of Judaism, Christianity and Islam. King states that the first use of the Latin term *spiritualitas* is found in a letter of St. Jerome from the early part of the 5th century. Increasingly it was used as a counter to *materialitas* (materiality) and in many ways is seen so today. Jews, who have an approach which connects the individual, family and society (see Sacks, 2005) speak of *ru'ach*, which means not simply a passive essence but very much a term to do with invigorated life. The Qu'ran speaks of Allah breathing God's *ruh* into human beings. Some professions such as occupational therapy (see Johnston and Mayers, 2004) and psychiatry (see Cook et al., 2009: 4) have developed agreed definitions. The new guidelines for staff in mental health services (see Gilbert et al., 2008) define spirituality as:

- Our life force.
- What makes me, me and you, you – our uniqueness as a person.

- Allied to our connections and connectedness to other people, nature, animals, sport and exercise, art, music and drama, the transcendent.
- Our life pilgrimage and quest.
- How we channel our desires.
- Our creativity.
- A search for hope, harmony and wholeness.
- What makes us tick.
- What keeps us going when times are tough.
- A belief in something or some being(s) other than ourselves and the material world.
- A vocation or calling.
- What gives our life meaning.

While again this may be open to criticism for being too broad in its approach, an increasing awareness of and research into our sense of the transcendent and our connectedness with others makes it unwise to be too definite at this stage. Neuropsychiatrist, Peter Fenwick, in his work on near death experiences and other aspects of life (see e.g. Fenwick, 2009) is a case in point, and while in the leadership sphere people like Goleman have written about 'emotional intelligence', physicist, Danah Zohar and psychiatrist Ian Marshall, in their book on 'spiritual intelligence', open up a whole range of new ways of thinking about the human experience (Zohar and Marshall, 2000).

It is increasingly common to hear people to say: 'I am not religious, but I am spiritual'. People often feel that: 'there is more to life than this' or 'there is something there'. The Australian David Tacey has written that:

> But the ideals of secularism, however well intended, are inadequate for life, since our lives are not rational and we are hugely implicated in the reality of the sacred, whether or not that is acknowledged.
>
> Tacey, 2004: 13

Zoologist David Hay, in his fascinating research in the East Midlands throws up the fact that an increasing number of people feel that there is 'something there' even though they find it difficult to define it and wouldn't necessarily categorise it as a religious belief or experience (see Hay, 2006). This does not, however, mean that there is some neat dividing line between spirituality and organised religion. Many people have moved between belief and unbelief; between religious systems; from belief to unbelief to belief again – especially in a crisis of physical or mental health. What Gordon Lynch calls 'progressive spirituality' (Lynch, 2007) may avoid some of the accoutrements of some aspects of much of organised religion, e.g. authoritarian paternalism and an overemphasis on structure and rigid rituals; but may not give the sense of solidarity that many people crave. Jean Davison's autobiography shows the dilemmas many people face when they lose a system of belief or a framework for life and are left without a sense of meaning or a moral code to guide them:

> But when I lost my religious beliefs, everything began to seem pointless ... But with nothing left to believe in on what should I base my morality?
>
> Davison, 2009: 12

This is an issue brought home by Jonathan Sacks (2005 and 2007) in his writing, and also in discussions I have with service users, carers and staff in mental health settings across the UK.

John Swinton, in his seminal work: *Spirituality and Mental Health Care: Rediscovering a 'Forgotten' Dimension* (Swinton, 2001) characterises spirituality as having three main elements:

- Intra-personal – a quest for inner connectivity, self knowledge and self awareness.
- Inter-personal – the relationships we have between other people and within communities.
- Trans-personal – reaching beyond the self and others into transcendent experience, which may involve a sense of connection with nature, the universe, a cosmic spirit, or God.

The increasing prevalence of Buddhist thought, spreading out into mindfulness approaches, may point to our need to reconnect with ancient philosophies and less materialistic ethos; but not merely individualistic but connected to a world view (see Coyte et al., 2007).

Chief Rabbi, Jonathan Sacks is probably the most persuasive advocate for the importance of faith and faith communities in modern society:

> The great Jewish institutions – the home, the synagogue, the community and the school – are all like this. They are environments in which we are bound to one another not by transactions of power or wealth but by **hessed**, covenant love, these are the places where we learn the intimate grammar of reciprocity, the delicate choreography of ethical intelligence, the knowledge that love given is not given in vain, and that by sharing our vulnerabilities we discover strength ... A community is where they 'know your name' and where they 'miss you when you are not there'. Community is society with a human face.
>
> Sacks, 2005: 54

Figure 22: The relationship between spirituality and religion

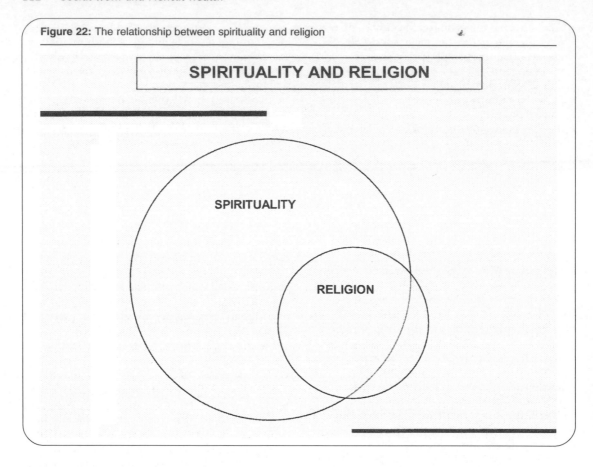

The definition of religion given in the CSIP/ Staffordshire University booklet is that it encompasses the aspects of spirituality, usually in the context of belief in (and perhaps a sense of personal relationship with) a transcendent being or beings, with an over-arching story. This narrative seeks to explain the origins of the world and those living in it, and the questions which we face as human beings around life, suffering, death and re-awakening in this world or another.

Religion can provide a world view, which is acted out in narrative, doctrine, symbols, rites, rituals, sacraments, a moral code, and gatherings; and the promotion of values and ties of mutual obligation. It creates a framework within which people seek to understand and interpret, and make sense of themselves, their lives and daily experiences (Gilbert et al., 2008: 4).

The relationship between spirituality and religion may helpfully be seen in Figure 22 above. Spirituality and religion are not necessarily the same, but they often overlap and intertwine.

Because, as the Department of Health has recently made clear in its guidelines on religion and belief (DoH, 2009e) Britain is a multicultural and multi-faith society. Mental health trusts will need to provide staff with at least some straightforward guidance around the nature of spiritual care in mental health (see e.g. Barber, 2009) and the main connections between belief systems (including Humanism) and mental health. A number of trusts have produced such guides, and the most comprehensive study is that published from the Staffordshire University multi-faith conference in 2006: *Nurturing Heart and Spirit* (see Gilbert and Kalaga, 2007).

Because it is almost impossible to know everything about a belief system, and most religious traditions have a number of distinct facets e.g. Calvinism and Catholicism within Christianity, staff can easily feel overwhelmed. It is important that all staff are enabled, through an education programme to feel confident in staying with people if they share their spiritual and/or

Figure 23: Identity and spirituality

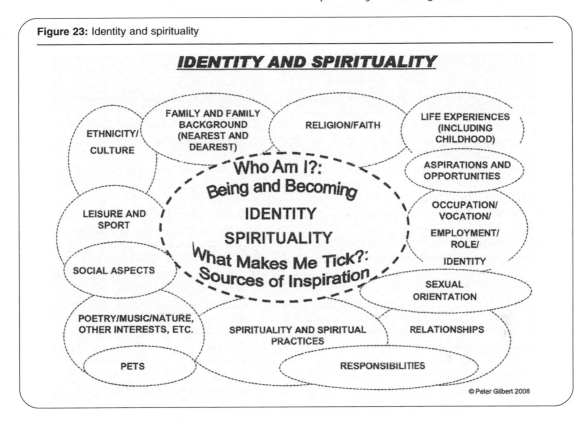

religious beliefs, and are aware of when to turn to the spiritual and pastoral care/chaplaincy team for specialist advice (see Aris and Gilbert, 2007).

It is important for organisations to give staff time to explore their own spiritual dimension before using that awareness within the service. The CSIP/Staffordshire University guidelines have a diagram which enables people to 'map' aspects of their spirituality and identity for themselves, or with others, see Figure 23 above (see also Gilbert et al., 2011, forthcoming).

Why has social work been so resistant to the concept of spirituality?

Ian Matthews, in his new book: *Social Work and Spirituality* (Matthews, 2009) addresses a major paradox as to why social work 'often seems to be oblivious' of spirituality as agenda whereas psychiatrists, occupational therapists and nurses have been discussing spirituality and bringing it into practice over recent years. Social work, at least in this country, which prides itself on being

an holistic profession, seems to find it a very difficult subject to grapple with. Matthews argues that 'social work is impoverished because of its lack of engagement with spirituality' and within a framework around the National Occupation Standards, addresses how social work can address this gap.

Margaret Holloway and Bernard Moss (Holloway and Moss, forthcoming) demonstrate that social work in North America like their complimentary partner professions has been addressing this issue over many years (see Canda and Furman, 1999). Holloway and Moss believe that the social work profession's journey towards official recognition and acceptance both within higher education and the professional communities of practice, in the UK, has necessitated a careful articulation of social work's value base and the theoretical concepts that underpin its work (see also Furness and Gilligan, 2009). As an emerging secular professional discipline it needed to distance itself from any religious frameworks or world-views, even though many of the roots of social work came out of Christian social concern and many members came into the profession as a result of their religious faith. Of course, some early social work theorists such as Biestek (1961) and Halmos (1965) drew on religious insights to inform their writings, but a perfectly justified suspicion of some aspects of organised religion and Freudian and Marxist analyses of religion and society created an atmosphere of suspicion and mistrust of religion and spirituality. Holloway and Moss believe that religious world-views were seen to be beyond the boundaries of the new professional remit, or perhaps worse, seen as being 'part of the problem' (see Holloway and Moss, forthcoming).

Social work emphasis on anti-discriminatory practice (see Thompson, 2006) may have increased that sense of suspicion. But equalities legislation allied to the broader personalisation agenda and an increasing emphasis on holistic approaches, and the recovery movement, makes it imperative that social work brings the spiritual dimension into play, and considers people's religious beliefs, while at the same time being aware of aspects of inequality in the way some religious traditions have panned out.

Recent research in 2009 in the Birmingham and Solihull Mental Health Trust and its local authority partner, Birmingham City Council, has demonstrated the importance professionals are now placing on spirituality; the overwhelming sense that professionals should attend to people's spiritual needs but also concerns about how to address those needs (Parkes, Milner and Gilbert, 2010);. The case study of 'Mrs A' by a social worker, acting as an ASW under the 1983 Mental Health Act just prior to the new legislation coming into force, exemplifies the need for patient and sensitive work with individuals, families and faith communities to gain the best outcome for the service user.

Case Example 10: Mrs A

Mrs A is a black Afro-Caribbean woman in her late thirties, she has two young children (approx five and nine years old) and a supportive partner. She and her family are evangelical Christians. She has been under the care of the mental health services for some years following the birth of her children when her mental health began to deteriorate. She had been supported by her CPN for some years who provided monitoring and anti psychotic medication.

Mrs A was referred initially 27/8/08 to me as an Approved Social Worker in the Home Treatment Team for an assessment under the Mental Health Act 1983, with a view to an urgent hospital admission. It was felt by the mental health professionals at this time that this was the only option. I had been told that her partner had moved out of the family home with the children as he could no longer cope with her bizarre and demanding behaviour, it was also stated that she had been verbally abusive and physically threatening towards her partner. There were concerns regarding her continued refusal to accept medication, consequently Home Treatment could not be used.

During the assessment it was clear that she was mentally unwell but that she stated that she was refusing medication stating that her faith would cure her. It was evident that her mother and wider family also felt this strongly. Both GP and the Psychiatrist present felt that she should be admitted under the Act for treatment, my colleagues Home Treatment Team also felt that there was little point in persisting as it was not thought likely that she would change her mind. She did not want to go to hospital. I agreed to delay that admission (losing the bed!) given that she had agreed to stay at her mother's house with her sisters and that she would be visited daily by Home Treatment, where she felt safe. The risk of harm to others or herself was limited and minimized by this. I visited daily and discussed the matter further with her family and her, who all felt very adamant that her faith would heal her and that medication was a 'bad' thing. Her partner felt that medication would improve things as it had in the past, he accepted that going to hospital would be destructive for her but if it was the only way of getting the family back together then that would be necessary. Home Treatment struggled on visiting her daily and attempting to engage her and her family. I had made attempts to contact the family Pastor which I felt could be helpful in enabling the family to see that medication can have a role to play in improving Mrs A's mental state. However, I did manage to speak at length to the mother's family Pastor who clearly felt that medication could not be of any help. Eventually out of frustration I discussed the case with a senior social work colleague who understood the importance of faith, as she has her own faith, who recommended that I contact the Pastor who is attached to the Mental Health Trust. The Trust Pastor was able to work with the family Pastor who in turn, was able to work with the family – attending reviews and meetings. Over some weeks this resulted in Mrs A accepting medication. It was a change in culture for mental health services to include different perspectives at reviews, but I felt strongly that the work we have to do with Mrs A and her family is long term. If we do not include the wider family and the active part that their faith plays in her life we run the risk of alienating the lady and her family, this ultimately would be detrimental not just to her well-being but to the community as a whole.

This was a long and drawn out process that took place over three months (August–November), when hospital admission was suggested twice more and Home Treatment found it difficult to provide support at times. However, with the support of the Trust Pastor and building a genuine rapport with Mrs A and her family (both her mother and her husband) it was possible to avoid hospital admission. Her care has been returned to her CPN and the community team; she continues to accept medication and lives with her husband and children once more. Her faith continues to be a vital aspect of her life.

Catherine Myers, Senior Social Worker

What the research tells us

It is vital that social work is constantly in touch with evidence-based practice (see Chapter 10 in this book) and that The Social Care Institute for Excellence constantly adds to our knowledge of a wide range of health and social care. As John Swinton has pointed out, however, much of the research stems from North America (see Swinton,

2007). Research undertaken by those such as Harold Koenig (see Keonig, Larson and McCullough, 2001) focuses primarily on religious commitment and its implications for health and human well-being, with the emphasis on specific practices associated with organised communities of faith. These communities are also mainly Christian and Jewish ones, and branches which are structured towards social solidarity. It is interesting to note that *Time* magazine devoted a major part of a recent issue to looking at the scientific evidence for health benefiting from religious faiths and spirituality; a debate between two psychiatrists and a chaplain; and religious practices across the globe (see Kluger, 2009).

Robert Putnam's famous study *Bowling Alone* (Putnam, 2000) charted the decline in community solidarity within North American society; utilising the striking image of the change over decades where groups of workers used to go to bowling alleys as a social group, but now often people 'bowled alone'. Putnam saw religious communities as often providing the social solidarity that human beings need for at least part of their lives to survive and thrive, and his current work is around the mega-churches in the United States, which may well be quite alien to us in Britain, though the fast-growing Pentecostal churches are mirroring some aspects of them. Crucially these mega-churches do not just feature a massive, and emotional Sunday service, but also break into small community groups meeting specific needs (see Gilbert, 2010b).

Koenig and colleagues' research demonstrates a number of physical and mental health gains, and Andrew Sims summarises what accounts for the benefits as follows:

- Social benefits: a sense of belonging.
- Trust in God and a sense of 'rightness' and the security this gives.
- Internal levels of control – e.g. the spirit of the divine and/or moral purpose within me helps me to assert my own will to do better.

See Sims, 2009

Swinton (2007) would add a number of other aspects to Sims' list notably:

- The provision of social resources.
- The promotion of positive self-perception.
- The provision of specific coping resources, not least through the signs, symbols, rituals and narratives which faith communities provide to give a framework for life.

- The generation of positive emotions e.g. love and forgiveness.

Psychologist Pargament in his article: *The bitter and the sweet: an evaluation of the costs and benefits of religiousness* (Pargament, 2002) concludes:

- The efficacy of religion depends on the degree to which it is well integrated into people's lives. Swinton (2001: 30) makes a distinction between 'intrinsic' religion, providing 'a meaning-endowing framework in terms of which one's self and one's life experiences are interpreted and understood' and where the individual extends their religion 'beyond the boundaries of a specific service of worship into every aspect of their life'. On the other hand 'extrinsic' religiousness is a form of comfort and social convention, which primarily meets the self-centred needs of the individual.
- Religious faith may be particularly helpful in more stressful situations. It is noticeable that when a train or plane crash or other civil disaster happens, many people, without necessarily any particular religious faith, state that they prayed. Pargament quotes an old adage 'There are no atheists in foxholes'. In a mental health setting, many people may well turn again to a religious faith, or at least tradition, which they have known in the past but not adhered to.
- Religiousness may be more helpful to socially marginalised groups. Richard Reddie's study of young black people in the UK converting to Islam is instructive here (see Reddie, 2009).

Research in the United Kingdom is at a much less advanced stage, and perhaps the largest study, taking a very broad sweep (see King et al., 2006) actually raises more questions than it answers. Perhaps one of the most interesting aspects of this survey is that is seems to indicate that people with an acknowledged spirituality, but not part of a developed community, may be more vulnerable to common mental disorders, than those who avow to no specific belief or a faith community. The common sense reaction to this might be that people with a high degree of sensitivity, but without a formed group in which to express their experiences and have them sympathetically received, may feel more alone and vulnerable. It may well be, that in a society that is far more secular than that of the USA, we need to have a greater ability to form groups which are sympathetic to people's experience of mental

distress. In Birmingham work has already taken place with Imams, in conjunction with Rethink (Rethink/CSIP/UCLAN, 2007) a major Sikh community in the city; black Pentecostal churches; and at the time of writing work with a Hindu community, it is intended to work with all major faiths. Because a number of people in my running club, Black Pear Joggers of Worcester (see Gilbert, 2005) have been open about their experiences of mental distress, it is much easier for other people to share their vulnerability and gain strength from the community as well as the physical and transcendent benefits of running.

Birmingham and Solihull Mental Health Foundation Trust launched a research programme, with the backing of the Medical Director, in October 2008 (see Parkes et al., forthcoming) which focuses on a number of specific areas of research:

- The development of a 'Personal Recovery Scale' which seeks to incorporate existential elements of recovery and can be used as a psychometric tool.
- The provision of a spirituality discussion group for young people with psychosis.
- Work on developing mutual understanding between the mental health trust and faith communities in the city, and reducing the stigma of mental illness within a number of religious groups, so as to enable early intervention to be brought into play.
- Researching professional attitudes (see Parkes and Gilbert, forthcoming).
- The placing of spiritual care advisers into teams.
- The rolling out of a training programme for all staff across the Trust.

Clearly more research is required to ascertain what works in what circumstances. For example the work with young people, described above, seems to be more effective in in-patient units, in that the gathering of a widely diverse group of people across various communities simply doesn't provide enough consistency. To become less dependent on research in the USA and gain a view of evidence-based practice in the United Kingdom is one of the major challenges for the next decade.

A new UK-wide research association considering the relationship between spirituality, religion and health in general (The British Association for the Study of Spirituality – BASS) was launched January 2010, with a new journal being launched in 2010, which will provide a helpful source of research for practitioners.

The national spirituality and mental health project

It was Professor Antony Sheehan, then Chief Executive of the nascent National Institute for Mental Health in England (NIMHE), who intuited the need for an approach to spirituality, as a response to the traumatic and iconic events of 9/11 in America and the widespread effects on a huge range of people, especially, of course, of Muslims in western countries; and also, a groundswell of opinion from service users, carers and survivors, that their spirituality should, in the words of the Somerset Spirituality Project, 'be taken seriously' (Mental Health Foundation, 2002). From 1 April 2009 the Project is managed by the National Spirituality and Mental Health Forum (see Aaron, 2008).

The Project focuses on two main issues:

- Spirituality as an expression of an individual's essential humanity, and the wellsprings of how they live their lives and deal with the crises, which can leave us drowning, rather than waving! It is, therefore, an essential element in assessment, support and recovery, for users and carers in a whole-person and whole-systems approach. It is also vital in the approach to staff, in order to create genuine person-centred organisations.
- The establishment of positive relations with the major religions, at a time when an harmonious construct between statutory agencies and faith communities is essential; and when research studies are indicating the benefits to physical and mental health and longevity, for those who are members of inclusive and supportive faith communities.

This is aligned with the imperative for greater social cohesion and the positive role faith communities can play in family and community life (see Cox et al., 2007).

The aims and objectives of the Project (see NIMHE/Mental Health Foundation, 2003) follow closely on the two main foci, in that the Project aims to:

- Chart what is known about the role of spirituality in mental health; the role of religion; and the role of faith communities.
- Identify areas of good practice.
- Build coalitions of individuals and groups.
- Develop and create linkages with other programmes.

- Set up Pilot Sites, linked to the regional development centres, which would learn from, test, develop and promote positive practice.
- Bring together the growing body of research evidence on the importance of spirituality in mental health and stimulate further research.
- Influence curriculum formation for all professional groups and to strengthen staff development at a front-line level.
- Support the role of chaplains (from all faiths) as part of the multi-disciplinary team.

Over the years, the Project has built constructive links with religious groups and foundations. It has been important to liaise with national umbrella organisations, such as the Inter-Faith Network and the Three Faiths Forum. Maintaining effective links with the Church of England's Home Affairs Advisor, has been important, not least because of the national church's links with other faiths. Relationships have been patiently built with the nine major faiths with which the Government liaises: Bahá'i, Buddhist, Christian, Hindu, Jain, Jewish, Muslim, Sikh, Zoroastrian and also the Humanist Society. A multi-faith conference (*Nurturing Heart and Spirit*) was held at Staffordshire University in November 2006, which engaged all 10 belief systems, with a strong user voice to focus on the difficult issues around mental health and belief, e.g. suicide, possession, etc; and also consider the synergies between belief systems (see Gilbert and Kalaga, 2007). A second conference on 8 January 2008 (Gilbert, 2008) on end of life issues (*From the Cradle: To Beyond the Grave?*) was followed by a third in 2009 on *The Flourishing City: The Role of Spirituality in Regeneration*.

Considerable work has been done on individual spirituality and engaging in faiths, through the National Spirituality and Mental Health Forum which had its provenance back with the health promotion charity, Mentality, and became a registered charity in 2006. The Project also kept in touch with the then Prime Minister's Adviser on Faiths, John Battle MP.

The Project never forgets that many people will not be signed up to a specific belief system. They may, in fact, have a faith in The Divine, but no adherence to a particular religious system. Many people move in and out of belief and different communities. One of the products of a diverse cultural society, is that people will move from one faith to another, or one denomination of a faith to another; or from faith to no faith and back again – especially at times of crisis! Some of the most desolate stories are from those who say that they have lost their faith and desperately want to believe, but belief is no longer with them.

In 2004 the Project produced a framework for what were called Pilot Sites, or the Spirituality Collaborative (see www.nimhe.org.uk) which involved Mental Health Trusts and their community partners signing up to a permissive framework, stressing adherence to local needs and culture. Bradford Care Trust, for example, has a project around those Muslims who feel that they are possessed by a *jinn*, or spirit, while such an approach may not be so relevant in other parts of the country. A national symposium was held for the Pilot Sites/Collaborative at Lincoln University in May 2006.

Work has been carried forward at a Government level in England, Scotland and Wales. In England work has been taken forward with the Department of Health and the Department of Communities and Local Government; liaison is maintained with the Scottish Executive, which has followed up its 2003 policy document with an update in October 2006 (NHS National Services Scotland, 2003 and 2006) and the Welsh Assembly Government is working on a policy on spiritual care. A growing number of university centres interested in spirituality, have now joined together to form a research association. The partnership work between NIMHE and the Mental Health Foundation produced a literature review in 2006 (Mental Health Foundation, Cornah, 2006).

Support has been provided to professional groups wishing to bring the spiritual dimension into their curricula. The Royal College of Psychiatrists is moving on this, and spirituality formed a part of the Chief Nursing Officer's review of mental health nursing in 2006 (DoH, 2006b paragraph 5.4.7 and recommendation 10). Social work's more de-centralised arrangement for education and training has meant some detailed work by Professor Bernard Moss from Staffordshire University, Professor Margaret Holloway from Hull University and others (see e.g. Moss, 2005; Furness and Gilligan, 2009; Matthews, 2009; Holloway and Moss, 2010). Christine Mayer, from Occupational Therapy, has also written extensively on the subject (see Johnston and Mayer 2005).

The importance of spirituality in social work

In 2007 a government minister announced that:

> *The role of faith-based groups in ensuring people have access to welfare services will be of growing importance over the coming years . . . (and) faith-based groups offer an individual link into communities.*
>
> Murphy, 2007

Dinham and Lowndes (2009) see faith-based groups being welcomed to the public table in at least three important ways:

- Faiths are increasingly seen as repositories of resources – buildings, staff and networks in a mixed economy of welfare (Home Office, 2004). A good example would be the Sikh community in Soho Road, Birmingham. As well as having a temple as a place of worship, the Sikh community provides *langar* or meals to a large number of people (of all faiths and none) every day of the week. They have also built a community/health centre, which is used for a wide variety of community-engagement projects, again with everybody in the neighbourhood, not just people from their own faith. They are also engaged in educational programmes, employment initiatives and charitable work oversees (see Singh and Gilbert, 2009).
- Faiths are recognised by governments by having a potentially important role in building 'community-cohesion'. Inter-faith networks have been identified as vital brokers in building better relationships between different communities and social groups.
- Faith communities are increasingly involved in Local Strategic Partnerships (LSPs).
  Dinham and Lowndes, 2009: 5–6

An increasing number of people in this country affiliate themselves, however loosely, to religious faith, and for those who don't, there is still the human need to provide a sense of transcendence with oneself and the material world – especially in times of crisis. Speaking with and listening to so many people within mental health services over the years, many express themselves very similarly to Jean Davison:

> *As a teenager I wanted badly to find the meaning, a purpose, a pattern, a God. To think as I started doing then, that there might be none of these things, was hard for me to take. Over the years I have leant to live with ambiguities, uncertainty, the possibility of never knowing. But*

It seems that 'something' of my leanings towards spirituality never left me. Not completely.

Davison, 2009: 360

As an avowedly holistic profession, social work really needs to catch up with this dimension of the human condition, and fast (see Moss, 2005; Matthews, 2009; Furness and Gilligan, 2009; Holloway and Moss, 2010).

An increasing amount of writing around the subject is taking place, with major publications such as Coyte et al., 2007 and Cook et al., 2009. Journals such as *Mental Health, Religion and Culture* (Routledge), *Ethnicity and Qualities in Health and Social Care* (Pavilion) and the forthcoming BASS journal on spirituality are important sources of knowledge an understanding.

For many people their spirituality or religious faith is 'An anchor for the soul' (Croydon Mind, 2005). Engaged with the fullness and complexity of the human condition is social work's role. But we also have to be aware of the darker side of spirituality i.e. that someone's animating spirit may be profoundly damaging to themselves or others. Our motivating force may lead us forward to positive achievements, it can also drive us to distraction. This is not simply a religious issue, a large number of people are driven along a path, which may be helpful initially, but is a road to self-destruction (see Miller, 2009).

In terms of faith communities it is important that individuals and organisations gain as much understanding as possible. Recent controversies over Muslim women wearing the veil require careful understanding (see Dhanda, 2008). The British and French (see Kedward, 2006) societies have taken radically different approaches to this issue.

As we have seen from the research, many people gain huge support, comfort and development from their religious belief and membership of a faith community. In a number of instances, however, there is a cultural overlay on the initial tenets of the faith itself. Muslim and Christian scholars, for example, would argue that the founders of both religions articulated a greater equality between the genders than might be evident today. A number of practices are culturally-based not spiritually-based. But these cultural overlays may be very powerful, and the recent study of South Asian women living in Derby, and subject to *izzat* (the importance of maintaining family honour and identifying with it) has created considerable pressures on a number of women in that community (see Gilbert, Gilbert and Sanghera, 2004).

Many within immigrant communities, over time experience what Khan and Waheed term 'acculturative stress' (Khan and Waheed, 2009, see also Arif, 2002; McKenzie, 2007). This 'acculturative stress' may be evident in staff as much as service users and carers. While it is most important not to exploit staff from a particular cultural group, as a cheap way of avoiding bringing in advice and translation services, staff groups themselves recognise that they are not always taking the time and trouble to learn from each other (see Box 6 from Zubia Arif).

Box 6: Personal and professional identity

I am a woman. I am someone's daughter, someone's sister and someone's wife. I am Muslim in religion, I live in a British society and my roots stem from a Pakistani background. So is this my identity I wonder? Or is it a part of it?

I work as a children's social worker in a learning disability and mental health team.

So what is it like?

Well this job offers me the opportunity to do what I have always wanted to do: work with children in a therapeutic way. However, time after time I face parents who are riddled with guilt. They wonder why their child has a learning disability or mental health issues. Their questions vary from wanting a medical explanation of the diagnosis to wanting to explain it all from a more religious perspective. For example, 'God has sent him/her to me as a test'.

So as a practitioner where your professional and personal values and attitudes need to be clearly distinguished, it can be difficult to help or reach out to that parent. I say this because my role as a social worker is defined by the guidelines set out by the General Social Care Council (GSCC) and my practice has to follow the policies and procedure of the team and the agency that I work for. These guidelines and procedure are obviously universal to all social work practitioners; however, they seem to neglect the 'person' that the practitioner brings to the job.

At the beginning I tried to define or explain my identity, and it is important, I think, to note that I bring all of this to my job. The parents that I face on a daily basis see this 'identity' first rather than the processes that dictate my practice. Consequently they will act according to what they perceive of me. Thus a South Asian family may be more open about certain topics to me than to my White or Black colleagues, as they feel that there is already a mutual understanding of the subject due to the shared ethnicity and religion.

Explanations that require a medical answer are easy. For example I can provide boundless information on diagnoses such as Asperger's Syndrome that can be explained medically, but when a parent is asking me for more than that, for example 'Why me?', 'Is this a test?' I cannot help but look at what I would do if I was in their position. I know that as my religion is very important to me I would most likely see the child as a gift from Allah (God) that has been given to me for a purpose. I would try to take comfort in knowing that while I may not see what the overall plan is, I would do my best to care and love this child to the best of my ability.

So if I feel that the parent would be able to understand this then I should simply tell them. The times that I have done this, irrespective of what religion or belief the parent adheres to, it seems that they take it as a type of solace. I guess it's another way of working coming from a different viewpoint. A viewpoint I hasten to add that gets neglected a lot of the time in our work.

It seems that we work in an environment where if our practice is influenced by a spiritual or religious viewpoint then this is frowned upon. However, I would argue that such work is critical as initially it may be the only thing that connects you to the family, and regardless of whether you believe in it or not if the family does then why cannot this be supported.

Zobia Arif, Senior Social Worker

Social workers need to practise self-awareness and attune themselves to their own spiritual

dimension. It is helpful if organisations give people time to explore the self in small 'safe' groups.

Learning from colleagues is important, and a wider gaining of understanding of the issues in relation to the personal, cultural and political aspects of this dimension of humanity. The CSIP/Staffordshire University guidelines are a helpful tool in this respect (Gilbert et al., 2008).

Social workers need to start where the individual is, as always, and look to undertake an assessment of the individual's needs with their whole context (see Chapter 7 in this book).

Clearly one of the major difficulties confronting social workers and other professionals, is the number of dimensions which need to be assessed. To suggest carrying out a full spiritual history (see Culliford, 2009) which may be very helpful at some stage, is simply not realistic all the time. But some reference to the basic questions of 'what makes you tick?' 'What keeps you going when life gets tough?' 'What are your sources of hope, meaning and connection?' and 'Do you have any spiritual or religious framework?' may be helpful in the initial stages and lead onto something more sophisticated later on (for a good example of guidance for staff see BSMHFT (Barber) (2009) and Figure 24 below.

It may be very important to know whether the service user has a religious faith. For example a Muslim may well wish to pray five times a day and have some dedicated space in which to do that (some trusts have developed 'sacred space' for people of all faiths and none to find a place for prayer and reflection). A Roman Catholic may need to see a priest so as to receive the sacraments of their faith. The challenge is, however that asking the closed question: 'Do you have a religion?' tends to elicit a yes or no answer. Open questions are likely to lead onto a broader range of issues, as well as eliciting a person's religious affiliation if they have one. Many service users might well describe themselves as a 'cultural Jew', a 'cultural Christian', but faced with an existential crisis, the belief that they held at one point in their life may come back with considerable emphasis, as Davison puts it:

My views on religion have not basically changed since I questioned, and lost, my beliefs in my teens. It would be pleasant to believe that we are watched over by a wise, caring God who will one day reveal to us what we cannot now understand.

Davison, 2009: 359

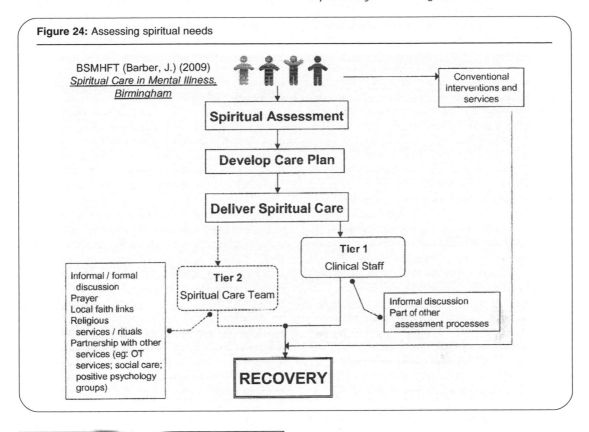

Figure 24: Assessing spiritual needs

Case Example 11

Gary is a young man who hears a voice, which he believes to be Jehovah. His conviction in the belief that this voice is Jehovah is very strong and cannot be shaken. Because of the strong belief system, Gary sets himself physical endurance tests in order to please God: not eating, drinking little water, praying excessively etc. Staff worked with the chaplains to assist Gary in joining a local Jehovahs Witness community so that he could develop his faith in its community context and therefore avoid the excessive penalties he was imposing on himself.

Despite this, Gary tended to shut himself away in his lodgings, and staff became convinced that this isolation would intensify his tendency to self-punishment. Gary's key worker, a Muslim, worked closely with a local Christian chaplain, and through the latter's theological knowledge, used Gary's Bible, to demonstrate that Adam, in the Book of Genesis, only becomes a person when joined by Eve in a reciprocal relationship. This spiritual/ theological explanation helped Gary to begin to integrate better with his peers.

From the CSIP/Staffordshire University (Gilbert et al.) Spirituality Guidelines, 2008

When time becomes more available it might be helpful to explore with the individual the following aspects of spirituality:

- *Identity*: what are the components which make up an individual's identity, nurture and nature, ethnicity, values, belief systems (including possibly a religious faith) and how has that identity travelled and might still be travelling?
- *Belief and meaning*: what are the beliefs that give meaning and purpose to a person's life and the symbols that reflect them?
- *Sources of strength and hope*: where does the individual derive their strength from and what gives them hope?
- What helps in a time of crisis?
- *Love and relatedness.*
- How does the individual relate to those intimate with them. Assumptions that families will be helpful or unhelpful are particularly dangerous here. Are there fractured relations which need healing?
- *Vocation and obligation*: what sense of calling and obligation does the person have in their life, and how are these expressed in relationships?

- *Affirmation*: does the individual feel affirmed by their past and present experiences and relationships?
- *Experience and emotion*: how does the experience of illness and the associated feeling relate to the individual's life meaning? How are 'negative' feelings handled? e.g. anxiety, guilt and anger.
- *Courage and growth*: how has the individual coped with crises?
- *Transcendence*: what provides an individual with their sense of transcendence? This may or may not involve relating to a divine entity, but may be through engagement with nature, art, spirit etc.
- *Rituals and practices*: exploring the rituals, which support the person's life meaning, and how they are being used in the present situation. Rituals may be present in either a religious and/or secular sense, they may provide a structure for people's life journey.
- *Community*: how does the individual relate to their significant community? If the community is important and helpful, how can links be maintained? Chaplaincy services may be particularly vital here.
- *Authority and guidance*: where does the individual look for guidance about life meaning in moments of stress? Is there a need for 'mediation', e.g. through an Imam or priest, and would it be helpful to involve chaplaincy services?

From Edwards and Gilbert, 2007: 154–7,
see also Culliford and Eagger, 2009

While scarce chaplaincy resources would be completely overstretched if they were called on every time everyone expressed a spiritual and/or religious need, the specialist assistance of chaplaincy services, and their relationships with community groups will be of vital importance.

Organisations need to support staff in dealing with all dimensions of the human being. The provision of specialist support is vital to provide the appropriate supervision and support for staff in their daily practice and development. One of the most difficult aspects of work is for those employed staff who then experience an episode of mental ill-health, as in the case of Linda Hart (1996). (See Chapter 5).

Case study 7 in the CSIP/Staffordshire University guidelines, features a CPN who experienced mental ill-health, and for whom her motivating force was the care of others. When she became ill it was as though her whole life had lost its meaning. Organisations need to create cultures of affirmation and shared learning (see Aris and Gilbert, 2007 and Merchant and Gilbert, 2007).

The range of human experience is vast. As Matthews puts it: 'We also need to acknowledge that the struggle to find spiritual hope and the journey of spirituality can be intensely difficult, even painful' (Matthews, 2009: 106). Human beings search for transcendence in individual and group senses. The cathartic experience of group worship and expression is linked way back in the history of humankind (see e.g. Waller, 2009).

As individuals we sometimes wish to be as individualised as possible, standing on our own; but other times we wish for group solidarity. Sometimes we desire our freedom, at others we search for security. Natascha Kampusch, the Austrian woman who was kidnapped on her way to school and held captive for eight and a half years, recently spoke of the difficulties in coming to terms with her freedom. This may seem highly paradoxical, but as Kampusch puts it:

In my cellar, I was perfect, self-contained and complete. Today I feel like people have taken away my ability to be myself.

Connolly, 2009

Social work must deal with the complexity of the human condition, the paradoxes of human existence and all dimensions of the human person.

CHAPTER 10

Research for Mental Health Social Work Practice

Nick Gould

*The days of stating an opinion as a professional judge-
ment, without explaining the evidence, are now quite
rightly behind us and in order to retain credibility social
workers are required to use and demonstrate evidence-
based approaches in their work.*

Bogg, 2008: 28

Why is research important for mental health social work?

Good practice in any social work setting blends
practice wisdom, skill and knowledge. Within
social work the definition of terms such as
'knowledge' and 'evidence' has become deeply
contested, with some commentators seeking to
locate social work within the Western scientific
tradition that emphasises observation,
measurement and experimentation, and others
who would emphasise the moral and practical
dimensions of knowledge developed through
practice and reflection (Trevillion, 2000). At some
levels this debate has become rather esoteric and
obscures the common ground that can usually be
agreed that practice should be informed by the
best-available knowledge that is appropriate to
the problem being addressed. Social work's
apparent insecurity about its relationship to
research and evidence may in part be attributable
to the lack of a tradition and culture of locating
decision-making within an expectation that
intervention will be justified in terms of known
research findings. This situation is reinforced by
the comparatively weak emphasis (particularly
compared to health professionals) on training in
research methods within qualifying and
post-qualifying social work education (Tew,
2002). As Webber has observed:

*Increasingly social workers are called upon to justify their
practice to their health colleagues whose training is
founded on empirical research evidence from within a
scientific paradigm. As social work practice is traditionally
derived from theoretical schema rather than empirical
research, this can lead to a number of misunderstandings.
In the worst case, the profession is perceived as lacking in
credibility as it struggles to articulate its evidence base.*

Webber, 2008: 1

Alongside this apparent or perceived deficit in
social work's relationship to research, the mental
health policy agenda has pushed towards all
professionals locating their practice within a
knowledge-based perspective. In the years
immediately following the election of New
Labour there was a succession of initiatives
announcing the modernisation of health and
social care including mental health services.
Three reports published in 1998 are particularly
noteworthy: *Modernising Health and Social Services*
(DoH, 1998a) established the case for improved
co-ordination of services through partnerships
between stakeholders, more consultation with
service users, and a stronger evidence-based
approach; *Modernising Social Services* (1998b)
established a new framework of governance for
social care, including the creation of the Social
Care Institute for Excellence to promote the
knowledge base and *Modernising Mental Health
Services* (DoH, 1998c) espoused the integration of
services for people with mental health problems.
Crucially, the *National Service Framework for
Mental Health* (DoH, 1999) provided a set of
benchmarks or standards for service
development that were explicitly evidence-based.
Part of the rationale for the NSF's standards was
that these would raise standards nationally to an
imposed level and so reduce postcode variation
in services.

One aspect of the thrust of the modernisation
process has thus been to engender a greater
research-mindedness in mental health social
workers and the creation of a knowledge-based
culture in integrated services. This also creates
the platform for the emergence of what Webber
(2008) has characterised as the 'advanced
practitioner 'in mental health social work, defined
as someone:

*... who has an explicit and articulated knowledge base
that is theory-driven and research-based and who can
create new forms of social work knowledge that inform and
shape policies and practice.*

Nathan, 2002: cited Webber, 2008: 179

Values and mental health research

It is a theme and message of this book that social work is a value-laden form of practice, some would go so far as to argue that social work is defined primarily by its value base. It is consistent with this perspective that research for mental health social work should reflect in its choice of methods the value assumptions of social work. This author collaborated with a group of service users, practitioners and academics to produce a report (Tew et al., 2006) articulating the values that should inform the production of mental health research. We began by identifying a set of fundamental questions that needed to be answered, such as:

- Who has been involved in deciding what needs to be researched?
- Who has relevant knowledge and expertise that may be used to guide the research?
- Who is going to be participating in the research and how do they give informed consent?
- Who is it hoped will benefit from the research and in what way?
- How will research findings be used and who will have access to them?
- Do all stakeholders in the research process have equal power and influence, or are some privileged with respect to others?

From one perspective these are practical questions about how research will be conducted, but the nature of the answers they provoke gives clues about the orientation that researchers have towards their activity. Within mental health, and particularly within most medical psychiatric research, the implicit answers would suggest that:

- People are passive objects that are *done to* by the technologies and practices of expert professionals.
- In order for research to be rigorous, it is better if people are ignorant of what is being done to them and why.
- Questions of meaning, categorisation and significance are to be determined by the researchers and not the researched.
- It is the individual, rather than their social/economic/political context that is problematic and needing to change.

Tew et al. 2006: 3

This approach is in many ways inimical to social perspectives in mental health that embrace principles of recovery, partnership and social inclusion. An alternative perspective on research values that 'goes with the grain' of social models of mental health has been proposed by the Social Perspectives Network, an alliance of mental health professionals, service users and carers, and academics:

- People are active participants or partners in their own recovery.
- People are experts *on* their own experience and *by* their own experience.
- The research agenda must be as much about promoting social change (attitudes, opportunities . . .) as it is about individual recovery.
- Service users, carers and practitioners who consent to participate in research must be fully informed about the purposes of the research and, if they wish, be given the findings of the research in a form that is accessible to them.
- If service users and carers are to be treated as experts by experience within therapeutic relationships, then it is vital that they are accorded a similar status with regard to the research process – and social research has the potential to be at the forefront of such developments.

Similarly, positions around other current issues in mental health, such as empowerment and valuing diversity, also need to be reflected in the value base of research – if research is to deliver evidence and findings that are actually going to be relevant to the diverse social and cultural contexts in which people are living (Social Perspectives Network, 2003 cited Tew et al., 2006).

Kinds of research and the questions they address

There are many methods for conducting research and each contains implicit assumptions about the kinds of knowledge that they produce. For example, experimental research is based on an assumption that generalisations can be produced that are applicable to the populations that are represented in the research, e.g. findings from an experiment to determine the effectiveness of cognitive behavioural therapy in reducing the auditory hallucinations of people living with schizophrenia might be assumed to be applicable to all people with schizophrenia experiencing these kinds of symptoms. In contrast, qualitative research explores the subjective experience of individuals or groups but its proponents are much more tentative about whether any findings are applicable beyond the particular context within the research has been conducted; interviews with African-Caribbean men living in London about their experiences of compulsory admission to hospital may not produce findings applicable to members of other ethnic groups living outside metropolitan areas of the UK. It is not possible within this chapter to review all the philosophical and methodological debates that are implied by these generalisations about research methods. However, a pragmatic approach suggests that there are 'horses for courses'; the type of research that we draw upon has more or less utility according to the nature of the question we wish to answer (Gould 2006 and 2008). Though it is a simplification, it may be helpful to illustrate this point further by considering four research approaches: qualitative, experimental, survey and mixed-method.

Qualitative

Qualitative research refers to structured inquiry that collects and analyses data in non-numerical form, usually text-based such as interview transcripts, accounts of partipant observation or documents. Usually qualitative research seeks to explore subjective experiences of individuals or groups and to understand how they construe specified aspects of their social world. An example would be Bodil Karlsson's (2009) study of the narrative account of a man who heard voices and had been diagnosed as schizophrenic. The research is based on detailed analysis of an extensive diary (over 100 pages) kept by the individual describing how his life had been since he began hearing voices, seeing visions and perceiving hallucinatory tastes and smells. Karlsson concludes:

> The voice hearer wanted to initiate dialogue with his readers, including professionals such as social workers. They should not simply dismiss a person as schizophrenic before listening to the story of one troubled by his voices. This study offers one possible way of using language within social work to communicate with the client about his condition.
>
> Bodil Karlsson 2009: 83

Most of the earlier qualitative work on the 'careers' of mental health service users was undertaken by professional academic researchers, primarily sociologists and anthropologists, but increasing recognition is given to the emancipatory research undertaken directly by service users (Beresford, 2003 and see below). There is, of course, no inalienable reason why standpoint research, i.e. research that is explicit in its epistemological and value positions and committed to progressive change, has to be qualitative though, to date, this has been the approach which has been dominant. An interesting example of qualitative research undertaken in partnership with service user researchers is described by Tew (2008) where individuals were interviewed about their experience of being compulsorily admitted to hospital. Analysis of the interviews elicited a number of themes, such as the stigmatisation people who have been sectioned feel on inpatient wards, seeing themselves as 'punished, helpless, hopeless and alone' (Tew 2008: 283). Qualitative research, unlike quantitative approaches, captures the subjective experience of people *in their own words*.

Experimental

Those who argue that social science should emulate the methods of the natural sciences ('positivists') claim that causal processes can only be dependably established by research that follows an experimental design. The core feature of this is that an intervention is applied to a so-called experimental group, and effects compared to a control group which either does not receive an intervention other than normal treatment, or receives a placebo. Ideally, subjects will be allocated randomly between the experimental and control groups, thus controlling for any confounding variables (perhaps age or gender) that might influence the results of the experiment. This research design is called a randomised controlled trial and in evidence-based practice is conventionally regarded as the 'gold standard' for research. A classic series of studies that has been influential in practice has been a series of experiments evaluating the effect on relapse in schizophrenia of psycho-education for families. Individuals diagnosed with schizophrenia who lived with their family had fewer relapses and hospital admissions if the family received a structured educational programme to reduce their level of their 'expressed emotion' (critical and negative attitudes), compared to families in the control group (Leff et al., 1982; Mari and Streiner, 1999).

Critics of positivism argue that in the social sciences it is often ethically unacceptable to randomly assign some people to a non-intervention, control group. Also, they would argue that there are so many variables present in real life that simple randomisation cannot control for all the factors that might impact on the effectiveness of an intervention. For these and other reasons, social work does not have available to it the number of experimental studies of the effectiveness of interventions that exist in other clinical disciplines such as psychology and psychiatry.

When several high quality studies exist that address a specific method of intervention these may be meta-analysed, i.e. the data from all the studies pooled identify whether there are consistent lessons to be learned. One example is the NICE-SCIE appraisal of the effectiveness of parent-training programmes in the treatment of children's conduct disorders (Gould and Richardson, 2006). An important initiative to create a resource bank of systematic reviews in medical research is the Cochrane Collaboration (http://cochrane.co.uk/en/index.html) which includes a number of studies relating to psychosocial interventions in mental health, and the more recent Campbell Collaboration (www.campbellcollaboration.org) which focuses on psychosocial interventions in social welfare. Both are important resources for social workers.

Survey-based research

Another research method which primarily is reported in terms of statistical analysis employs survey methods (though surveys may also contain open-ended questions that invite qualitative responses). Surveys are useful for evaluating satisfaction with services, but they also enable important explorations to be made of social factors that are associated with mental health problems. In the UK there have been two important surveys of mental health in the community undertaken for the Office for National Statistics (see Meltzer et al., 2002). These provide a wealth of information not only about the prevalence of particular diagnoses amongst the general population, but also a great deal about the social circumstances of people with mental health problems.

Survey data contributes significantly to our understanding of the social nature of mental distress, and is the basis of much of our understanding of concepts such as social capital and social exclusion in relation to mental health. However, it is important to remember that single surveys provide a snap-shot of factors correlated with mental health, but cannot provide causal explanations of why mental health problems arise. A survey cannot show the direction of causation, e.g. whether unemployment causes depression, or whether depression places individuals at greater risk of becoming unemployed. These kinds of causal questions require longitudinal or panel surveys, where the survey is repeated over time with the same individuals so that the changes over time can be tracked and causal hypotheses tested.

Mixed methods and case studies

Sometimes it may be beneficial to design a research study that combines the strengths of quantitative and qualitative research methods. The logic of this can operate in at least two directions: the generalised findings of a quantitative study can be explored in greater depth through in-depth qualitative inquiry, or the issues identified in a qualitative study can be explored quantitatively to examine their applicability to larger populations. An example of such a mixed methods study is O'Leary and Gould (2009) which researched the mental health outcomes for men who had been sexually abused as children, in particular their suicidality. The study comprised a survey of men who had been sexually abused which was compared with a survey of non-abused men to identify how the mental health of abused men differed. A sub-sample of men were then interviewed in depth to draw out at a finer level of detail the subjective views of men about how they dealt as adults with memories of childhood abuse.

Mixed methods are also useful in case studies where the research topic may be a complex entity such as an organisation or project, where more than one method is necessary to capture the various dimensions of the case study. In an organisational study of a mental health agency, for example, an online survey of managers, practitioners and service users may be augmented by in-depth interviews with a small number of key personnel as well as scrutiny of strategic policy documents. A notable example of this kind of approach was Peck et al.'s study of service integration in Somerset to create a joint health and social care partnership trust (Peck et al., 2001).

Service users and carers as co-researchers

The values perspective that emerges then from the social perspective in relation to mental health stresses the status of the service user as an expert in relation to their own experience. The extension of this position in relation to the doing of research is the desirability of participation of experts by experience in the research process as researchers in their own right. There has been, in recent years, a growing recognition that this is not just a moral issue but also contributes to the methodological rigour of research. Fisher (2002) has usefully pointed to some of the advantages that service users and carers bring to the research process at all stages:

- *Specifying the research problem.* Identifying and refining the research question is the critical act that launches a research project. If service users or carers have no input to this initial stage then research may not provide knowledge that users of services find relevant or helpful to their situation. Professional researchers may be oblivious to the subtleties of the experience of people who use services and misdirect research projects away from important areas of inquiry.
- *Defining outcome measures.* Not all, but much research evaluates the outcomes or impacts of treatments or other forms of intervention. This may be undertaken in the form of an experiment, comparing outcomes for those who receive the new intervention compared to an equivalent group who do not, or they follow a 'before and after' design. Experts by experience are able to discriminate, as with research questions between measurements that are relevant and helpful, and those that seem less relevant or even insensitive.
- *Analysis and interpretation of data.* Research initially collects raw data that may include statistics derived from surveys, material from interviews, direct observation of situations, extracts from documents and so on. This data

needs to be interpreted, often 'coded' into themes or categories that summarise or simplify the raw data and support findings that answer the original research question. Even in quantitative research, analysing statistical data, there is an interpretive element to the production of research findings. Again service users and carers may be alert to significant findings that are not evident to professional researchers, who may miss nuances within the data.

It is clear that experts by experience can bring added value to all stages of the research process. This includes the very preliminary stages of prioritising, commissioning and funding research, helping to make certain that the limited level of resource that is available for research is channelled towards areas of inquiry that are perceived as important and relevant to service users and carers. It is increasingly the case that major funders of research such as the Department of Health, the Joseph Rowntree Foundation and the Economic and Social Research Council are co-opting representatives of service users and carers into the research commissioning process.

Although the inclusion of experts by experience into the research process can be demonstrated to be a 'good thing', there are still the vexed questions of how participation can be made meaningful, going beyond tokenistic and symbolic incorporation that legitimises the research but without real sharing of power and responsibility? Tew et al. (2006) suggest that a genuinely emancipatory research approach includes:

- Academic researchers and practitioners listening to and learning from service users' and carers' views through setting up opportunities for dialogue.
- Service users and carers having opportunities to learn about research methods including quantitative as well as qualitative approaches.
- Service users and carers developing their own research groups and support networks, theoretical and methodological perspectives, and negotiating the terms of their collaboration with other groups involved in the research process.
- Academic researchers and practitioners transforming their own practice – and not just abdicating the field to service user and carer researchers.

- Formation of new partnerships and collaborations – including academic researchers participating in service user or carer-controlled research projects.

Going beyond paying lip service to emancipatory approaches to inclusive research practice means that service users and carers are likely to have training, development and support needs which are taken for granted by university-based researchers. They may also face practical obstacles to participating as researchers, for instance facing disqualification from welfare benefits because their availability for work is compromised. All this requires changes in thinking about how social research is funded and practised.

Building research capacity and identifying priorities

If the case is accepted that we need to take action to produce a stronger research culture in relation to mental health and social work then the next questions to be asked concern the means to build capacity to undertake more research, and identifying the areas of research that should be given priority. There is a particular need to develop larger-scale research that has sufficient validity to be a dependable basis for developing effective practice and for service development. This is a view put forward by the Mental Health Research Network:

> *Until now mental health research has not led or supported practice development. Reliance on small, localised studies has prevented researchers from drawing valid general conclusions ... As a result, research has failed to inform policy, lacking coherence, relevance and crucially credibility with users and professionals.*
> Mental Health Research Network http://www.
> mhrn.info/index/about/why-need.html

The author and colleagues undertook a survey, commissioned by the Department of Health, of practitioners, service users and academics (Gould et al., 2007) to ask them what they thought should be done to increase capacity for social research in mental health. The following are the main themes identified from their responses:

- Support more service users to become involved in research, including the provision of training.
- Support the development of research-mindedness amongst practitioners, including

strengthening the research elements of the qualifying degree for social workers, including requirements to undertake research in job descriptions, and research mentoring within agencies.
- Build stronger links between service providers and universities, including the creation of joint fellowship schemes.
- Provide greater representation of social researchers on research ethics committees to create greater understanding of the nature of social research.
- Develop more imaginative methods for disseminating research findings to practitioners, given the pressures on the latter and problems of accessing journals.
- Create local research networks linking the different constituencies within the research process and supporting those who are less experienced.

Respondents to the survey were also asked what they thought were the highest priorities for further research. The clearest indication from our findings was the emergent consensus across a wide cross-section of interests, that *social inclusion, social capital, social networks* and *social factors that enable resilience and recovery* were the highest priority topics for research. These suggestions are congruent with policy emphases on social inclusion and recovery commented on elsewhere in this book.

Sources of knowledge

Increasingly, research evidence is available for mental health practitioners through the internet. Although publishers of academic journals protect their commercial interests by making access to original papers conditional upon subscription, there are increasing numbers of institutes providing rigorous reviews of research evidence that provide a digestible and quicker form of access to research findings that are relevant to practitioners. Also, government departments and voluntary organisations frequently publish research studies they have commissioned on their own websites. Social workers need to use discretion in discerning websites that are reputable; there are too many to review them all but the following are some important repositories of knowledge for mental health practitioners.

Social Care Institute for Excellence (www.scie.org.uk)

SCIE was established in 2001 to identify and spread knowledge about good practice in social care. It undertakes systematic reviews of published research into all areas of practice including mental health, and also undertakes 'practice reviews' to identify and disseminate examples of good practice in action. All of its products are available as free downloads and includes good practice in relation to numerous areas of mental health social work including assessment of the mental health needs of older people and working with parents who have mental health problems. SCIE also hosts Social Care Online, the UK's most extensive free database of social care information which includes summaries of research briefings, reports, government documents, journal articles, and websites.

National Institute for Health and Clinical Excellence (NICE) (www.nice.org.uk)

NICE is part of the National Health Service but has an independent status and produces national guidance on the promotion of good health and the prevention and treatment of ill health. It has produced practice guidelines in relation to all the major forms of mental disorder. Although its guidelines are directed at practitioners within the NHS (and some critics regard its guidelines as too conforming to the medical model) its guidelines synthesise research evidence in relation to causative social factors implicated in mental disorder and review the effectiveness of psychosocial interventions. Its guideline for dementia care was jointly undertaken with SCIE, recognising the interdependence of health and social care services in meeting the needs of people with dementia and their carers (Gould and Kendall, 2007).

Social Perspectives Network (www.spn.org.uk)

The Social Perspectives Network (SPN) is a coalition of service users / survivors, carers, policy makers, academics, students, and practitioners interested in how social factors both contribute to people becoming distressed, and play a crucial part in promoting people's recovery. The SPN website provides links to a range of online resources including papers that have been delivered at study days, discussion paper on aspects of mental health policy and the deliberation of SPN's own research group.

Department of Health (www.dh.gov.uk)

The Department of Health is the UK government department responsible for public health, the NHS and social care. Its website is an important resource for locating health and social care policy, guidance and other official publications including research commissioned by government. The mental health page (http://www.dh.gov.uk/en/ Healthcare/Mentalhealth/index.htm) brings together links to recent policy and consultation documents, implementation guides and good practice examples.

National Mental Health Development Unit (http://www.nmhdu.org.uk/)

This Unit has replaced some of the national activities previously carried out by the National Institute for Mental Health England, the latter having been an arms-length body of the Department of Health responsible for leading modernisation of mental health services. Its website is a repository for resources including research and good practice guidelines, including evidence-based care pathways.

Sainsbury Centre for Mental Health (http://www.scmh.org.uk)

The Sainsbury Centre for Mental Health is a voluntary organisation that more recently has focused on employment and the criminal justice system, but this is augmented by additional work on mental health and public policy. It produces in-house and externally commissioned research that can be downloaded or ordered from its website.

Mental Health Foundation (http:// www.mentalhealth.org.uk)

The Mental Health Foundation is a leading UK mental health charity that for many decades has commissioned and published research across a range of issues for policy and practice. Most of its reports can be downloaded free from its website.

Alzheimer's Society (http:// alzheimers.org.uk/site/index.php)

The Alzheimer's Society is one of the principal charities active in the fields of dementia and older people's mental health. The Society places a strong emphasis on research, which it promotes under the themes of cause, cure and care. It has commissioned numerous important studies, including *Dementia UK*, an important study of the prevalence and economic costs of dementia.

CHAPTER 11

The Value of Social Work in Management and Leadership

Peter Gilbert

The **Personalisation is about whole system change**, *not about change at the margins. It will require **strong local leadership** to convey the **vision** and **values**, which underpin it and to reach beyond the confines of social care.*
DoH, 2008: 5, *Transforming Social Care*, quoted in Allen, Gilbert and Onyett, 2009

Why Should Anyone be Led by You?
Rob Goffee and Gareth Jones, book title (2006) posing the essential question for leaders

What makes a significant difference to the performance of an organisation is the quality and competence of front-line managers.
Denise Platt, then Chief Inspector of the SSI, Annual Report, 1999

Leadership is the vital spark in creating and maintaining value-based and effective services at a time of unprecedented change.
Jo Williams, ex DSS Cheshire and CEO, Mencap, 2005

In this life you have to be your own hero. By that I mean you have to win whatever it is that matters to you by your own strength and in your own way.
Jeanette Winterson, 2000: 155

Leadership has been the neglected element of the reforms in recent years ... that must now change ... Leadership will make this change happen and facilitate meaningful conversations which transcend organisational boundaries.
Lord Darzi, DoH, 2008b

*We want to be led by **real** people!*
Gareth Jones, speech to ADASS Spring seminar, April 2009

Figure 25: Management and leadership combined.

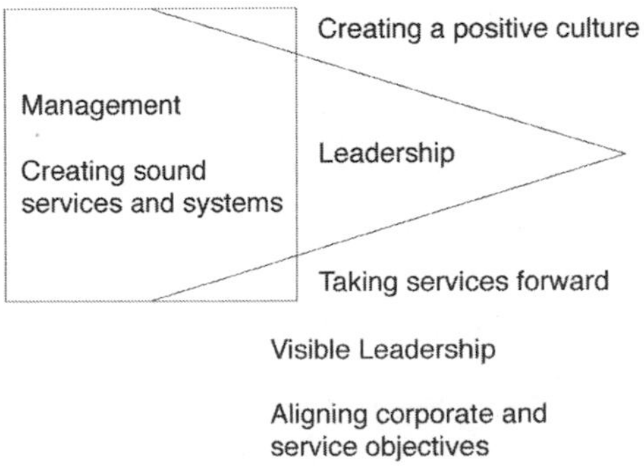

Creating a positive culture

Management
Creating sound services and systems

Leadership

Taking services forward

Visible Leadership

Aligning corporate and service objectives

The leadership challenge is how leaders mobilise others to want to get extraordinary things done in organisations.
Kouzes and Posner, *The Leadership Challenge*. 2007

Having been a practitioner, a frontline manager and a senior manager in organisations, I find it both sad and infuriating when practitioners and managers engage in postures of mutual incomprehension. As Terry Scragg and I made clear in our publication *Managing to Care*, practice and management are two sides of the same coin (Gilbert and Scragg, 1992). Practitioners, especially those who work in organisations, delivering statutory and organisational requirements, and working to help their clients negotiate complicated routes through society's systems, have to be good at managing themselves, managing the therapeutic relationship (and I don't mean controlling it!), and managing the environment. Social workers in the mental health field have to manage their own personal system; work/life balance, emotions, the balance between the emotional, the cognitive, the creative, the spiritual and the physical; they need to be able to manage their time and to interact in an effective way across a range of partnerships. Their management of the therapeutic relationship is not one of control but of clarity in agreeing shared outcomes, and enabling a vulnerable and perhaps chaotic individual to stick to those agreed objectives. As Gerard Egan has written:

Helpers are seen as competent because they are active, because they listen intently ... talk intelligently ... are understanding, genuine and respectful.

In all this, Egan argues that:

*helpers must be able to **deliver**.*
Egan, 1986, quoted in Gilbert and Scragg, 1992: 112 (my emphasis)

The Greek Xenophon (writing in the 4th century BCE) believed that there was small risk of a leader being 'regarded with contempt ... if whatever he (sic) may have to preach, he shows himself best able to perform'. In this respect, leadership in the multi-disciplinary setting is complex, as managers with training in one discipline will be leading staff from other disciplines. Managers do not have to be the most proficient practitioner, but they have to have and demonstrate empathy with the end users (whether we're talking care service or business) with their frontline staff and managers and backup staff. The larger and more complex the organisation, the wider the range of professional experts there will be who have to be nurtured and directed to work towards the goals of the organisation. Flamholtz and Randle (1989) set out three key requirements for playing the inner game of management successfully (see also Gilbert and Thompson, 2010, forthcomoing):

1. Being able to manage your own self-esteem so that you derive satisfaction from the things managers are supposed to do, that is enabling rather than doing.
2. Being able to manage your need for direct control over people and results. People in strategic management positions who keep micro-managing minute details are clearly out of their depth.
3. Being able to manage your need to be liked so that it does not interfere with performing the managerial role.

Chris Payne, in a short article, which still is an excellent read for frontline managers, comments that:

It is a sad fact that there are many residential managers who interpret their role either in terms of 'doing' all the things for which their staff are paid to do or who become administrators pure and simple. Instead of which they should be building on their knowledge and understanding of practice to take a more rounded and prospective view of the services being offered; to initiate sensitive programmes of, for example, staff recruitment and selection, development, supervision, training and stress management; to create a sound 'foreign policy' for their establishment; and most importantly to offer skilled professional leadership to staff.

Payne, 1988

If practitioners sense that their manager is not a leader in the real sense of pathfinding with individuals and groups towards common goals (see Gilbert and Thompson, forthcoming) but rather has their eye purely on the bottom line, especially if it's the bottom line of their own ambition, then they will be disinclined to see them as authentic leaders and to follow them.

One of the major interactions between practice and management is at the frontline manager level; in this instance the management of community mental health teams, day opportunity services, supported living services etc. Forging genuine two-sided coins of practice and management is an essential function of senior management. Frontline managers are in a potentially very creative, but also possibly very invidious position, and must be helped to blend the best of practice and management together.

When one looks at the conclusions from the findings of research into the integration of health and social services in Somerset (Gulliver, Peck and Towell, 2002; see also Bogg, 2008) it is very evident that it is vital to ensure that leadership is seen as a concept for all staff and for all partners in the enterprise. Especially if one looks at the management of risk that practitioners and managers have to engage in, leadership is an essential component here.

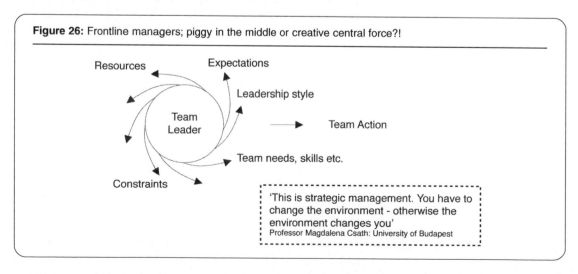

Figure 26: Frontline managers; piggy in the middle or creative central force?!

Resources

Expectations

Leadership style

Team Leader → Team Action

Team needs, skills etc.

Constraints

'This is strategic management. You have to change the environment - otherwise the environment changes you'
Professor Magdalena Csath: University of Budapest

Case Example 12

Dangerous liaison

Declan Henry faced a tough task in trying to rehabilitate a murderer and habitual drug user. His client, who stabbed his father to death, refuses to acknowledge that he has a mental illness, and is expressing a hatred of his mother.

Case notes
The name of the client has been changed.
Practitioner: Declan Henry
Field: Deputy manager of a forensic rehabilitation unit for mentally disordered offenders
Location: London
Client: George Kemp, aged 36.
Case history: Kemp has been diagnosed with paranoid schizophrenia and has a paranoid personality disorder. He also has a long-standing habitual drug problem. In 1988, he murdered his father, stabbing him 26 times. He said he felt emotionally abused by his father, who had become an 'object of hate' in his life. On being discharged from hospital, Kemp lived for two-and-a-half years in the community. But in 1997 he was recalled to hospital after his mother reported him for growing marijuana in his back garden, since when he has been detained in a medium secure unit (under section 37/41 of the Mental Health Act 1983). Efforts to implement his deferred conditional discharge have failed since November 1999 owing to his refusal to follow his care plan and his continued drug misuse.
Dilemma: Kemp's unrealistic expectations and, at times, limited view of reality may well set him up to fail, but – given his institutionalisation – may also be deliberately contrived precisely to fail.
Risk factor: Kemp's inability to accept his mental illnesses, drug misuse, and his growing hatred towards his mother may put himself and others at risk of serious harm.
Outcome: Kemp's overnight stays at the rehabilitation unit have been successfully completed without attempts to sabotage the care plan and with signs of drug use.

When Declan Henry became the keyworker to George Kemp, a murderer with diagnosed paranoid schizophrenia and a paranoid personality disorder, and attendant drug habit, he knew he had his hands full.

Not just because of the challenge presented by Kemp's case, but also because he was a murderer – or rather, because of his murder victim. Henry, deputy manager of a voluntary-run forensic rehabilitation unit, had recently suffered the trauma of his own father's death through natural causes, and here was a client who, in 1988, had brutally murdered his father by stabbing him 26 times: 'The loss I was feeling for my own father clashed with the sometimes cavalier attitude that he had towards killing his father,' Henry recalls.

His own feelings aside, Henry identified three main risks with Kemp: his habitual drug-taking, his violent history, and his lack of understanding of his mental illness.

'Since being accepted in September 2001, he has sabotaged his placement by taking crack cocaine on at least three occasions,' says Henry. 'And if he was able to get hold of crack cocaine in a medium secure hospital, out here the opportunity is considerably greater. It's not a restricted unit. Clients have their own front-door key. Kemp will have to reside here at night in line with Home Office restrictions, but can come and go as he pleases.'

Kemp finally began his 'afternoon leave' in January. Again, the omens were not good. 'On his return from his first unescorted visit,' recalls Henry, 'he tested positive for cannabis and possibly another substance. We gave him a final warning – any more and the offer of a placement would be withdrawn.'

Henry considers that his sabotage tactic may be deliberate: 'Maybe there is a lot of anxiety about coming out of an institution,' he says. But this is where the unit usually comes into its own. 'We work with very difficult clients and we have a heavy emphasis on life skills, which we teach them so they can move on to less supported accommodation or an independent flat,' says Henry. 'Ideally, they stay with us for between 18 months and two years. We don't usually look at clients moving on until they have been here at least a year.'

Kemp's perception of reality was, not surprisingly, blurred. He had monthly depot injections (see Factfile, page 41) but complained that they caused trembling as a side-effect. 'He doesn't feel he has a mental health problem and wants to stop having the injections,' says Henry. 'He feels he was mentally ill at the time of his father's murder, but that his psychotic illness was induced by drugs. He says he is remorseful about the offence but does not feel responsible because he was unwell at the time. At other times he is not remorseful.'

The forensic psychiatrist recommended Kemp's medication remain unaltered given the major change about to happen in his life. 'We felt a review would be more appropriate later on depending on his progress,' says Henry.

Kemp's violent history was also a crucial factor. He had been violent towards fellow patients but not staff. He hadn't spoken to his mother after she informed on him, since when she has replaced his father as his new object of hate. She is 'in hiding' in France.

Kemp – who has attempted suicide twice and has self-harmed at least three times over the past 10 years – was very capable of hostility. 'My first experience came when I attempted to address his drug problem,' says Henry, who admits his forthright tactics were possibly stirred by memories of his own father. Kemp's initial response was: 'I no longer have a drug problem – it's in the past.' But Henry knew he had taken drugs six weeks previously, and had spent over £28,000 on crack cocaine (he rented out a flat he owned) and was in debt with a bank loan. 'In retrospect,' says Henry, I feel I went too far,' he concedes, 'and our relationship deteriorated. He was angry with me for challenging him and I felt inadequate as a practitioner by his response to my approach.'

At a three-way clear-the-air meeting Henry, his manager and Kemp discussed these difficulties, with Kemp eventually accepting that Henry would remain as his keyworker.

The relationship has clearly improved. Kemp, aware of the expectations placed upon him, has begun his twice-weekly overnight stays and has remained drug-free. Henry is confident that Kemp's full-time trial period will soon begin. 'Our main source of work from now on will be containment. It doesn't sound like much, but given the complexity of a client like this, it will be an achievement,' says Henry.

Arguments for risk

- Kemp has displayed an ability to live in the community in relative safety, but was unable to deal effectively with his drug use. Targeted work within this area could lead to a successful transition.
- He has, at times, shown remorse for killing his father and has blamed his mental illness for his actions.
- Kemp has been institutionalised for a long time and the thought of having to deal with the outside world may be at the root of his attempts to sabotage his community placement. Skilled help could see him overcome this fear.
- Kemp is stable and well. Henry is confident that he is capable of making a focused effort to deal with his situation positively.
- Living in an environment that permits freedom of movement (excepting the need to remain at the unit at night) allows Kemp some independence and choice that would be denied him in hospital.

Arguments against risk

- Kemp is a murderer and habitual drug user. He has at times displayed a less-than-remorseful attitude to the murder. He has also, time and time again, relapsed into drug use from cannabis (which is potentially harmful considering his mental health and medication) to crack cocaine.
- He can seemingly obtain drugs relatively easily – even when a patient at a medium-secure hospital. Moving him into a more independent lifestyle will only raise the temptation and access to drugs.
- Kemp is very able to scheme and manipulate. Challenged by Henry, he demanded that he be removed as his keyworker. This could indicate an unwillingness to tackle his behaviour constructively.
- If living more independently, there is a real risk that Kemp will stop his depot injections.
- As the new object of hate in his life, his mother is clearly at risk from harm. Although she is in hiding, she may return or, indeed, Kemp may try to find her.

Independent comment

Henry's approach demonstrates the value and centrality of a therapeutic relationship, writes Tom Dodd. It is understandable that the weight of Kemp's history alone (it has been 14 years since he killed his father) would tip the balance in favour of a containing and less-flexible regime.

The experience of paranoid disorders often means that the individual is less likely to take responsibility or see their role in the detrimental things that happen in their lives. Kemp may find it difficult to get pleasure from relationships, he may construe any comments as criticisms and blame the 'persecutor'. As his keyworker, Henry will need to take a cautious but intensive approach, while at a pace that is acceptable to Kemp because he is likely to disengage easily. If the aim of intervention is to modify Kemp's beliefs and behaviour, then he is less likely to fail.

The service's relationship with Kemp is likely to be over a period of years. To maintain opportunities for Kemp, the keyworker will need continued and comprehensive support from the multidisciplinary team. The care package is complex and will need a detailed rationale, with contributions from a number of sources. Such decision-making requires transparency and clarity from everyone involved. The more risks that are evident – and this case highlights many – the greater the imperative to take a team approach, sharing decision-making, accountability and responsibility.

Tom Dodd is co-ordinator for assertive outreach at the Sainsbury Centre for Mental Health.

Reprinted by kind permission of *Community Care*, 11–17 July, 2002.

The above case example demonstrates just how much leadership is involved in enabling people with potential to harm themselves or others to lead as independent a life as possible. A former Director of Social Services and Chief Executive of a major voluntary organisation perceived the dichotomy between practitioner and manager as one that is often artificially constructed:

Social workers have to take very tough decisions . . . All of this is a strong school for decision-making. Social worker skills are eminently transferable to a management environment.

quoted in Fielding, 1989

Managers in mental health services need to be aware of the major environmental factors affecting the work that they are undertaking, without becoming overwhelmed by those same factors. The STEP process, enables one to chart the major influencing factors (see Gilbert and Thompson, forthcoming, for more detail):

- Sociological
  - increased consumer power
  - demographic changes
  - multiculturalism and culture/creed tensions
  - marginalisation of some groups
- Technological
  - faster (but not always better) communication
  - technological innovation
  - cross-fertilization of ideas
  - need for quicker responses across a range of areas
- Economic
  - a knowledge-based economy
  - market uncertainty, post Enron, and the 2008/9 credit crisis
  - increasing role of private sector finance
- Political
  - new political alliances post 11th September 2001
  - dangers of polarisation
  - tensions between classic liberal capitalism and communitarianism

All of this takes place in a globalised market place with increased opportunities and increased threats.

Change and faster change appears to be endemic, and there is a widespread belief that structural change will produce better performance, but as Mark C. Scott demonstrates in his study of business organisations, the major structural changes have produced increasingly small returns (Scott, 2000: 6) and as he states:

The problem with knowledge for most businesses and their boards is that it is intangible . . . it is personalised. It tends to walk out of the building each night!

Roger Harrison in his study of organisational culture is clear that:

. . . the organisation is a living organism . . . and the more you ask it to change, the less energy it will have available for its daily work. It behoves us to intervene no more 'deeply' than is required to obtain the desired competencies.

Harrison and Stokes, 1990

This is a message also reinforced by Edward Peck from the Institute for Applied Health and Social Policy, in his commentary in *Managing Community Care* (10: 3, June 2002) on the previous issues study of case studies in integrated health and social care, namely that the lesson both from the private and the public sector is that mergers and acquisitions do not always bring tangible benefits for users and carers.

Over the past century, there have been different ways of considering organisations and how one needs to run them.

Zohar and Marshall propose five generations of business models:

1. the organisations as machines
2. organisations as systems
3. organisations as organisms (living systems)
4. organisations as emotional/social systems
5. organisations as fully human systems

Zohar and Marshall, 2000

The best businesses and health and social care agencies have left the first evolutionary model – the organisation as machines – behind, but the culture within organisations varies markedly and has a profound effect on how organisations deliver services to the people they serve. Sadly some health and social care entities think that setting remote performance targets is what leadership is all about – it isn't! Organisational culture is sometimes described as: 'the way we do things here' and in those simple terms one can often touch the culture within a team, ward, house, day service – or even within an organisation as a whole. Edgar Schein, the doyenne of studies in organisational culture defines it as:

A pattern of basic assumptions – invented, discovered, or developed by a given group as it learned to cope with its problems of external adaptation and internal integration – that is worked well enough to be considered valid and, therefore, to be taught to new members as the correct way to perceive, think and feel in relation to those problems.

Schein, 1985: 9

In his 2004 edition, Schein develops further this theory of the interaction between leaders and the cultures of the organisations they lead (for a fuller discussion of the subject, please see Gilbert, 2005; Mannion et al., 2005; Gilbert and Thompson, forthcoming).

In her study of culture in the public sector, Newman states that culture is learned and passed on from individual to individual or group:

Culture is like language: we inherit it, learn it, pass it on to others, but in the process we invent new words and expressions – it evolves over time.

Newman, 1996: 17

Charles Handy famously described four cultures and labelled them with the names of Ancient Greek gods (see Handy, 1979 and 1985; Harrison and Stokes, 1990):

1. The power culture – frequently found in small entrepreneurial organisations. The system depends on a central power source (one person or a small coterie) 'with rays of power and influence spreading out from that central figure' (Handy, 1985: 189).
2. The role culture – central and local government departments fit the description for Handy's role culture. Its strengths are its stability and predictability, but at a time of change, that is its weakness as well.
3. The task culture – job or project orientated. Accent is on performance with a bringing together of the right people from any level in the organisation, with appropriate resources and setting them to get on with the task in hand.
4. The person culture – in this the individual is the central point. The structure exists only to serve and assist the individuals within it. Consultancies, barristers' chambers and architects' partnerships, are the type of organisations which Handy quotes as appropriate here.

Some general practitioner practices might well have fallen within the fourth culture, but in many ways, the formation of primary care groups and then primary care trusts were clearly created in part to bring GPs more into the organisational ring.

Cultures will change over time but they are notoriously slow to do so. Johnson and Scholes have a very helpful section on what they call the

cultural web of an organisation based around a central 'recipe' and the ingredients comprising: rituals and myths, power structures, symbols, organisational structures, control systems and routines. To change the recipe in a large organisation is extremely difficult, though by changing some of the ingredients under the headings described will eventually lead to a modification, at least, of the recipe itself (see Johnson and Scholes, 1989: 37–47, text and case studies).

Edgar Schein makes clear that, in his opinion: 'the only thing of real importance that leaders do is to create and manage culture' (Schein, 1985: 2). If a newly arrived manager is aware of a service focused around organisational concerns rather than focused on positive outcomes for users and carers, or an organisation that is 'institutionally racist', then the leader's role is to change the recipe. Leaders, therefore, must:

● Identify the cultural recipe and how malleable it is.
● Diagnose its features and its layers.
● Ascertain how appropriate the recipe is for the desired strategy.
● Use transformational values and skills to mould the culture, by acting on the ingredients within the recipe. For example, managers going 'back to the floor' and working with frontline staff.
● Will not only inspire by example (walk-the-talk) and learn a great deal, they will also begin a weaving of stories (Bates and Gilbert, 2008) and relationships which create a powerful force for positive development.

Just as organisational theory was changing, so were the issues around management. Before the Second World War, there was a focus on 'administration' as an approach. This was characterised by mistake avoiding; rarely measuring performance; long hierarchies and limited delegation; risk avoiding; conformity and uniformity.

From the 1960s onwards, there was more of a focus on 'management', with objectives stated as broad strategic aim; performance measurement; shorter hierarchies and increased delegation; an active approach with a greater acceptance of risk and an accent on independence.

In the 1980s, 'leadership' theory was evolved to cope with an increasing environment of rapid change. Sir John Harvey-Jones makes a point which connects leadership and social work; in his words:

Table 6:   The balancing foci of management and leadership

The manager focuses on systems and structure	The leader focuses on people
The manager maintains	The leader develops
The manager asks how and when	The leader asks what and why
The manager concentrates on planning and budgeting	The leader sets a direction and aligns people
The manager has his eye on the bottom line	The leader has his eye on the horizon
The manager is deductive and rational	The leader is inductive and intuitive
The manger ensures the accomplishment of plans by controlling and problem solving	The leader achieves goals through motivating and inspiring people
Good management copes with current complexity	Leadership is about coping with change
The manager does things right	The leader does the right thing

Gilbert, adapted from Kotter, 1990

Management and industrial leadership is an art, not a science. Each of us approaches the problem from a different background, and each of us is dealing with a different situation, and a different culture, and from a different starting point.

Harvey-Jones, 2003: 27

It might well be said that leadership is now being overstressed at the expense of management. Leadership is indeed required to take an organisation forward, but management is essential if the organisation is to work. Somebody once said that management and leadership are all about three interlocking activities: getting things right; keeping things going, doing new things. I tend to follow John P. Kotter who asserts that 'the real challenge is to combine strong leadership and strong management, and use each to balance the other'.

It is not always easy to combine the attributes of management and leadership in one person, though that may well be the ideal. If it's not possible then management teams need to be balanced to make sure that the correct skill mix is there:

What makes a significant difference to the performance of an organisation is the quality and competence of frontline managers. They manage the primary tasks and activities of the organisation. They have a key role in determining whether standards of practice are consistently maintained, in supporting staff engaged in complex, personally demanding practice, and ensuring that staff are continually developed in knowledge-based practice.

Denise Platt, then Chief Inspector of the SSI, Annual Report 1999

There are a number of theories of leadership:

- Leaders are born not made – charismatic leadership.
- Situational leadership which views leaders in the context of:

 – their own character and qualities
 – those of their subordinates
 – the situation at the time
- Theories based on the functions of leadership.
- Handling the creative tension between 'transactional leadership' (management) and 'transformational leadership' (leadership) (see Kotter, 1996)
- Distributed or shared leadership – leadership at all levels
- Leadership being about leading change through 'the never-ending white water of change' (Charles Handy, quoted in Alban-Metcalf and Alimo-Metcalfe, 2009a) and redefining organisation goals through that change.

Leadership is fundamentally about working through others to achieve a vision for a better future.

The characteristics of a leader could be viewed under the following headings:

1. Personal: self-belief, self-awareness, a desire to drive improvement and integrity. The persona being made up of personal and professional qualities and values, and experience. Learning from challenges, and indeed our mistakes, is crucial.
2. Demonstrating competence and a willingness to draw in others with additional competencies.
3. Setting direction: vision, intellectual flexibility, political astuteness and a drive for results.
4. Engaging staff and partners in a common cause.
5. Delivering improved services: leading change in an open and inclusive way, holding people to account and empowering others. Developing the workforce.

6. Building both human and social capital.
   Alban-Metcalfe and Alimo-Metcalfe, 2009b

Jim Collins, in his study of enduringly successful organisations (and I stress enduring as opposed to the quick fix approach) points to leaders whose ambition is for the organisation and the service of their end users and not for themselves (Collins, 2001). The collapse of Enron and Worldcom and the corporate scandals in America have led many business thinkers and business schools to go back to fundamental issues such as values and consider what makes an organisation successful over a considerable time period. Jim Collins and Gerry Porras put it like this:

> *Contrary to popular wisdom, the proper first response to a changing world is not to ask, 'how should we change?' but rather to ask, 'what do we stand for and why do we exist?' This should never change. And then feel free to change everything else. Put another way, visionary companies distinguish their timeless core values and enduring purpose (which should never change) from their operating practices and business strategies (which should be changing constantly in response to a changing world).*
>
> Collins and Porras, 2000

The 2008/9 credit crisis brought on by reckless and poorly regulated 'casino capitalism' has reinforced this message. In this context Social Work has a great deal to offer leadership both today and in the future. The Hay Group's *Leadership Competencies for Foundation Trusts* (Hay Group, 2009) have many congruencies with social work approaches.

> *The leader looks out of the window to give praise and looks in the mirror to accept blame.*
> Jill Garrett, formerly European Director of Gallop

1. Integrity and a sense of values

When interviewed for Community Care on her appointment as President of the ADSS, Jo Williams spoke of a 'fundamental' belief in equality, and treating everyone with the same respect as integral to her way of working both as a practitioner and as a senior manager. 'It's just part of me – how I am', is how she put it (*Community Care*, 28 October 1999). People who worked with Jo Williams as a social worker and a manager say that's exactly how she is. In management-speak she 'walks-the-talk'; unfortunately a number of people in senior positions are perceived as only being able to 'talk-the-talk'. They march to a different drum, that of their empty ambition.

> *It is not good enough just to preach the doctrine; you have to live the life.*
> Victoria Woodhull, US presidential candidate, 1872

Stephen Covey in his work on principle-centred leadership argues for a congruency of personal, managerial and organisational principles:

Level	Principle
organisational	alignment
managerial	empowerment
interpersonal	trust
personal	trustworthiness
	Covey, 1992

As we have seen in Chapter 5, 'genuineness' is one of the prime attributes of the effective social worker. This is true for business leadership as well. Collins and Porras speak of 'core values' as the 'organisation's essential and enduring tenets – a small set of timeless guiding principles that require no external justification; they have *intrinsic* value and importance to those inside the organisation' (Collins and Porras, 2000: 222).

Collins, in his studies of leadership, is clear about a value-driven approach, concentrating on the good of the organisation, not the ambitions of the individual (Collins, 2001 and 2009). Kouzes and Posner (1990) in their overview of *The Credibility Factor: What Followers Expect From Their Leaders* (see also Kouzes and Posner, 2007) found that the responses to their survey of managers put integrity (trustworthiness), competence (capability and effectiveness) and leadership (direction-setting and inspiring) as the three most pronounced responses in that order (Kouzes and Posner, 1990). Jack Welch, one of the most admired business leaders of his generation, recalls being asked how he could hold a particular belief system and be an effective businessman at the same time. Welch says that he answered emphatically that he could – 'the simple answer is', he stated, 'by maintaining integrity, establishing it and never wavering from it, supported everything I did through good and bad times. People may not have agreed with me on every issue, and I may not have been right all the time – but they always knew they were getting it straight and honest . . . I never had two agendas. There was only one way – the straight way' (Welch, with Byrne, 2001: 381. See also leadership case studies in Gilbert and Thompson, 2010; Gilbert, forthcoming).

I have largely been very fortunate in the people I've worked for, but occasionally one comes up against somebody who can't even spell integrity let alone act with it. These are the 'hollow men' (and women), the 'Teflon' characters, who devalue the enterprises they and others are engaged in. They are not committed to the role and the organisation they are meant to be serving, but are intent on furthering their own career.

My favourite fictional/philosophical author, Ursula Le Guin, portrays such an individual in one of those children's books which have a lot to say to adults, *The Farthest Shore*. Cob, who had formerly been a mage engaged in doing good, had been corrupted by a desire to prolong his own life at the expense of others. His own rapacity for immortality was beginning to suck the life and colour out of the fabric of the universe. The mage who promotes life, Ged, challenges him in these words:

> *You exist, without name, without form. You cannot see the light of day; you cannot see the dark. You sold the green earth and the sun and the stars to save yourself. But you have no self. All that which you sold, that is yourself. You have given everything for nothing. And so now you seek to draw the world to you, all that life and life you lost, to fill up your nothingness. But it cannot be filled. Not all the songs of earth, not all the stars of heaven, could fill your emptiness.*
>
> Le Guin, 1973: 189

At a time when business and business schools are having to re-evaluate their value-base in the light of the business and accountancy scandals in the United States, and the world-wide banking crisis, which saw the CEO of the Financial Services Authority, Lord Turner, attack some banks, in the summer of 2009, for the lack of social utility; a profession which has a clear value-base and code of ethics, has a great deal to offer in today's world.

2. Managing oneself

As I said at the beginning of this chapter, practitioners, to be effective and helpful to others, have to manage themselves. They need to be self-aware, self-motivated, organised, dependable, and with a focus not only on positive outcomes for users and carers, but an awareness of their motivation for acting in a particular way.

As is the case in medicine, so it is for social work, the first injunction is to do no harm.

> *Think about the leaders you've been impressed with over the course of your working life. Almost without exception they will be people with high self-esteem, whose actions are congruent with their espoused views, who understand their own beliefs and values and who have a strong sense*

of their own direction. To be truly effective as a leader, you've got to be comfortable with who you are and what you are about. Essentially, concentrating on leading yourself is a powerful way to grow your ability to lead others.
Chris Lake, Programme Director, *Developing Leadership Potential*, Roffey Park Management Institute

Sydney Finkelstein (2004) in his study of why previously successful leaders failed when confronted by new situations, points to a lack of self-awareness and a denial in learning lessons (or learning the wrong lessons!) which leads to a 'rabbit in the headlights' approach when new circumstances and challenges arise. There are challenging transitions from practitioner to manager and from operational manager to strategic roles. Terry Scragg's book for frontline managers (2009) is essential reading for that vital first transition.

3. Assessing situations

One of the prime social work tasks is assessing the needs of individuals and care systems in a holistic manner. Social work assessments are not purely about an individual therapeutic relationship, as we have seen, they look at the individual in the context of their relationships and social circumstances.

Assessment of situations and possible consequences of actions or non-action is an essential part of leadership.

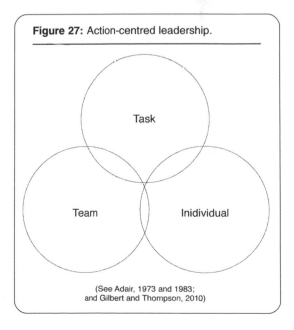

Figure 27: Action-centred leadership.

Task

Team

Inidividual

(See Adair, 1973 and 1983; and Gilbert and Thompson, 2010)

4. *Direction-setting*

When I joined the Army in the late 1960s, they had just engaged John Adair, to consider the interaction between historical and experiential views on leadership and the theoretical base. One of the simple models used by Adair and his successors and still very relevant today, is that of the famous three circles as set out in Figure 27.

There is no doubt of the primacy of the mission or task; but of course it is usually groups of people who are required to fulfil the mission, especially if it is complex and requires bringing in a number of specialists (Finance, IT, HR, etc.) at the same time the team is only as strong as the weakest or least focused individual and specialists may be brilliant in their own field but not particularly good 'team players'. The most effective social workers have to bring into play, co-ordinate and influence a whole range of people from different professions and agencies. This is a good school of management. People with severe and enduring mental health needs,

such as those surveyed in the Westminster Study (MacDonald and Sheldon, 1997) require a co-ordinated care package over a considerable period. Managing services which may be much dispersed and often out-sourced from the commissioning organisation, with staff out-posted and difficult to communicate with directly, require the manager to be extremely robust in making connections.

In Staffordshire with a staff group of about 6,000 people, with some of our most vital staff, home carers, at the end of a long line of management and communication, we spent considerable time when I was Director of Operations there, in ensuring a direct link between listening to our users, carers, and frontline staff, managing strategically and involving those who were carrying out the day-to-day caring role.

In Worcestershire as DSS, a financial crisis immediately following on from local government reorganisation and the national budget freeze of 1997/8, led to us creating a radical coalition of

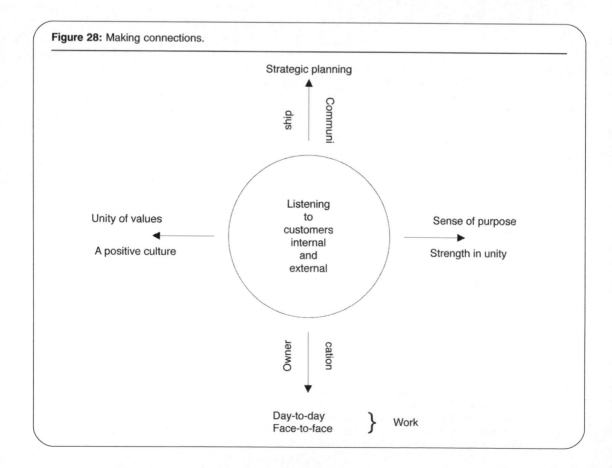

Figure 28: Making connections.

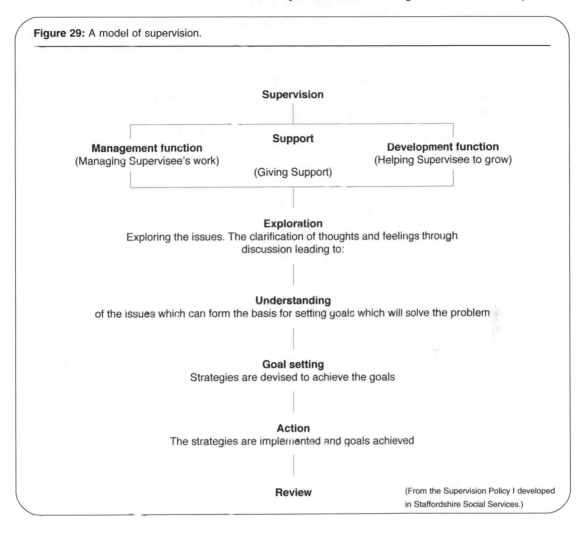

Figure 29: A model of supervision.

Supervision

Management function
(Managing Supervisee's work)

Support
(Giving Support)

Development function
(Helping Supervisee to grow)

Exploration
Exploring the issues. The clarification of thoughts and feelings through discussion leading to:

Understanding
of the issues which can form the basis for setting goals which will solve the problem

Goal setting
Strategies are devised to achieve the goals

Action
The strategies are implemented and goals achieved

Review

(From the Supervision Policy I developed in Staffordshire Social Services.)

users and carers organisations, and statutory and voluntary agencies to produce a partnership approach to riding the white waters of change.

One of the main ways of ensuring performance is managed and evaluated, comes through the supervision process, which has been a common model for social work staff for many years, but is not so well known in other professional groups. Supervision integrates aims and tasks with the necessary development of attitude and aptitude within the staff member. Again, practice teaching, which is a well developed art in social work, and supervision, are good management attributes. Improved supervision for staff is a strong recommendation of the Social Work TaskForce, which reported to the Government in late 2009 (DoH/DCSF, 2009).

5. Creating a positive culture

To operate successfully, social workers have to engage with people's cultural milieu – not only in terms of race and creed, but in the cultural web which we all weave within ourselves, around ourselves, within our immediate and extended families, and in the wider neighbourhood and society. The social worker has to understand what McLean and Marshall term 'a web of understanding' (McLean and Marshall, 1988: 11) and how various ingredients interact with the recipe as a whole. Tom Peters is often quoted as saying that 'managing at any time, but more than ever today, is a symbolic activity' (see Peters and Austin, 1985, and Peters, 1989) while Smith and Peterson (1988) assert that the art of leadership resides significantly in the mediation of cultural messages between leaders and led.

In the complex organisational world of today, where public sector organisations are often vertically or horizontally linked with other public sector or private sector entities, the effectiveness of the leader lies in his/her ability to make activity meaningful for those around them.

Hence, the diagram below which moves action-centred leadership forward into today's world:

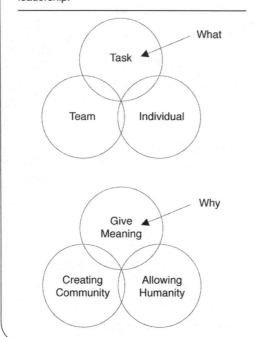

Figure 30: The progression of action-centred leadership.

In an organisation which depends ultimately on interactions between people, then, as Charles Hampden-Turner points out in his book *Corporate Culture* (1990) leaders need to model behaviour for their staff. A number of service industries went to the public sector to gain ideas over caring for employees; now it may be that public sector organisations have to go back to learn from service industries. Goran Carstedt, who turned around Volvo France in the 1980s, expressed his belief that:

You won't get your people to care about customers unless you show your people that you care about them. They'll pass on your concern. You don't 'motivate' your em-

ployees, you show them the concern you want them to express to customers.

Quoted in Hampden-Turner, 1990: 167

Case Example 13

Barry, who had long-term enduring, and at times, acute paranoid schizophrenia, leading to a very chaotic lifestyle, had a poor relationship with his current care co-ordinator, erratic compliance with medication and viewed intervention as oppressive. His mental health deteriorated to a point where he was compulsorily admitted to hospital.

The medical and nursing views were that residential/nursing care was required at point of discharge. Following a social worker's assessment, it was felt that, although residential care would meet some of his needs, it would mean that he would have to give up his home, which he would find very difficult as he was attached to it – it was where his wife had died.

An alternative plan was sought which included seven-day home support, with support from a new care co-ordinator, who was a social worker. Barry was at first wary, but over time, established a trusting relationship. His previous problems of being exploited, poor financial management and therefore financial stresses, and having an insufficient diet were addressed, thus managing the stressors which had significantly impacted on his mental well-being.

Barry's view of the mental health services has now changed, to one of partnership, and he readily agrees to continue taking medication, thus assisting his continued residence in his own home, attending community resources.

---

6. Partnership and communication

It is a sad fact that sometimes positive and productive relations at the front line are sabotaged either by secrecy or conflict at a senior manager level between or within organisations, or at times good working relationships at a senior level which never get passed down to frontline staff through the middle management tier.

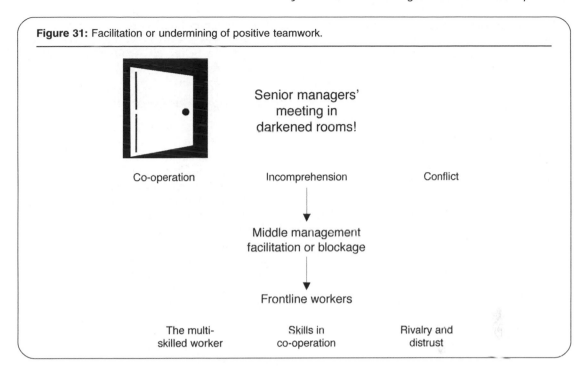

Figure 31: Facilitation or undermining of positive teamwork.

Organisations can 'guard' their reputations so secretively that none of the essential learning both within and between organisations occurs. Commenting on both the Baby 'P' (L.B. Haringey) and Mid Staffordshire Acute Hospital scandals in 2009, Jo Webber of the NHS Confederation wrote:

> *A successful organisation is one where the board is endlessly curious and challenging in fulfilling its ultimate responsibility for performance ... Haringey and Mid Staffordshire senior managers and board spent too much time distracted by more easily attainable targets, which told them they were doing well, and not enough seeing what occupied people's minds on the frontline.*
> Webber, 2009

Social workers, because of their need to bring in partners within families, neighbourhoods and agencies to assist their service users and their carers, have strength in communication and partnership working.

Because of the level of historical distrust which often exists within and between organisations, there is a need for courageous communication and co-working. Leadership has to be 'embodied'. As one commentator has argued:

> *Our post-modern world makes it all the more important that we communicate with one another, build consensus, from a basis of strong conviction.*

And again:

> *This is about being visceral, passionate and embodied – speaking from the gut and the heart as well as from the head. For with this goes openness, honesty and earthiness.*
> Webster, 2001: 3

7. Planning, managing and deploying resources

The care management process, which we considered in Chapter 5, is an excellent micro-management system. Though many social workers were resistant to care management as a concept, for many of the same reasons as a number of GPs were resistant to fund holding, i.e. that the management of a budget could constrain their assessment of need and battle for the appropriate resources.

Whatever the ins and outs of the ethical dilemmas, however, care managers have to plan efficiently, deploy resources economically, and manage and evaluate the care package effectively (see Figure 17).

Factors found to promote modernisation:

- Clear and credible leadership with visible and active support of senior managers.
- A known and understood joint vision.
- Engagement in focused planning and implementation structures which include representation from all stakeholders.

- Addressing basic management issues in joint services such as conditions of service, and line management and supervisory arrangements.

- Effective representation of wider social services responsibilities in planning (particularly childcare responsibilities).
- Application of performance management regimes.
- Services and care practice which place service users at their centre and which promote independence.
- Valuing diversity (particularly promoting culturally competent services).
- Robust and evidence-based approaches to risk assessment and management.
- A commissioning approach applied to all relevant services.
- Clear responsibility for co-ordinated care arrangements and a 'Whole System' approach which is performance managed.

From SSI, *Modernising Mental Health Services*, June 2002: 5

8. Empowerment and accountability

Thurstine Basset, one of my many very helpful correspondents while writing this book, mused that one of the paradoxes of being a member of a profession with an accent on facilitating, enabling and empowering is that it is difficult to broadcast success:

> It is hard to point out the positive contribution when the contribution is centred on empowering others.
> conversation with the author, 13 February 2002

This empowerment, however, has to be a clear part of the management role. Delivering services to people through people, especially in a diversity of settings, cannot be done in a command and control manner. People have to be orientated, educated, trained and supported to work independently to promote people's independence.

Accountability is a matter for the manager and for the staff member jointly. Devolvement of responsibility by managers at any level must never be shelving or a shirking of responsibility. Devolution is not about abrogating responsibility.

Managers also need to role model 'followership' as well as 'leadership' (see Kelley, 1988). Good leaders demonstrate that they can follow as well as lead, and Martin Brown, who oversaw the introduction of the NSF for Mental Health, gives as a prime bit of career advice: 'First learn to follow before you aspire to lead' (quoted in *Health Service Journal*, 18 July 2002).

9. Building enduring organisations

One of the factors which strikes one from the Westminster Study, which I've used extensively in this book, is that of the sheer 'stickability' of social workers in the face of extreme deprivation and distress. Organisations require stickability as well, and too often in the public sector there is a sense of panic if things don't appear to be going according to plan, and long-term corporate health is sacrificed for short-term wins.

Again, to quote from the commercial sector, Collins and Porras demonstrate that companies who have survived and generated enduring success have not necessarily been consistently successful: 'Indeed, all of the visionary companies in our study faced setbacks and made mistakes at some point during their lives, and some are experiencing difficulty as we write this book. Yet – and this is a key point – visionary companies display a remarkable *resiliency*, an ability to bounce back from adversity' (p4).

Public sector organisations particularly should take note of Collins and Porras' dictum that while strategies and tactics have to change to meet changing circumstances in a fast-changing world, core values should remain a constant.

Conclusion

There is an increasing emphasis on competency frameworks in management approaches and education. This is welcome, but it is only a facet of the whole. As Alban-Metcalfe and Alimo-Metcalfe (2009) point out, it only takes us part of the way. People who are in management positions and those who take responsibility for leading on issues without perhaps holding an actual, defined position of responsibility, need to draw on their personal values and qualities and express those through competencies and what the Metcalfes call 'engaging leadership behaviours'. Sound values without effectiveness and engagement leads nowhere; competence without engagement result in isolation; a direction without values may lead to disaster.

Sometimes images and stories (see Bates and Gilbert, 2008) can be most effective in portraying what practice and management is about.

It's only a story, you say. So it is, and the rest of life with it . . . I can change the story. I am the story.
Jeannette Winterson, *The Power Book*, 2000

Recently, a colleague of mine went white water rafting in America, and compared the experience to being a frontline manager in today's public sector organisations.

So to use this image, as a leader, at any level we have to:

- Set the direction in which we want to steer.
- Have expertise in negotiating both the surface water and the undercurrents.
- Have the ability to motivate and support the crew (as a group and as individuals) even when they are exhausted.

- Be able to negotiate obstacles.
- Work with people, not against them.
- Ensure that the boat is supplied with essential resources.
- Have the determination to complete the task.
- Celebrate success and learn the lessons of failures

Ours is overwhelmingly an individualistic society, but leaders have to be imbued with ideas of community and connection. We have to know ourselves, we have to lead ourselves, we have to be grounded in the present and able to look to the horizon of the future; to take people with us we must convey a message and a meaning. **Ultimately, we have to serve to lead.**

CHAPTER 12

Looking to the Future

Peter Gilbert

My social worker has been a constant presence throughout my illness and into my recovery. She has always held my hope for me even when I felt the flame had flickered out of my life.

service user to the author, 2009

Well, of course, I am still quite depressed and feel awful at times but I know that if things go wrong I can rely on my social worker. Out of all the people involved in my case, it is the social worker who is the best.

service user quoted in SSI, *Modernising Mental Health Services*, 2002: 12

I believe that social care has such a pivotal role in promoting well-being in our communities that it must go with the community leadership role of local authorities . . . This is the heart of citizenship for the future.

David Behan, Director General, DoH, in his presidential address to ADSS, 2002

If you do not know which port you are sailing to, no wind is favourable.

Seneca, Roman philosopher

By 2020,most adults will understand the importance of mental well-being to their full and productive functioning in society . . . People with mental health problems, and those at risk, will receive personalised care packages designed to meet their individual needs. They will be able to make decisions about their care, treatment and goals for recovery, as well as to monitor their own condition.

DoH, *New Horizons*, 2009

Social work, unlike other disciplines, does not have a tradition of relying upon consulting rooms or physically invasive intervention. The easy chairs, the pills and the needles have not been there as a signifier that something is being done to the mental health service user. This is a significant issue for people from black and minority ethnic groups. The feeling of being 'subjected to' something or someone undermines the experience of black and minority ethnic mental health service users, who collectively have a history of being in that position. Social work offers interventions based significantly on building a relationship with the service user in a physical and psychological context of empowerment. Social work offers a mechanism for building trust with those who receive cues from society and from within mental health services, that institutions must not be trusted.

Former SSI inspector and social care director of a mental health trust

The necessity for social work

The irony of the current position is that social circumstances would seem to make the need for social work even more evident and imperative, and yet social work, at least in its current form and host organisation is often looked at askance. My philosophical eldest daughter once remarked in some perplexity, following changes at her primary school, that: 'nothing ever happens until it's actually happened'! And it must feel like this for many social work and social care staff who are being pulled in different directions, and may experience what Sir Roy Griffiths once remarked about community care that it is 'a poor relation; everybody's distant relative but nobody's baby' (Griffiths, 1988).

A publication on mental health policy asserts: 'Mental health and well-being are issues of everyday life and should be of interest to every citizen and employer, in addition to all care, education and administration sectors. Mental health is influenced (enhanced or jeopardised) in families and schools, on the streets and in workplaces – where people can feel safe, respected, included and able to participate, or maybe in fear, marginalised or excluded' (Jenkins et al., 2002: 3).

All the evidence from user research demonstrates a requirement to meet people's emotional and practical needs in a human way, and that a purely 'psychiatric response', as Cliff Prior, former Chief Executive of Mental Health Charity Rethink (formerly the National Schizophrenia Fellowship) calls it (*Guardian Society*, 3 July 2002: 11) often institutionalises people almost as thoroughly as the old mental hospitals.

It is important that the old debates between medical and social care approaches are not allowed to damage genuine attempts to provide services which are more flexible, responsive and accountable. Social care complements health intervention by ensuring that social experiences are considered and dealt with – such factors as racism, sexism, unemployment, difficulties in personal relationships, are key to the overall well-being of the individual. Social care has a great deal to be proud of in having brought these issues to prominence.

social care director

Kathleen Jones in her seminal history of mental health services charts a thematic wave of trends – a series of overlapping circles that progress with recurrent themes and challenges. Jones (Jones, K., 1972 and 2002) saw the 1890 Act as 'the triumph of legalism', and following that a build up towards a more medical and treatment-orientated approach. 'It is only now', at her time of writing in the early 1970s, 'when the social services have developed a comparable professional status, which the social approach is coming into its own again' (p153). Ironically, it may be that the social approach is arriving sans social workers? Denise Platt, former Chief Inspector of Social Services and Chair of CSCI, in an address to the National Institute for Social Work, expressed her concerns thus: 'I think social work is becoming a lost art – not to practitioners but to organisations, and as we lose it we realise what a contribution it has made.'

It is certainly clear to me that the social perspective, social work and social care are even more important now than they were. When social work commenced in its roots in the 19th century, it grew through campaigners such as Mary Stewart, in the London Hospitals, where they refused to be boxed into a purely individualistic approach but insisted on reaching out to the community and seeing people in a holistic and whole systems way. Modern society is much more complex and deprivation increasingly visible. Despite strenuous efforts by Government, a number of social think tanks are indicating widening gaps between rich and poor in terms of health, housing, income, pensions etc (see Friedli for WHO, 2009). England is now no longer considered purely in terms of historical comparators, but as against Scotland, with its very different approach to some aspects of social welfare, and the continent as a whole (see Woodward and Kohli, 2001).

With the decline in feelings of solidarity with and responsibility for our fellow citizens; the removal of many effective powers from local authorities, the building up of what Simon Jenkins calls 'the new magistracy' (see Jenkins, 1995) and the social dislocation caused by the Credit Crunch and resulting recession, many people are increasingly excluded, and have difficulty in finding recourse. 'Modernism' with its often over-weaning optimism, has given place to 'post modernism' where 'we are our own little story-tellers, living among the ruins of our former grand narratives' (Harvey, 1990; see Bauman, 2007). This may be fine if our innate sense of self is strong and we have confidence in our own stories, not so promising for those who have become lost and detached from their own inner reality and from other people.

Mental distress may be caused or compounded by poor living conditions and difficult personal circumstances. The role played by social workers can therefore be crucial to recovery from mental illness precisely because their focus is personal, giving practical support and help to resolve problems of living that might otherwise appear insurmountable to someone who is also trying to deal with his/her mental distress. This type of support not only contributes to recovery from a period of illness, it can also help to reduce the likelihood of a further episode recurring.

Michelle Rowett, former Chief Executive, Manic Depression Fellowship, 2003

The situation for people from black and ethnic minority communities is particularly acute, as made clear by the statistics in earlier chapters of the book. The Sainsbury Centre's review of the relationship between Mental Health Services and African and Caribbean communities, *Breaking the Circles of Fear* (SCMH, 2002: 64) speaks of services that fail to match the needs and aspirations of users and their families. Within all of this, 'culture is an important but much misunderstood and complex entity' and it is clear that the social work perspective of understanding somebody as an individual, but within their cultural and community context, but existentially again as an individual in their own right, is absolutely vital (see Sewell, 2009; Bennett, 2009).

One of the National Institute for Mental Health in England's first national programmes was one on 'Equalities', around issues of citizenship and social inclusion (see NIMHE, 2002; Morris, 2001). Users of mental health services do not wish and see no reason why they should accept a concept where they are citizens one minute, and then, when they experience a mental illness, unlike those undergoing a physical ailment, are apparently removed from the society of citizens. Rachel Perkins, a director with South West London and St George's MHT, who has overseen a major expansion in employing staff with a user experience, highlights in her talks how she has to use staff washrooms one day and the patients' ones the next!

Users wish to be treated as fellow citizens, worked with in a human and empowering way;

have their emotional and practical needs taken seriously and addressed; and given hope for the future.

Too many people have been allowed to sink into a chronic state, and as Topor asserts:

> *The cause of chronicity, which has long been sought within the individual (biological or psychological characteristics) is not inherent in the illness itself, a part of the natural order, but rather is clearly connected with the person's life in society.*
>
> Topor, 2000

Just as Care Management in the 1990s required Social Work values and practices to make it both effective and humane, so Personalisation will also require professionalism, but one which takes empowerment to new levels and is better at balancing the individual choice and social issues, or as Ivan Lewis, the government minister most identified with the advent of personalisation, put it, we have to balance 'independence' with 'interdependence'. In his article balancing the pros and cons of current approaches, Jon Glasby (2009: 28) quotes social work and social policy lecturer Peter Scourfield, as saying:

> *In the rush to both 'hollow out' and contract out the public sector, too many of its functions and responsibilities are being pushed towards the individual.*

This sentiment is resonant in all Bauman's work, and is currently being played out in the USA debate on healthcare.

While fully acknowledging the strengths, expertise and courage of other professions, it has often struck me during my time as a practitioner and manager that it is social workers and social care workers who are willing, and adept at hanging onto the coat tails of the most deprived service users facing the greatest social dislocation. Society faces a number of dangerous fissures and fractures, like a land beset with earth tremors; it is the social worker who grapples with the whole picture. George O'Neill's fascinating study of role differentiation between CPNs and Mental Health social workers, points to the primary focus of CPNs on the individual, and the social worker on the individual and their systems (see O'Neill, 1997). But the challenge over the past decade was that social work has been squeezed into a care management and legalistic box and is in danger of losing its skills in managing systems and building bridges in communities.

Just as it is dangerous to view people from ethnic minorities as of a homogeneous group, it is equally so with carers, as Michael Bainbridge demonstrates in an article for *Mental Health Today*, where he sees 'friends and families as innocent secondary victims of illness (the 'Medical Model') where they are relegated to an entirely tangential role' (Bainbridge, 2002: 24). People are not just their caring role, but are individuals in their own right. It is perhaps significant that legislation around carers has placed duties on local authorities in an entirely appropriate way, and this is not the only thrust of government policy which implicitly or explicitly stresses the need for skilled social work interventions. Repper et al. quote a carer as saying:

> *They (service providers) need to value my views, and believe my experiences. I am pro-active in calling them, so they can do their job better, but they see me as troublesome. We have the same goal (they and I want the best for my mother) yet they do not consider my contribution to her well-being.*
>
> Repper et al., 2009: 424

The small handbook on mental health social work produced by Oldham Social Services and Oldham NHS Trust describes the range of connections which social work makes:

Within the text, the authors make clear that:

> *Unchecked, the impact of a serious mental health problem will be very destructive of a person's quality of life. It often results in self-neglect, poverty ('social drift') social isolation, social exclusion (including institutionalisation) depression and suicide. Mental Health social workers aim to work with individuals, carers, families, social groups and other related professions to counter these effects and to promote a greater sense of well-being, value and social inclusion.*
>
> 2002: 7

Modernising mental health services

In June 2002, the SSI published its findings of its national survey of 19 authorities across six regions in England. In many ways the report is positive:

> *Much direct work with service users was valued by them. This was particularly true where work recognised their abilities as well as their needs and where it acted as a lifeline at a time of difficulty and as a passport to a range of helpful services. In all councils, most service users expressed generally positive levels of satisfaction with the way that they were treated by staff. There were also examples of innovative services which promoted independence and positive lifestyles. These were particularly valued by users.*
>
> SSI, 2002: 1

Figure 32: Where does mental health social work fit.

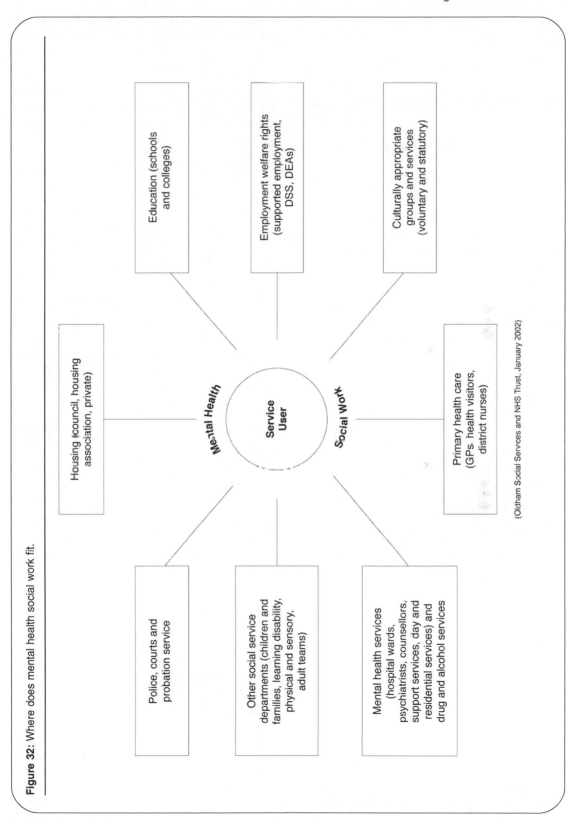

Education (schools and colleges)

Employment welfare rights (supported employment, DSS, DEAs)

Culturally appropriate groups and services (voluntary and statutory)

Housing (council, housing association, private)

Mental Health

Service User

Social Work

Primary health care (GPs, health visitors, district nurses)

Police, courts and probation service

Other social service departments (children and families, learning disability, physical and sensory, adult teams)

Mental health services (hospital wards, psychiatrists, counsellors, support services, day and residential services) and drug and alcohol services

(Oldham Social Services and NHS Trust, January 2002)

There were also, however, a number of cautionary signs:

- Good practice was often 'the result of past opportunistic development . . . stimulated and maintained by local champions', rather than it being the result of a more strategic approach.
- There was an insufficient strategic and practice link between mental health and children's services. This was being exacerbated in certain circumstances where structural change had seen a separation out of services for children from the traditional social services departments, and likewise mental health workers from social services transferring into mental health trusts.
- Black and minority ethnic communities were not well served even in 'councils with a robust general approach to equality issues, mental health services performance was poor' and this was especially true in joint services where the SSI 'found that there was an informal "division of labour" under which equality and diversity issues were regarded as being the business of social services and not of the service as a whole' (p24).
  Sadly, I've sometimes found component parts of the NHS have struggled with issues around user and carer involvement and promoting culturally competent services. It is an area to which social services staff working with or transferred into trusts can bring considerable expertise.
- The CPA was not always as user-focused as it could be. Common problems included:
  - Viewing the CPA as a review mechanism rather than as a systematic approach to identification and meeting of needs.
  - Not placing the service user at the centre of arrangements for their care.
  - Lack of attention to diversity issues.
  - Failing to address the needs of children and carers.
- Changes in structures were clearly major issues, and recent structural change, the lack of common boundaries, and a history of poor partnership arrangements clearly reflected in worse outcomes for users and carers.
- Social care needed a clear 'champion' within the system.
- Focus on the National Service Framework was essential, but so also was attention to the wider policy context.

A social care perspective adds significantly not just to the direct provision of services but to the strategic approach adopted within mental health services by taking this beyond a narrow focus on assessment and treatment of individuals.

Former NIMHE Development Centre Director

The *Future Vision of Mental Health* report by the Sainsbury Centre (in partnership with NHSC, LGA and ADSS) looks to a vision in 2015 where sound mental health is promoted at all ages and at all levels, and with maximum possible control and choice for service users (SCMH, 2006). Vision and essential practice need to go hand-in-hand; reviewing the NST, ten years on, Adam James points out that only 40 per cent of services users in community settings have a copy of their own care plan! (James, 2009).

Change is not necessarily loss

I came into social work three years after Seebohm, and its introduction of social services departments, and the apparent misunderstanding that Seebohm's recommendation of the generic departments meant having generic workers.

It is easy to romanticise the past. The passing of the old mental welfare officer was much lamented, but picking up a number of cases from them in the early seventies, some people had clearly been offered routine monitoring rather than assessment and intervention suited to their specific needs.

In the 1990s the advent of care management was seen by many as an undermining of traditional social work, but where it was allied to traditional social work values and skills, there were often benefits for service users and carers in procuring more personalised services.

The move towards care management as a function, and the continuing financial and demand pressures on Social Services meant that in many places the creative community role of social work was largely lost, to the extent that in a recent lecture David Morris, when leading NIMHE's programme on equalities, stated that other professions are moving into the gap that social work has left.

When we are educating and training social workers we are endeavouring to equip them with knowledge and understanding of a range of theories and perspectives, all of which will be relevant to their work in mental health settings. This includes professional perspectives, which will help them to work effectively in multi-disciplinary teams. It includes a wide range of theories, e.g. medical models of mental illness so that, although social workers may not use these models in their approach to their work, they can understand what they are and how to recognise them. It also includes service user perspectives, which will help them to become fully conversant with issues of diversity and inequality in relation to the provision of services.

Social work educator

When I am not feeling defensive about my age I sometimes admit to having been a generic social worker! The value of course of the generic approach was its breadth, and the ability to transfer knowledge across the client groups and age ranges; the disadvantage, of course, was that it was just too broad and it was very difficult to attain and retain specialist knowledge across such diverse groups, and I must admit that I personally found it a relief to specialise in mental health and learning disability in the 1980s, though generic training and practice was extremely helpful when my management remit broadened in the 1990s. Specialisation has brought greater job satisfaction to social workers and increased appreciation of their work in specialist fields, but organisations such as Young Minds have expressed concern about the 'general level of awareness amongst social workers of mental health problems as they manifest themselves in children and young people, as well as a lack of awareness of prevalences', while acknowledging that there are 'outstanding examples of where . . . social workers are highly skilled in working with the psychodynamics of families and children' (conversation with the author, April 2002).

In 1982, the Barclay Report argued for a greater community focus for social work, while one of the minority reports by Professor Pinker argued strongly for a focus on a professional and statutory approach. The imperatives of work with people with mental health needs are for attention to both perspectives.

New organisations

There are clearly considerable merits in the formation of specialist Mental Health Trusts, especially in their ability to provide a co-ordinated service to users and carers, with the right skill mix of staff, and economies of scale. The caveats are also obvious:

- The new trusts must avoid the isolation from the broader aspects of mental health policy and practice. The SSI report of June 2002 raises some warning notes similar to the issues Kathleen Jones identifies in her studies of institutional approaches in her historical sweep of mental health services.
- There are concerns that a purely medical model may re-exert its dominance, though there are also hopes that the new structures will actually assist a social and environmental perspective.
- It is vitally important that primary care and secondary care are closely aligned and interlinked. The necessity for the long-term health of the organisation in involving users, carers and minority groups, and involving frontline staff must be really internalised in the NHS mindset (see ADSS/NIMHE, 2003).

I have remarked earlier about the tendency to seek structural solutions to complex challenges. The Northern Ireland model of integrated health and social care is often held up as a shining example, but Terry Bamford, who has managed services in both Northern Ireland and England at a Chief Officer level has warned about a too sanguine look across the Irish Sea (Bamford, 2000). Gulliver, Peck and Towell's study of The Somerset Integrated Approach, is clearly saying that the case for such change shows promise but is not yet proven (Gulliver, Peck and Towell, 2002) and increasing numbers of studies of change management in the private and public sectors counsel caution in instituting major structural change unless the arguments for such change are overwhelming.

During structural change, people inevitably turn inwards, worry about their own positions, lose contact with some of their networks which bring about positive outcomes for users and carers, and suffer stress and exhaustion. Liam Hughes, a former Director of Social Services for Bradford and now Chief Executive of one of the Leeds primary care trusts, in a mainly positive article about change (Hughes, 2001, in Allen, 2001) quotes Burke and Cooper (2000) who identify a range of dysfunctional reactions to change which is not well managed.

Hughes goes on to say that in many cases 'organisational memory has been lost and employees find it difficult to get their bearing. Loyalty is undermined, and pride diminished. These organisations have become unhealthy and anxious places' (Hughes, 2001: 74).

On the other hand, companies/organisations that do better have taken time to:

- Align and affirm their core values.
- Over-manage change.
- Communicate with and involve internal (staff) and external partners as much as possible.

> *Health and social care have operated under separate management and spending systems since the 1970s, but with increasing recognition that working collaboratively, both informally and formally, improves patient care. The initial mutual suspicions have given way to a mutual recognition of the value of the joint approach. It is particularly encouraging that most health care professionals now more than acknowledge the value of the skills of social care staff and have come to understand that the social model of care, with its emphasis on the individual, and daily living skills, enables people to achieve a better quality of life. The integration of health and social care is the last major barrier to bring down and should bring about major change for the better.*
>
> Project manager, Development Centre

When I went to Staffordshire in 1992 as Operations Director, Adult Services, the imperative to bring the National Health Service and Community Care Act into operation for the 1 April 1993, was one of the strongest challenges I have ever experienced. While meeting practical targets at all points, the team also desired to bring about a wider cultural change, and affected this by building on an initial change process over the next five years. I have met managers who genuinely believe that they have brought in much more far reaching changes than are evident, and this is because the ground is not laid for long-term, but is like a landscape hastily prepared, washed away by the first heavy rain. I have recently been working on a ten stage change process, building on John Kotter's work and that of Ann Proehl (Gilbert, 2005).

Successful leadership in multi-disciplinary settings requires:

- An understanding of a variety of perspectives and an ability to shape these to the needs of the service.
- Cultural sensitivity.
- An understanding of professional expertise and sensitivities, and an ability to align these with the good of the service, not to the narrow dictates of any one profession.
- Making the best use of the skill mix.
- Ensuring that all channels of communication are functioning.

- Ensuring that a whole systems approach is created and maintained.

Bob Hudson, from the Nuffield Institute, who has been researching the Health Act's flexibilities, concluded in a recent article (Hudson, 2002: 10) that it was unclear where the care trusts constitute an answer to the causes of fragmented service delivery:

> *The fixation with structure has led to a preoccupation with the **means** of integrated working, and a neglect of the **ends**. Organisational change is only a proxy for the achievement of better outcomes . . . The best way the debate can progress is to have more emphasis on definitions of quality of life from the perspective of individual service users and their carers.*

Bogg, in her overview of integration in mental health services of health and social care, reflects that integration is not so much about structures as about shared values and principles, learning together and a focus on outcomes which reflect an improved quality of life for users and carers (Bogg, 2008, Chap. 13).

New professionals

George Bernard Shaw once said: 'All professions are a conspiracy against the laity', and we know in our hearts that there's a great deal of truth in this. The challenge is to become as professional, in the best sense, as possible while not building up the boundary fences which are so forbidding to users and carers.

Tony Russell, NIMHE Core Group colleague and user champion has always argued forcefully for a uni-professional so as to break down boundaries and increase co-ordination and the strength of relationship between professional and user. As a champion for the STR worker (Support, Time and Recovery) Tony is clear that this development comes from what users want.

On the other hand, other people I have spoken to believe it important to have the different perspectives, education and expertise of a range of professionals, especially those that counterbalance a biochemical approach where that is dominant. My own view is that it would be unwise at this stage to attempt to merge all the professions. What should be happening is a focus on better outcomes for users, and a non-defensive approach by professions as to who is the best person to assist in achieving those outcomes at any one time. My own experience of working in a multi-disciplinary team in the 1980s is that this is perfectly possible. It is usually inadequate leadership and professional insecurity which leads to inappropriate professional defensiveness. Multi-disciplinary working, with the appropriate use of well-orientated and skilled support workers can provide a rich mix of skills which gives the service user and their carers more choice and access to a range of expertise.

As the above case study demonstrates, in well functioning teams, perspectives and skills are being shared, so that it is not always obvious who is a community nurse, an occupational therapist (as in the example above) a social worker, psychologist, psychiatrist etc. In the multi-disciplinary team I worked in, people were confident in their professional identity and became increasingly confident and competent in their team identity. Professionalism was sought and attained but not used as a mask to blank out those we were working with, either users, carers or members of the public. Hughes calls this 'an identity of interest' (Hughes, 2001: 75). He points to new professions emerging as alliances grow, with some new features e.g.

- Dual qualifications becoming more common, especially in mental health and learning disability.
- The possibility of a new profession around the assessment, care management and rehabilitation of older people, including those with mental health needs.
- New professions gradually emerging out of the new team services such as YOTs, Sure Start, regulatory services etc.
- The establishment of Connexions building bridges between careers, youth work, education, social work, residential work and after care.

Organisations and professions have an inbuilt tendency to serve their own internal needs. This is no longer acceptable.

The hidden social worker

One of my correspondents during this project, Thurstine Basset, raised the interesting concept of 'the hidden social worker'. Some years ago it would have been unlikely to have seen anybody move from social work into a different organisational setting; chief executives of local authorities, for example, were almost all from a

legal or financial background. Increasingly now, however, people with a social work background are becoming chief executives of Local Authorities, Mental Health Trusts, PCTs, moving into different aspects of government and related organisations such as the LGA.

It is to be hoped that social work with its perspective on the individual and on wider society will have something particular to add.

> *There will be other storms to face. Social work is a difficult and complex task; we will never know enough, or have enough resources, or work for sufficiently competent organisations for the job always to be done as well as the client deserves and the social worker wishes. I do not expect social work to be popular. It deals with people society would usually prefer to forget; unwanted, stigmatised, dependent. It does not do so quietly, but acts as an irritant by standing up for their rights and needs.*
> Sir William Utting, former Chief Social Work Officer, DHSS

Possible pathways

> We shall not cease from exploration
> And the end of all our exploring
> Will be to arrive where we started
> And know the place for the first time.
> T.S. Eliot, *Little Gidding* (1888–1965)

Jane Lewis, in her collection of essays (Allen 2001) remarks on the positive feelings amongst many social work and social care staff when they moved from a health-based organisation to the new social services departments in 1971. It should be said, however, that this was not a universal expression; many people from a mental health background whom I met when I came into social services in 1974, were strongly of the opinion that being under the auspices of an able and energetic medical officer of health gave them an advantage in building up resources which looked at a whole community approach; and certainly when one looks at some of the outstanding medical officers of health, their concept of individual and public health and their mutual congruence were certainly influential in promoting approaches which we would now put under headings such as social inclusion, health promotion etc. (see Dickens and Gilbert, 1979).

Since 1971, organisational approaches have swayed this way and that, but some of the most productive for users and carers, and the most satisfying for social work staff and their colleagues in other disciplines, have been where

Case Example 14

Success in the last chance saloon

A young Asian woman diagnosed with schizophrenia was on the verge of losing her 'last chance' place in a residential unit. Then Marianne Thomas and her team stepped in at the 11th hour to give her more autonomy – and keep her out of hospital

Case notes

Practitioner: Marianne Thomas

Field: Occupational therapist and outreach worker, assertive outreach team, mental health

Location: London

Client: Kashmira Narayan (not her real name) is a 24-year-old Asian woman who has been known to social services for seven years and has a diagnosis of schizophrenia. She also has a history of substance misuse, particularly solvents but other soft drugs also. She has been sectioned on several occasions.

Case History: Four years ago, following another spell under section in hospital, Narayan's family took her back to India to be married – hoping this would cure her illness. It made matters worse. Within months she returned to England without her husband, now estranged, because she was so unwell. She moved back in with her parents but this soon became untenable. The house was overcrowded, added to which Narayan's father, who drank excessively, was verbally and physically abusive towards her. A number of residential placements subsequently failed because Narayan was very chaotic, difficult to engage and challenging, while her solvent misuse escalated, endangering her health. She was also being exploited by a succession of boyfriends.

Dilemma: Narayan, a bright and articulate young woman, was proving very vulnerable to sexual and financial exploitation.

Risk factor: Supporting Narayan to become more independent may lead to more failure and see her sectioned again.

Outcome: Narayan is making slow but sure progress in taking control of her life.

Nine months ago a young Asian woman's hopes of getting a flat or a job seemed a lifetime away. Kashmira Narayan (not her real name), diagnosed with schizophrenia, was challenging her health and social care services to the limit. Already sectioned a number of times, there were serious doubt that she could function healthily in the community. A challenging behaviour unit was emerging as the final option.

On the verge of having her last-chance residential care placement terminated, Narayan received a boost following the creation of a new assertive outreach team. With promised intensive support from the team, the residential home agreed to Narayan staying.

'While an in-patient she was aggressive and verbally abusive,' says outreach worker Marianne Thomas, who began working closely with Narayan. 'When we got to know her, a lot of the outbursts in the ward seemed part of a negative cycle. She'd have leave, would have an outburst, have leave stopped and so on.'

There was also concern about her solvent misuse and that she took cannabis regularly. 'This meant she felt that she was being locked up as 'a naughty girl', and felt she was being punished,' adds Jo Fuller, the assertive outreach team manager. It was explained to Narayan that although she might think that cannabis-taking was part of a 24-year-old's lifestyle, it has a negative effect on her condition.

'Because she felt she was in what seemed to her like prison,' adds Thomas, 'she was reacting to that. We saw our role as focusing on her as a person.' It was a focus that began to change her life. Although looking long-term, Thomas concentrated on getting Narayan established away from hospital and into the residential unit.

'We knew it could all go wrong,' says Fuller, 'but there really was something engaging about her.' Thomas agrees: 'There were a lot of practical things we could help with. She was very vulnerable. There was financial exploitation which was out of her control, which if eliminated would reduce the risk for her.'

Thomas arranged for Narayan's money to be managed by social services. 'She now gets an amount each day, which means that she doesn't have books that people can take and cash,' says Thomas. Although this action could be construed as controlling, Narayan agreed to it and is now relieved at the arrangement: 'It helped her realise what was happening. There was one person she was having a relationship with but who now doesn't want to see her because the money's not there.'

The outreach team work 365 days a year including weekday evenings, making themselves more available for Narayan. 'The big thing for her,' says Thomas, 'was seeing her as a person. Rather than focusing on "are you taking your medication?" we'd go to the hairdressers or go swimming.' Realising that she can work with the team rather than kick against it, Narayan is responding well, particularly as she can see progress, albeit slowly, being made. 'She is attending an adult education class,' says Thomas, 'but still wants that normal life – that job, that flat. That's some way off but it seems a possibility now.'

Thomas, recognising Narayan's fractured relationships with family and boyfriends, focused on building trust. The 'everything up for negotiation' approach, belief in her possibilities for advancement, advocating on her behalf with other services ready to give up on her, and consistency in her life are delivering rewards. 'She's just asked if she can have a mobile phone,' smiles Thomas, 'so that when she's out or stays out she's able to keep in touch. Also she feels confident enough to tell us she's feeling unwell or hearing voices again – I think she knows that if she tells us things, we can work through it and stop her being sent back to hospital. So I think that trust is really working.'

'For years,' adds Fuller, 'she's either been in hospital and contained, or out and been completely chaotic. This is the first time she's been settled for years. And it can still all go wrong – she has a history of things going wrong, after all. But for every month that she's out and managing and coping, that's a positive thing – and all down to positive risk taking.'

For Narayan, having her own flat and a full-time job may still seem a lifetime away. But for now she's living safely in the community and Thomas is exploring the possibility of Narayan taking on some voluntary work for a couple of hours a week. It may be some years before there is light at the end of the tunnel – but at least they're in that tunnel and travelling the right way.

Arguments for risk

- The team were sure that with the right support it would be possible for Narayan to live in the community. Narayan deserved another chance to experience more independence and the improvement in the quality of life that goes with that.
- For the first time in years, Narayan was achieving some stability and building trust in her life and the time was right to make progress on that.
- Although Narayan argued cogently against nurse-injected medication to convince the team that she should use replacement oral medication, she has shown maturity by understanding that she needs some sort of medication and that if the new system fails to work she will resume with the injections.
- Narayan's residential home has worked well with the team despite ambivalence from some care staff about giving Narayan one more chance. This has provided a permanent base for her – adding to the consistency in her life.

Arguments against risk

- Narayan's recent history would indicate the possibility of misusing drugs again. The more she felt she was living a normal life, the more she might be tempted to take drugs – something she considers part of a normal lifestyle. The scale of her solvent misuse had caused worries about possible brain damage, with cannabis also having a negative effect on her condition.
- As Narayan enjoys more independence, there is the possibility that she may cut off contact and revert to her old lifestyle. This may result in her being sectioned again.
- Given the team's open and non-restrictive approach to working with Narayan, she might consider that the team are condoning her actions.
- At her last care plan approach meeting it was agreed, although not without reservation, that rather than a nurse administered system, she would receive replacement oral medication, which, although managed by the staff in her care home, would give Narayan more opportunity to avoid taking it.

Independent comment

The family's arrangement to have Narayan return to India is a typical response when an individual presents delusional and bizarre behaviour, the belief being that local healers can erode the spirits that are causing the behaviour, writes Raj Jhamat. It is also a common response to have a woman married off without fully detailing her mental health difficulty to her future husband and in-laws. This more than often leads to young women being traumatised by abusive in-laws and subjected to domestic violence.

The support Narayan requires appears to have been identified in clinical terms but there is a missing element around independence. Within Asian communities, connections to family and the community are far stronger than those of the white population. Isolation can lead to further mental health difficulties.

At Sahayak befriending service in Kent, we offer support to people rebuilding lives outside of the family. We also seek to build bridges back to the community.

Mental health promotion helps families and community leaders understand the complexity of mental health difficulties and to remove taboos. Gaining the community leaders' support opens up referral channels that would otherwise avoid existing statutory services.

The complex difficulties facing Narayan must be faced by a multi-agency team approach along with support for the family, enabling her to feel secure in her rehabilitation.

Raj Jhamat is a National Schizophrenia Fellowship community mental health worker.

Reprinted by kind permission of *Community Care*, 21–27 March, 2002.

social workers have worked in multi-disciplinary teams, but had strong links with their own profession. Part of the unease currently is to do with some aspects of organisational culture within the NHS – for example, one major trust being criticised by an inner CHI report for focusing on performance targets and its financial deficit rather than clinical governance, clinical outcomes and service planning. It is not reassuring to social work and social care staff to hear one of the apparently leading trusts in the country admitting that it needed 'to give clinical quality as much priority as money and activity'! (see *Health Service Journal*, 15 August 2002: 4). The crisis at Mid Staffordshire Acute General Hospital in 2009 resulted again from an inappropriate concentration on certain targets rather than considering care in an holistic way, including partnership with carers. The possible resurgence and reassertion of a medical model is another cause for concern, and this is ironically more likely in Trusts, allied to medical schools, with a strong emphasis on medical leadership; so much depends on how psychiatry defines itself in the future and educates and trains its practitioners. A recent focus on Spirituality by the Royal College of Psychiatrists (see Cook et al., 2009, and Chapter 9 in this book) is most encouraging.

Links back to the wider social work profession, local government and professional guidance are also crucial; a number of transfers of staff by Local Authorities do not appear to have effectively retained these links and this commissioning strength, so that staff are effectively cut adrift.

> *As a qualified social worker and now as Chief Executive of MIND, I know that social work has been key in developing a broader based and more holistic approach to mental health than was previously the case when it was exclusively in the hands of the medical profession.*
> Richard Brook, former Chief Executive, MIND

Possible routes for social work could be:

1. Social workers as part of integrated teams in mental health trusts or care trusts. This would be an extension of current trends under the Health Act flexibilities. The social work role remains substantially as it has been historically, but there are huge opportunities for enunciating and promoting social perspectives and the value-base of social work as a profession, while at the same time taking on board the perspectives, skills and values of

other professions. Duncan Double, a consultant psychiatrist and honorary senior lecturer with the University of East Anglia, writes cogently of this kind of approach (Double, 2002) and Martin Webber, a social worker/care manager in a community mental health team in the Borough of Kingston-upon-Thames, speaks of the 'invigorating' climate of working in a multi-disciplinary setting (*The Independent*, 25 February 2002).

Gulliver, Peck and Towell's warning in the light of their evaluation of the integration of health and social services in Somerset, is that a focus on structures as opposed to outcomes and how to ensure these, can lead to unreal and unrealised expectations (Gulliver, Peck and Towell, 2002). These caveats around structural change are also there in the debate around the future shape of children's services. Jane Held, Co-chairperson of the ADSS Children and Families Committee, and Director of Camden Social Services in 2002, cautioned that:

> . . . it is crucial to remember that child protection is at the centre of working with kids. It is also everybody's responsibility. If you separate it out and give it to a new agency, it becomes somebody else's responsibility and that magnifies rather than reduces risk.
> Community Care, 29 August, 2002

The tragedy of Baby 'Peter' in Haringey in 2009 demonstrated that some new Children's departments may have been over-dominated by educationalists, with inadequate concentration on child care; and that Ofsted did not have the depth of knowledge of either SSI or CSCI.

This will be a problem for the mental health trusts if they separate themselves from the wider social inclusion agenda and for local authorities if they fail to honour their commitment to mental health in all its manifestations.

Social services departments will need to ensure that there is a champion for social work and social care within the new organisations, and proper commissioning and professional connections maintained and nurtured. In 2009 some local authorities had withdrawn their staff from trust bodies as they felt that the social care/social work agenda was being neglected. Whatever the structures, however, integrated working is essential and inter-professional education at qualification level will also be a necessity.

There are generalised feelings being expressed that the role of social work and that of the Approved Social Worker is not understood or valued. This seems particularly highlighted when social workers are in teams where there is a manager from the Health Services rather than from a social work background – though this is not always the case – much seems to depend on individual managers and their approach to and willingness to understand the social perspective and the role which social work can play.

Social work educator

2. Part of a new unified profession.
The introduction of STR workers and other front-line workers, who will be alongside service users in the way that the latter have expressed a need for, and the many research studies across client groups which have shown an impatience and confusion with the range of different professionals entering people's homes gives some indication that we may be moving towards a single profession. Certainly joint training courses are coming more into vogue, but in the past joint professional awards have not always been given the required recognition, and it is to be seen whether the new organisations are more forthcoming.

One concern would be that the new support workers could become over-professionalised and lose the 'whole person, whole life' approach that has been particularly appreciated by service users. On the other hand, the different professions could lose something in their integration, and so could service users. In a conversation with a nurse manager recently, he told me 'I don't feel the fully generic worker will give the quality and range of experience and skills that users need' (conversation with the author, 2002). This was echoed in a conversation that I had with a social work team, who also felt that the particular professional training, skills and values which the different professions brought, when properly co-ordinated, gave a greater richness to the service users and carers they served.

3. Social workers in primary health care teams.
One of the most beneficial approaches in recent times has been the increasing propensity to place social workers in primary care settings. While this is no panacea, and resources and specialisation create a number of challenges, general practice/primary care is so crucial to the health of the majority of the population that better communication between the professions, increased access for users and carers, and a shared understanding of the benefits of different approaches and perspectives has produced better outcomes for all concerned (see Griffiths, 2010).

I have already quoted the Worcestershire approach (Le Mesurier and Cumella, 2001), and the *Health Service Journal* carried an enlightening article around the approach in Hull (see Banyard et al., 2002: 24–5). In most inner cities, there is a heightened incidence of single-handed general practitioners, which creates additional challenges in terms of communication and resources. Many singleton GPs who I worked with as a practitioner, especially in my role as an ASW, were considerably more problematic to work with than those within a group practice. It is interesting that at least one single-handed GP in Hull is quoted as saying that having a social worker attached was 'like the light at the end of the tunnel'. One can see that the presence of GP attached social workers, alongside the advent of the new primary care workers, will bring increased benefits to the delivery of mental health services.

Ultimately, the great strength of social work as a subject area lies in the sheer scope of the knowledge and experiences it draws upon. But its great weakness also lies in this wide scope, because without careful articulation of its aims and purpose, and a selective approach to deciding which theories best meet these aims and objectives in practice in particular contexts, then social work can seem an ineffective approach to bringing about change in people's lives.

Social work educator

4. The role of the Approved Mental Health Professional.
The role and practice of the ASW was one of the enduring benefits of the 1983 Mental Health Act. Successive Mental Health Act Commission biennial reports and the findings of mental health enquiries have shown the value of these well trained practitioners with a holistic, individual and social systems approach. The independent perspective dates back over the history of mental health services (see Chapter 8 in this book) and is of vital importance.

While both BASW and the ADSS accepted a need for change because of the shifting tectonic plates of society and organisations, all the relevant bodies and all professions saw an essential need to carry forward the skills and perspective of the ASW into the new system. This was most clearly articulated by Margaret Clayton, as Chairperson of the Mental Health Act Commission (see Clayton, 2002).

The British Association of Social Workers, in its response to the consultation on the Draft Mental Health Bill (BASW, 2002: 2) put it:

> It is essential that the official taking on the quasi-judicial element of the present ASW role should be trained to the same standard, should be capable of evaluating the social and environmental aspects of the case, and should above all be demonstrably independent of the health body which was proposing the use of compulsory powers.

Andrew McCulloch, Chief Executive of the Mental Health Foundation, saw the demise of the ASW as a potential loss to users and carers and the judicial system, if the independent perspective, so vital in British justice systems, was lost. The fact that this social work role was defined by statute, praised by independent bodies and colleagues, as well as users and carers, and had a link back with the wider local government agenda, is something that gave social work considerable credibility and prestige, though at times it meant that specialist social workers perhaps came to focus too much on this quasi-judicial role and lost sight of the wider community focus (see below).

> Approved social workers bring a healthy and independent view to the process of sectioning and compulsion ... Approved social workers provide an essential buffer between psychiatrists and individuals at the point of using compulsory powers, as long as ASWs are able to retain their independence.
>
> Richard Brook, former Chief Executive, MIND

The Mental Health Act Commission made it clear that the ASW had a wider role than purely reacting to requests for admission to hospital (Mental Health Act Commission, 2001) and this was echoed by Greg Slay, a Mental Health Practice Development Manager with West Sussex County Council, and a member of BASW's Mental Health Special Interest Group, when he wrote that: 'ASWs also need to be supported and valued in developing that wider role by their employing authority' (Slay, July 2002).

One of the problems BASW saw with the current ASW role was, just as in the case in a great deal of statutory childcare work, ASWs were being pushed into an increasingly functional, though valuable, task and not able to perform their wider therapeutic functions. Dr Double, a consultant psychiatrist, who is part of the Critical Psychiatry Network, and a supporter of social perspectives, sees that:

> ... the case for arguing that such a move could free social workers from the bureaucracy and officialdom of the ASW role to use their knowledge and skills more broadly in working with users and their families, allowing them to return to their traditional emphasis on the social model.
>
> Double, September, 2002

Research is required to ascertain how the broadening of the professional input to the post 2007 APMH role works, and whether social workers have been freed up to return to a more community-focused approach.

5. A return to community work model.

When I was practising as a generic social worker in the 1970s, our office had a community worker. The Barclay Report should have seen an extension of this community approach, but the pressures of statutory work have tended to diminish the availability of social workers to develop community resources.

> The people who will need social care remain however the pieces are moved around the board to try and ensure the best possible delivery of services to them.
>
> ADSS, Review of ADSS Needs, Structures and Resources, June 2002

John Pierson's recent work (Pierson, 2002 and 2009) demonstrates a need for social work and its current local authority host to rediscover this community dimension, and for social workers moving into Health and Social Care settings to promote this perspective.

In all of this, social work needs to feel valued as it gives value to those it works with. The Audit Commission Report (*Recruitment and Retention*, 2002) demonstrates starkly the workforce challenges and how critical a motivated workforce is 'to delivering the reform agenda and improvement of public services' the Government desires (the Audit Commission's Director for Public Services Research, quoted in *The Guardian*, 4 September 2002).

There is a concern that, at a time when social work is probably needed more than ever, it may be overtaken by events. No profession has an inherent right to survive, and while professionalism is always important, professions sometimes put up such walls around them that they are no longer permeable by outside influences, especially by those who use the service.

As a history graduate, I am always acutely aware of the issues around cultural identity and cultural transference. There is, for example, a theory that Anglo-Saxon culture flourished so quickly and profoundly because the Romano-Britons had been able to transfer their cultural achievements to social groups who brought a different, but also rich culture with them, leading to a new and creative cultural landscape. It may be that one of social work's major roles now is to carry the holistic and social perspectives into other settings and enriching those and other professions.

6. Other roles and perspectives
   If there is 'no health without mental health' then the social work, mental health perspective must reach into other areas. Palliative care (see Beresford et al. 2007; Reith and Payne, 2009) is one aspect where the mental health of those using palliative care services, and their carers, will be of prime importance. As we face death – the ultimate existential crisis (see Gilbert, 2008) – our mental well-being is of vital concern.

   In a global environment, international perspective will be of increasing importance (see Lawrence et al. 2009) and the World Health Organisation and World Psychiatric Association are working on bringing differing perspectives together to improve our understanding.

Power and empowerment

The love of liberty is the love of other people, the love of power is the love of ourselves.
William Hazlit (1778–1830)

Only connect ... and human love will be seen at its highest. Live in fragments no longer.
E.M. Forster, *Howard's End*

We need to work with clarity and pride with other professionals. After all, social workers are streets ahead with empowerment, advocacy and consultation, and participation with service users. Nowhere is a person-centred response more obvious ... Surely as professionals, if we truly believe in what we are doing, we will continue to promote and demonstrate such principles.
Margaret Reed, social worker, quoted in Reed, 2002

In multi-disciplinary settings, power relationships are both explicit and opaque. Thompson pinpoints three levels – individual, cultural and structural – with power as the common factor (Thompson, 2009). Relations between users and carers and staff members, or the team as a whole, and relationships between teams, can become corrupted and counterproductive if there are individual power struggles, battles within discourse – language and culture; and class, gender and other structural conflicts.

Unless services are sensitive to power issues then certain groups can see themselves as not just outside an ostensibly helpful system but oppressed by it. This is demonstrated very graphically in the Sainsbury Centre's review of the relationship between mental health services and African and Caribbean communities, *Breaking the Circles of Fear* (SCMH, 2002, see also Sewell, 2008) and issues for women (see e.g. Kohen, 2000). For some groups there are issues around double discrimination, e.g. for black women (see Chantler, 2002) older people, people with learning disabilities (Gilbert, 2006) etc.

Health service professionals are often found, quite rightly, bemoaning the discrimination of people experiencing mental distress, by other members of the community. But professionals themselves put up 'them and us' barriers. Rachel Perkins, Clinical Director of Adult Mental Health Services for the South West London and St. George's Mental Health NHS Trust, writing from the perspective 'of both a provider and a recipient of mental health services', states that the first requirement of helping 'people rebuild their lives' is 'to be able to form relationships with our clients that foster and maintain hope'. To do this, professionals need to be able to:

- Value the person for who they are.
- Believe in their worth.
- Listen to and heed what they say.
- Believe in the authenticity of their experiences.
- Accept and actively explore these experiences.
- See and have confidence in their skills, abilities and potential.
- Tolerate uncertainty about the future.
- See problems and setbacks as part of the recovery process.

The next requirement is to help people to make sense of what has happened and in taking back control. This involves helping people to:

- Reach an understanding of what has happened to them that makes sense to them and allows the possibility of growth and development.
- Mobilise their internal resources, especially their confidence and self-belief, and recognise their skills and ambitions.
- Gain control over their problems and to decide what they want to do in their life.

The third aspect is to enable people to access the roles, relationships and activities that are important to them, and the resources and support they need to pursue them. This involves providing assistance and support to:

- Maintain existing activities and relationships.
- Reduce the barriers that prevent people from accessing new things they want to do, and gain access to the material resources and opportunities that are their right.

Perkins ends by saying that:

> *Most of all, practitioners must learn from those whom they serve ... Perhaps the real challenge is to move towards a position where we put our expertise at the disposal of service users, rather than making decisions for them and doing to them.*
>
> Perkins, 2002, see also McPherson in O'Hara, 2009

> *An important and frequently very moving aspect of the user's voice is not uncommonly the experience of 'treatment' as some form of attack on the symptoms rather than assistance with the difficulties they are trying to negotiate. I am convinced that one of the reasons behind this disparity is a continuing failure to set patients' [sic] symptoms, difficulties and disabilities within their social context.*
>
> consultant psychiatrist

So much of the underlying attribute of the 'skilled helper' is that of an ability to use professional authority where appropriate, but eschew the easy recourse to the use of power. The use of power can never be neutral, while one person accrues power to themselves they inevitably remove power from other people.

> *For many black and minority ethnic mental health service users, a social worker represents a mental health professional who will reach out to build a relationship. The relationship is intended to ensure that the service user can get what they need (accommodation, benefits, work) rather than the social worker using the relationship to broker the right to do something to the service user. Black and minority ethnic people feel they have suffered too long at the hands of those determined to do things **to** them.*
>
> SSI Inspector, now Director of Social Care for a Mental Health Trust

I was struck, when reading Kay Redfield Jamison's autobiography, *An Unquiet Mind* (Jamison, 1995) by how she describes her psychiatrist. Jamison herself is a professor of psychiatry at the John Hopkins University School of Medicine, and experienced bouts of extreme and life-threatening manic depression. Jamison is very frank about her fight against the taking of Lithium to control her bi-polar mood swings, a reluctance based on a number of considerations, all of which were understood by her psychiatrist but, as she describes him, he was:

> *Very tough, as well as very kind, and even though he understood much more than anyone how much I felt I was losing – in energy, vivacity and originality – by taking medication, he never was seduced into losing sight of the overall perspective of how costly, damaging, and life-threatening my illness was. He was at ease with ambiguity, had a comfort with complexity, and was able to be decisive in the midst of chaos and uncertainty. He treated me with respect, a decisive professionalism, with an unshakeable belief in my ability to get well, compete and make a difference.*
>
> Jamison, 1997: 88

That ability to balance professionalism with the personal, complexity with a stable and clear-sighted view of the long-term goals, and authority without the abuse of power, is something that is absolutely vital for the practitioner and for the manager. As I said before, a great many of the issues for practitioners are also there for managers at whatever level. Work by Jim Collins (Collins, 2001, see also Goffee and Jones, 2006) focuses on what he calls 'level 5' leadership, which is essentially about the humility of great leaders who channel their ego needs into the greater good of the organisation, rather than into their own ambitions.

It is sometimes easier to get at these issues through literature or film. For me, the American writer, Ursula Le Guin, has an amazing facility for describing and encapsulating the individual's need to leave the world a better place than when they found it, without abusing their gifts or position, and without encroaching on the life and liberty of other people inappropriately. In *The Lathe of Heaven*, George Orr's ability to dream different realities is manipulated by his therapist, Haber. Haber appears powerful but:

> *The big man was like an onion, slip off layer after layer of personality, belief, response, infinitely as layers, no end to them, no centre to him. Nowhere that he ever stopped, had to stop, had to say here I stay! No being, only layers.*
>
> Le Guin, 1971: 80

Figure 33: The long journey out of the institutions for mental health services: Implications for leadership.

Approach to services	Theory base	View of people	Delivery systems	Roles	Knowledge/power locus	Leadership approaches
1840s–1970s: Segregated institutional care	Medical treatments Custodial and/or Asylum based	Lunatics cases, patients	Fixed sites: closed hospitals, asylums	Doctors, nurses, clergy, lay visitors	Doctor knows best	Charismatic Morally based Imperial Directorial and rigid Uni-professional reporting (medicine, nursing) Deeply hierarchical Containment and experimental-treatment focused
1980s–present day Community care	Multi-professional/ multi-disciplinary care and cure Organised duality of 'health' and 'social' care interventions	Clients and service users	Multi-disciplinary community teams, some hospitals, some cross sector partnerships, some third sector provision	Multi-disciplinary professionals	Professional knows best Manager knows best	Multi-disciplinary team based Translocational-management across health and social care Heroic-transformational style of change Ethics of compassion towards service users Activity and output focused
Emerging future: Recovery, personalisation and self directed support	Overarching Social model of disability Recovery approach	People/citizens: with rights, control, opportunities and entitlements	Emerging forums of new service across statutory, voluntary, user-led and private sectors. More diverse sources of support. More evidence-based treatments offered where indicated	Educators Advocates Peer-support workers Evidence-based practitioners	Co-production of expertise between person and service provider	Customer/consumer leadership Leadership at points within networks across sectors Host, facilitator and mentoring leadership Public service leadership emphasis demonstrating humanistic values Ethics or rights Governance driven/outcomes focused

Orr initially trusts Haber because he sees him as 'not an evil man. He means well', but what Orr objected to is Haber's 'using me as *an instrument, a means* – even if his ends are good' (p44, my emphasis). Orr begins to feel that the therapist is without a centre, without integrity 'The doctor was not, he thought, really sure that anyone else existed, and wanted to prove that they did by helping them' (p27).

In the end, Haber takes over the dreaming from Orr, in order to accelerate the move towards a perfect world as Orr sees it. But because Orr has no core to his own being, his dreams, far from creating a new reality, completely undo any kind of reality, creating a world which is literally insane and unbound.

Likewise, in the Earthsea Quartet, in the third book, *The Farthest Shore*, the desire of one man who has had magical powers to do good, but has now abrogated to himself the ambition to cheat death, is draining all life and colour and energy from the world around him. When the hero, Ged, confronts the man who is now neither dead nor alive, he challenges him that he sold everything to save himself, but now 'you have no self. You have given everything for nothing'. To try and gain everything he has created a nothingness, as did Haber with his empty dreams of ambition. Ged goes on to say:

> *And so now you seek to draw the world to you, all that light and life you lost, to fill up your nothingness. But it cannot be filled. Not all the songs of earth, nor all the stars of heaven, could fill your emptiness.*
>
> *The Farthest Shore*, 1973: 463

When Ged asks the other man what life is, the other's response is 'power'; and again in the answer to 'what is love?' again, he gives the answer 'power'.

To close the door between the world of the dead and world of the living, and to make it whole again, Ged has to sacrifice all his own powers for the common good.

> *Social workers, along with others, including service user groups, have been part of a strong coalition that has challenged traditional stereotypes in mental health. This has led to a greater emphasis on rights and more quality being seen in the relationships within mental health work as far as service users are concerned.*
>
> Richard Brook

Such things are repeated in Le Guin's extraordinary study of individuals and social systems – *The Dispossessed*. The physicist, Shevek, lives on a world without any explicit power structures, part of a group of people who emigrated from the host world where Le Guin depicts capitalist and totalitarian systems. But the community set up without power structures has been corrupted by a group who suppress ideas by ignoring them, by refusing to think, refusing to change. As Shevek's friend points out, the person who is suppressing his radical ideas:

> *. . . has power over you. Where does he get it from? Not from vested authority, there isn't any. Not from intellectual excellence, he hasn't any. He gets it from the innate cowardice of the average human mind. Public opinion! That's the power structure he's part of, and knows how to use. The unadmitted inadmissible government that rules the Odonian society by stifling the individual mind.*
>
> Le Guin, 1974: 142

Shevek faces this by undertaking a personal journey of self discovery and using his own centredness and integrity as a way of making new connections with people and helping them to confront themselves, not always successfully. At the end, in a common theme for Le Guin, he returns to where he started. Like the social worker who uses their own integrity to get alongside other people in distress: 'he had not brought anything. His hands were empty, as they had always been' (p319). Social workers create value with 'empty hands'. We do not have the prescription pad or the needle, we have to forge an ethos of hope from combining head and heart, from being professional and doing human.

Creating value

> *To a large extent, we're the keepers of each other's stories, and the shape of these stories has unfolded in part from our interwoven accounts. Human beings don't only search for meanings, they are themselves units of meaning; but we can mean something only within the fabric of larger significations.*
>
> Eva Hoffman, *Lost in Translation*, 1989: 279

> *It is time for social work to recover its ambition as an organised and cohesive force for good in society.*
>
> Bill Utting, former Chief Inspector, SSI, 2002

> *I have striven not to laugh at human actions, not to weep at them, nor to hate them, but to understand them.*
>
> Benedict Spinoza, born 1632

> *Everyone is interesting who will tell the truth about him (or her) self.*
>
> Quentin Crisp (quoted in Beresford) 2002

Running a half marathon around Wolverhampton I got into a conversation with a

Figure 34: The individual and the organisation

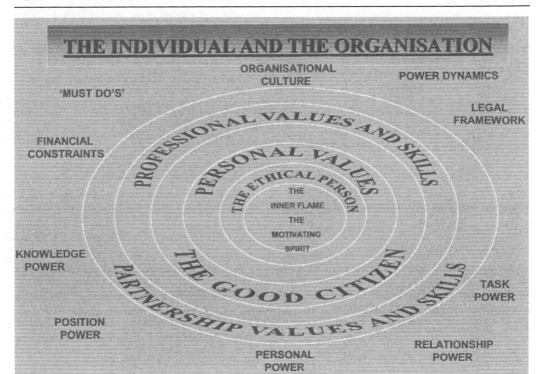

fellow club member who is an engineer. 'I don't envy you guys,' he commented, 'we're both in the business of risk, but when I am considering the strength of steel, I know what pressure I can put it under, what weights and tensions it will bear, before it breaks. You are dealing with human beings, who knows when they will break, whether it's at the point of greatest pressure, or when the pressure has seemingly been removed, and then some small straw causes the human structure to fracture. And at the end of the day, if you choose to intervene or not to do so, you are open to blame and very little praise'. Just as mental distress and mental ill-health is something that needs to be experienced at some level to gain a real insight (see O'Hara, 2009), though profound empathy can almost get there, so social work is a calling which needs to be experienced to gain an insight into its complexity. When I was a trainee social worker and social worker in an area office, we shadowed medical and nursing colleagues and the GP Trainee Scheme sent its doctors to shadow social services staff. This was enormously beneficial in long-term understanding and relationship building. I

directly experienced lives being saved through the understanding that was built up at this level.

In an article in *Community Care* (7 March 2002) a medical student shadowed social workers in Sheffield:

> *My view totally changed when I worked with social workers. I have a lot of respect for those doing the job. It is not a 9–5 job – it offers a 24-hour 7-day-a-week service. It's hard to switch off from some of the stuff they deal with when they go home. It takes a certain type of person to do it'. It certainly does!*

All the evidence from research, from talking to users and carers, from reading autobiographies like Kay Redfield Jamison's, tells us that people experiencing mental distress and mental illness, of whatever type, but especially that which is enduring or cyclical, require people of great integrity, sensitivity, resilience, skill and 'stickability' to work with and stay with those who are in Swinton's words 'hanging on' (Swinton, 2001).

As one of the most pertinent research studies demonstrates, that in Westminster, where many people were living in very diminished environments, MacDonald and Sheldon assert 'The role of specialist social workers was obviously pivotal in the system of care. They both arranged for services, and were a service *themselves*'. (An awkward principle for those who speak and write about 'services', as if these were always 'things'.) In this study, the social services staff emerged as individuals to be relied upon to provide emotional support and counselling, for a range of practical services and for their well-respected 'advocacy' function. This appears to have been carried out with a distinctive friendliness, openness and professionalism which, for the majority of respondents, was thought to be the best thing about the help they received' (MacDonald and Sheldon, 1997: 51).

Professor Peter Beresford of Brunel University, and who describes himself as a long-term user of mental health services, in a recent article speaks of, in our need to encourage care in communities, a need to focus on language and meaning; ourselves and our identities – keeping in touch with who we actually are; and between social settings and individuals (Beresford, 2002).

The language of distance, of dispossession, of dichotomy are well developed in our society. We prefer to talk about 'them' and 'us' rather than 'us' and 'us'. As Ian McPherson, head of the Government's National Mental Health Development Unit, points out, he had hoped, when he became a mental health professional, to draw on his experience to good effect, but was told that there were professionals and service users and never the twain should meet on common ground (see O'Hara, 2009). In an article in *The Observer* (1 September 2002) a feature on stress at work was very keen to emphasise that this was social distress and not mental distress, inviting us to think that if we suffer from mental distress, we don't need to identify with people who experience a mental illness. So much healthier are those people who took part in the recent exhibition where stories of well-known people exemplified the normality of moving through different states and stages of life. As Beresford puts it:

I am simply saying that if we start by seeking to understand and be honest about ourselves to ourselves, we may well be able to be more understanding and less judgemental of others and of madness and distress. What begins as a denial of who we are ends up as a denial of the rights of others to be who they are, just as surely as what

begins as the burning of books ends with the burning of people. We must start with ourselves.
Beresford, February 2002: 29, my emphasis

It is social work and social workers who are at the margins, walking the boundaries of the forgotten lands with forgotten people; raising their voices for the dispossessed; valuing the unvalued; combating stigma for those we stigmatise; working to empower those who are disempowered (see Figure 35).

The philosopher, William James, once wrote that he had 'done with great things and big things, great institutions and big successes, and I am for those tiny invisible molecular moral forces that work from individual to individual, creeping through the crannies of the world like so many rootlets, or like the capillary oozing of water . . .' Social work works to empower and transform (see Payne, 2002) and fight for justice for individuals and social justice; and this is especially pertinent in the role of the APMH and the area where the individual collides with the law.

Social workers have been part of the recognition that Mental Health is not just about hospital and medication but about care, support, rights and opportunities to be citizens on an equal basis.
Richard Brook

Social work is about recognising the individuality and innate dignity of each person, connecting with them, seeing the whole person in the context of their past and future aspirations, their family and neighbourhood, their community and connections. It is about building on integrity and creating trust and meaning, listening to and walking with, comprehending culture, race and creed, and engaging with the lived experience.

We are all complex individuals, living in a complex world (see Basset and Stickley, 2010). This complexity requires a response which is both direct and sophisticated. These skills are even more imperative today when we seem to be, like Ernest Shackleton and his team of Antarctic explorers, sailing out into the unknown and striding along uncharted shores. The historian, David Cannadine (Cannadine, 2002) speaks of a history of economics and sociology, of causes and explanation, developing into a history of psychology and anthropology, a cultural approach to history around meaning and understanding. Patricia Shaw in her *Changing Conversations in Organisations* (Shaw, 2002) speaks of horizons being so complex that 'we must

Figure 35: Walking the boundaries to add value

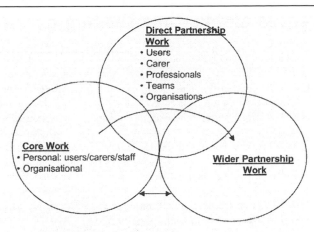

The Professional / Manager
has to walk the boundaries
to achieve positive change

Direct Partnership Work
• Users
• Carer
• Professionals
• Teams
• Organisations

Core Work
• Personal: users/carers/staff
• Organisational

Wider Partnership Work

Personal

• Acting with integrity
• Aiding recovery
• Ensuring safety
• Exercising discernment
• Integration past, present and future
• Developing new skills
• Assisting team formation

Organisational

• Maintaining the overall vision
• Hitting targets and P.I.s
• Reaching for wider corporate and L.S.P. goals
• Reconciling competing aims and targets
• Reaching out to wider coalition and partnership building

recognise that we are shaping the evolving meaning of living experience as an ongoing creative social endeavour. Our present sense-making acts back to reshape the meaning of the past which changes the possible meaning of the future – lively enquiry amidst diversity is key. We can never be in control and need to rethink what it means to be in charge' (Shaw, 2002, see also Parton and O'Byrne, 2000: Chap. 1).

When one looks at Daniel Goleman's work on leadership, one sees that his components of emotional intelligence at work: self-awareness, self-regulation, motivation, empathy and social skill (Goleman, 1998) speak very much to what social work is about. We are all explorers now of meaning, of diversity, of boundaries, of hope and aspiration.

Although the 2009 Government White Paper: *Shaping the Future of Care Together* (2009), is mainly focused on older persons, the *New*

Horizons document, out for consultation at the time of writing, echoes in its broad vision the partnership *Vision for 2015* approach set out by local authority, health and voluntary sector partners (SCMH et al., 2006). The accent is very much on inclusion, integration, hope and a partnership between those who use services and those who provide them.

As one service user put it, 'My social worker picked up that I was ready to explore sort of what was happening to me' (quoted in *Mental Health Foundation*, 2002).

Although the cross-party support for the recommendations of the Social Work TaskForce (DoH/DCSF, 2009) is encouraging we don't yet know the future for social work, so in the words of Dag Hammarskjold 'For all that has been – Thanks! To all that shall be – Yes!' (*Markings*, 1964).

References and Further Reading

Aaron, M. (2008) Spirituality, The Heart of Caring. *A Life in the Day*, 12: 4, 24–6.

Adair, J. (1973) *Action-Centred Leadership*. London: McGraw-Hill.

Adair, J. (1983) *Effective Leadership*. Aldershot: Gower.

Adair, J. (1986) *Effective Leadership*. Aldershot: Gower.

Adair, J. (1987) *Effective Teambuilding*. London: Pan.

ADSS/NIMHE (Gilbert, P. and Joannides, D.) (2003) *Positive Approaches to the Integration of Health and Social Care in Mental Health Services*. Leeds: National Institute for Mental Health in England.

Ahmed, M. (2009) Should I Pray or Should I Go? *Community Care*, 1 October 16–17.

Alban-Metcalfe, J. and Alimo-Metcalfe, B. (2009a) Engaging Leadership Part 1: Competences Are Like Brighton Pier. *The International Journal of Leadership in Public Services*, 5: 1, 10–18.

Alban-Metcalfe, J. and Alimo-Metcalfe, B. (2009b) Engaging Leadership Part 2: an Integrated Model of Leadership Development. *The International Journal of Leadership in Public Services*, 5: 2.

Alcock, P. (2008) *Social Policy in Britain*, 3rd edn. Basingstoke: Palgrave Macmillan.

Alford, J. (1998) A Public Management Road Less Travelled: Clients as Co-Producers of Public Services. *Australian Journal of Public Administration*, 57: 4, 128–37.

Allan, C. (2006a) *Poppy Shakespeare*. London: Bloomsbury.

Allan, C. (2006b) Defining Moment. *Society Guardian*, 19 April.

Allan, C. (2009a) My Brilliant Survival Guide. *Society Guardian*, 14 January 1–3.

Allan, C. (2009b) Is the Truth Out There? It Depends Who You Believe. *Society Guardian*, 6 May 6.

Allen, I. (Ed.) (2001) *Social Care and Health: A New Deal?* London: Policy Studies Institute/University of Westminster.

Allen, R., Gilbert, P. and Onyett, S. (2009) *Leadership: for Personalisation and Social Inclusion in Mental Heath*. London: Social Care Institute for Excellence. Position Paper 27, Nov. 2009.

Allott, P. and Loganathan, L. (2002) *Discovering Hope for Recovery from a British Perspective: A Review of a Sample of Recovery Literature, Implications for Practice and Systems Change*. Birmingham: West Midlands Partnerships for Mental Health.

Appignanesi, L. (2008) *Mad, Bad and Sad: A History of Women and the Mind Doctors from 1800 to the Present*. London: Virago Press.

Arif, Z. (2002) *Islam and Identity Among British Pakistani Youth*. Keele University, BSc Dissertation.

Aris, S.J. and Gilbert, P. (2007) Organisation Health: Engaging The Heart of The Organisation, in Coyte, M.E., Gilbert. P. and Nicholls, V. (2007) *Spirituality, Values and Mental Health: Jewels for the Journey*. London: Jessica Kingsley.

Armstrong, K. (2009) *The Case for God: What Religion Really Means*. London: The Bodley Head.

Audit Commission (2002) *Report to the House of Commons Health Select Committee on Social Care*. London: Audit Commission.

Bachrach, L. (1997) Lessons from the American Experience in Providing Community-Based Services. In: Leff, J. (Ed.) *Care in the Community: Illusion or Reality?* Chichester: Wiley.

Bailey, D. (Ed.) (2000) *At the Core of Mental Health*. Brighton: Pavilion.

Bainbridge, M. (2002) Carers are People Too. *Mental Health Today*. June.

Bamber, C. (2001) Modernising Crisis Services: What do Users Want from 24-hour Services? *The Mental Health Review*. 6: 1, March.

Bamford, T. (1982) *Managing Social Work*, London: Tavistock/Methuen.

Bamford, T. (2000) *Integrated Health and Social Care in Northern Ireland: Myth and Reality*. Paper for ADSS Seminar, August.

Banks, S. (1995) *Ethics and Values in Social Work*. London: Macmillan.

Banyard, R. et al. (2002) Social Skills. *Health Service Journal*. 29 August.

Barber, J. (2009) *Handbook of Spiritual Care in Mental Illness*. Birmingham: Birmingham, and Solihull Mental Health Foundation Trust.

Barber, P., Brown, R. and Martin, D. (2009). *Mental Health Law in England and Wales: A Guide for Mental Health Professionals.* Exeter: Learning Matters.

Barclay Report (1982) *Social Workers: Their Roles and Tasks.* London: NISW.

Barnes, D. and Brandon, T. with Webb, T. (2000) *Independent Specialist Advocacy in England and Wales: Recommendations for Good Practice.* University of Durham Centre for Applied Social Studies.

Barnes, M. et al. (2008) *Designing Citizen-centred Governance.* York: Joseph Rowntree Foundation.

Bartlett, P. and Wright, D. (Eds) (1999) *Outside the Walls of the Asylum: The History of Care in the Community 1750–2000.* London: The Athlone Press.

Bartley, M. (2006) *Capability and Resilience: Beating the Odds.* ESRC, available on line at http://www.ucl.ac.uk/capabilityandresilience/ (Accessed 19/08/2009).

Basset, T. and Stickley, T. (2010, forthcoming) *Voices of Experience.* Oxford: Blackwell/Wiley.

Bates, P. (2008) Connecting with Communities. Module 6, in Forrest, S. and Bradstreet, S. (2008) *Realising Recovery Learning Materials.* Scottish Recovery Network and NHS Education for Scotland.

Bates, P. (Ed.) (2002) *Working for Inclusion: Making Social Inclusion a Reality for People with Severe Mental Health Problems.* London: Sainsbury Centre for Mental Health.

Bates, P. and Gilbert, P. (2008) 'I wanna tell you a story': Leaders as Storytellers. *The International Journal of Leadership in Public Services,* 4: 2, 4–9.

Bates, P. Developing Socially Inclusive Practice: Module 6, in Basset, T., Lindley, P. and Barton, R. (2005, revised 2007) *The Ten Essential Shared Capabilities: Learning Pack for Mental Health Practic.,* London: NHS University.

Bauman, Z. (1998) *Globalisation: The Human Consequences.* Cambridge, Polity Press.

Bauman, Z. (2007a) *Liquid Times: Living in an Age of Uncertainty.* Cambridge: Polity Press.

Bauman, Z. (2007b) *Consuming Life.* Cambridge: Polity Press.

Behan, D. and Loft, L. (1999) Primary Care Groups: A Social Services Perspective. *Managing Community Care,* 7: 2.

Bell, A. and Lindley, P. (2005) *Beyond the Water Towers: The Unfinished Revolution in Mental Health Services 1985–2005.* London: Sainsbury Centre for Mental Health.

Benedict of Nursia (circa. AD 540) Translation Fry T. (Ed.) (1982) *The Rule of St. Benedict in English.* Minnesota: The Liturgical Press.

Bennett, J. (2009) Black and Minority Ethnic Issues, in Brooker, C. and Repper, J. (2009) *Mental Health: From Policy to Practice.* London: Churchill Livingstone/Elsevier.

Beresford, P. (2002a) Making User Involvement. *Professional Social Work.* June.

Beresford, P. (2002b) Encouraging Caring Communities. *Mental Health Today.* February.

Beresford, P. (2003) *It's Our Lives: A Short Theory of Knowledge, Distance and Experience.* London: Citizen Press.

Beresford, P. (2005) Social Approaches to Madness and Distress, in Tew, J. (Ed.) (2005) *Social Perspectives in Mental Health.* London: Jessica Kingsley.

Beresford, P. (2007) *The Changing Roles and Tasks of Social Work From Service Users' Perspectives: A Literature-Informed Discussion Paper.* London: Shaping Our Lives National User Network.

Beresford, P., Adshead, L. and Croft, S. (2007) *Social Work, Palliative Care and Service Users: Making Life Possible.* Philadelphia: Jessica Kingsley.

Biestek, F. (1961) *The Casework Relationship.* London: Allen & Unwin.

Biestek, F. (1976) *The Casework Relationship,* London, George Allen & Unwin (originally Published in 1957 by The Loyola University Press).

Bird, A. and Wooster, E. (2008) Personalise This! *Open Mind,* 153, September/October. Blackwell Press.

Boardman, J., Griffin, J. and Murray, O. (1986) *The Oxford History of The Classical World.* Oxford: Oxford University Press.

Bodil Karlsson, S. (2009) Schizophrenic or Occult Harassed? A Narrative Study of an Autobiographical Text about Auditory and Visual Hallucinations. *Qualitative Social Work,* 8: 1, 83–100.

Bogg, D. (2008) *The Integration of Mental Health Social Work and The NHS.* Exeter: Learning Matters.

Bolam, S., Carr, S. and Gilbert, P. (2010 Forthcoming) Learning from Experts by Experience: The Jersey partnership perspective, *The International Journal of Leadership in Public Services*

Boviard, T. (2007) *Beyond Engagement and Participation: User and Community Co-Production of Services.* Carnegie UK Trust.

Boyle, D., Clark, S. and Burns, S. (2006) *Hidden Work: Co-Production by People Outside Paid Employment*. York: Joseph Rowntree Foundation.

Bracken, P. and Thomas, P. (2005) *Postpsychiatry: Mental Health in A Postmodern World*. Oxford: Oxford University Press.

Braye, S. and Preston-Shoot, M. (1995) *Empowering Practice in Social Care*. Buckingham, Open University Press.

Brayne, H. and Martin, G. (1999) *Law for Social Workers*. 6th edn. London: Blackstone.

Brechin, A., Brown, H. and Eby, M. (Eds) (2000) *Critical Practice in Health and Social Care*. London: Sage/Open University Press.

Brewin, M. (1996) *Respectful Privacy, Dignity and Religious and Cultural Beliefs: The Needs of Patients From Different Ethnic Backgrounds*. Bath Health Promotion Unit/Wiltshire Health Authority.

Brindle, D. (2008) A Positive Spin on Mental Health. *Society Guardian*, 15th Oct.

British Association of Social Workers (1975, Amended 1986) *A Code of Ethics for Social Work*, BASW.

British Association of Social Workers (1977) *The Social Work Task*. Birmingham: BASWA.

British Association of Social Workers (2002) *Response to The Consultation on The Draft Mental Health Bill*. BASW.

British Association of Social Workers (2002, revised) *The Code of Ethics for Social Workers*, BASW.

Brooker, C. and Repper, J. (2009) *Mental Health: From Policy to Practice*. London: Churchill Livingstone/Elsevier.

Brooks, R. (Ed.) (2007) *Public Services at The Crossroads: Executive Summary*. London: Institute for Public Policy Research.

Brown, R. and Barber, P. (2008) *The Social Worker's Guide to The Mental Capacity Act 2005*. Exeter: Learning Matters.

Bucknall, B. (1981) *Ursula K. Le Guin*. New York: Frederick Ungar.

Bunting, M. (2005) *Willing Slaves: How The Overwork Culture is Ruling Our Lives*. London: Harper Perennial.

Burk, R. and Cooper, C. (Eds) (2000) *The Organisation in Crisis: Downsizing, Restructuring and Privatisation*. Oxford: Blackwell.

Burke, J. (2009) Divided Poland Falls Out Over Solidarity. *The Observer*, 31 May, 2009, 26–7.

Burleigh, M. (2006) *Sacred Causes: Religion and Politics From The European Dictators to Al Qaeda*. London: Harper Press.

Burleigh. M. (2006) *Earthly Powers: Religion and Politics in Europe From The Enlightenment to The Great War*. London: Harper Perennial.

Butler, A. and Pritchard, C. (1983) *Social Work and Mental Illness*. London: Macmillan.

Butler, I. and Drakeford, M. (2005) *Scandal, Social Policy and Social Welfare*. Bristol: Policy Press.

Butrym, Z. (1976) *The Nature of Social Work*. London: Macmillan.

Cable, V. (2009) *The Storm: The World Economic Crisis and What It Means*. London: Atlantic Books.

Campbell, J. and Mclaughlin, J. (2000) The Joined up Management of Adult Health and Social Care Services in Northern Ireland. *Managing Community Care*, 8: 5.

Campbell, J. and Oliver, M. (1996) *Disability Politics: Understanding Our Past, Changing Our Future*. London: Routledge.

Campbell, P. (1996) The History of The User Movement, in Heller, T. et al. (Eds) *Mental Health Matters*. Basingstoke: Macmillan.

Cannadine, D. (Ed.) (2002) *What is History Now?* Basingstoke: Palgrave Macmillan.

Canda, E. and Furman, L. (1999) *Spiritual Diversity in Social Work Practice: The Heart of Helping*. New York: The Free Press.

Carlisle, J. (2009) Women and Mental Health, in Brooker, C. and Repper, J. (2009) *Mental Health: From Policy to Practice*. London: Churchill Livingstone/Elsevier.

Carr, S. (2004) *Has Service User Participation Made a Difference to Social Care Services?* Bristol: Policy Press.

Carr, S. (2008) *Personalisation: A Rough Guide*. London: SCIE.

Carr, S. and Robbins, D. (2009) *SCIE Research Briefing 20: The Implementation of Individual Budget Schemes in Adult Social Care*. London: SCIE.

Carrier, J. and Kendall, I. (1997) Evolution of Policy, in Leff, J. (Ed.) *Care in The Community: Illusion or Reality?* Chichester: Wiley.

Cassam, E. and Gupta, H. (1992) *Quality Assurance for Social Care Agencies*. Harlow, Longman.

CCETSW (2000) *Guidance on The Implementation of Assuring Quality for Mental Health Social Work*. London CCETSW.

Challis, D. et al. (1990) *Case Management in Social and Health Care*. Canterbury: University of Kent Personal Social Services Research Unit.

Chantler, K. (2002) The Invisibility of Black Women in Mental Health Services. *The Mental Health Review*, 7: 1, March.

Cherish, B.U. (2009) *The Auschwitz Kommandant: A Daughter's Search for The Father She Never Knew.* London: The History Press.

Clark, C. and Lapsley, I. (Eds) (1996) *Planning and Costing Community Care.* Edinburgh: Jessica Kingsley.

Clarke, J. (Ed.) (1993) *A Crisis in Care? Challenges to Social Work.* Buckingham, Open University/SAGE.

Clayton, M. (2002) Valued Beyond Doubt. *Community Care,* 23rd May.

Coldham, T. and Spandler, H. (2005) Making Choices and Taking Control. *Openmind,* 132, 18–19.

Coleman, R. (1998) *The Politics of The Madhouse.* Gloucester: Handsell Publishing.

Coleman, R. (1999) *Recovery: an Alien Concept.* Gloucester: Hansell Publishing.

Collins, J. (2001) *Good to Great.* London: Random House.

Collins, J. (2009) *How the Mighty Fall,* London: Random House.

Collins, J. and Porras, J. (2000) *Built to Last: Successful Habits of Visionary Companies.* 3rd edn. London: Random House.

Commission for Health, Audit and Inspection (2005) *Count Me In: Results for The National Census of In-Patients in Mental Health Hospitals and Facilities in England and Wales.* CHAI.

Commission for Healthcare Regulatory Excellence (2008b) *Learning About Sexual Boundaries Between Healthcare Professionals and Patients: A Report on Education and Training.* London: CHRE.

Commission on The Social Determinants of Health (2008) *Closing The Gap in a Generation: Health Equity Through Action on The Social Determinants of Health. Final Report of The Commission on Social Determinants of Health,* Geneva: WHO.

Connolly, K. (2009) Kampusch: 'I May Be Free But I'm Still A Prisoner'. *The Observer,* 23 August 29.

Cook, C., Powell, A. and Sims, A. (Eds.) (2009) *Spirituality and Psychiatry.* London: Royal College of Psychiatrists.

Cooper, A. (2002) Keeping Our Heads: Preserving Therapeutic Values in A Time of Change. *Journal of Social Work Practice,* 6: 1.

Cooper, C.L. and Makin, P. (1984) *Psychology for Managers,* 2nd edn. Trowbridge, The British Psychological Society and Macmillan.

Cope, R. (1989) The Compulsory Detention of Afro-Caribbeans Under The Mental Health Act. *New Community,* 15: 3, 343–56.

Copsey, N. (1997) *Keeping Faith: The Provision of Community Health Services Within a Multi-Faith Context.* The Sainsbury Centre for Mental Health.

Copsey, N. (2001) *Forward in Faith: an Experiment in Building Bridges Between Ethnic Communities and Mental Health Services in East London.* Sainsbury Centre for Mental Health.

Cormack, D. (1988) *Team Spirit.* MARC.

Coulshed, V. (1988) *Social Work Practice: an Introduction.* London: Macmillan.

Cornah, D. (2006) *The Impact of Spirituality on Mental Health: A Literature Review of the Evidence.* London: Mental Health Foundation.

Cotter, J.P. (1990) What Leaders Really do. *Harvard Business Review,* May/June.

Coulshed, V. and Orme, J. (1998) *Social Work Practice.* 3rd edn. London: Macmillan.

Covey, S. (1992) *Principle-Centred Leadership.* London: Simon and Schuster.

Cox, J., Campbell, A. and Fulford, K.W. (2007) *Medicine of The Person: Faith, Science and Values in Health Care Provision.* London: Jessica Kingsley.

Coyte, M., Gilbert, P. and Nicholls, V. (Eds) (2007) *Spirituality, Values and Mental Health: Jewels for The Journey.* London: Jessica Kingsley.

Croydon Mind (2003) *Hard to Believe,* Croydon: Croydon Mind.

Crump, H. (2009) 'What's In A Name? PCT Branding Has a Long Way to Go. *Health Service Journal,* 30 July.

CSIP/Eastern Development Centre (2009) *Whole Life Workbook.* Colchester: Easter Development Centre.

CSIP/Rcpsych/SCIE (2007) *A Common Purpose: Recovery in Future Mental Health Services.* Joint position paper. London: SCIE.

Croydon Mind (2005) *Hard to Believe,* DVD.

Culliford, L. (2009) Taking a Spiritual History. *Whole Life Handbook.* Eastern Development Centre.

Culliford, L. and Eagger, S. (2009) Assessing Spiritual Needs, in Cook, C., Powell, A. and Sims, A. *Spiritually and Psychiatry.* London: Royal College of Psychiatrists.

Cummins, J. and Miller, C. (2007) *Co-Production, Social Capital and Service Effectiveness.* London: OPM.

Davies, M. (1981) *The Essential Social Worker.* London: Heinemann Educational/Community Care.

Davies, M. (1994) *The Essential Social Worker.* 3rd edn. Aldershot: Gower.

Davies, P. (2006) *The Goldilocks Enigma: Why is The Universe Just Right for Life?* London: Allen Lane.

Davison. J. (2009) *The Dark Threads*. Glamorgan: Accent Press.

Dear, M. and Wolch, J. (1987) *Landscapes of Despair: From Deinstitutionalisation to Homelessness*. Oxford: Polity Press.

De Bruijn (1993) PSI Psychology and Psychiatry. In Romme, M. and Escher, S. *Accepting Voices*. London: Mind.

DEFRA *Wellbeing Indicator 68*, www.Defra.Gov.Uk/Sustainable/Government/Progress/National/68.Htm (Accessed 19/08/2009).

Degan, P. (1992) *Recovery, Rehabilitation and The Conspiracy of Hope*. Keynote Address, Burlington VT.

Desai, S. and Bevan, D. (1998) Anti-Racist Practice: The Role of The Social Worker in Managing Different Perspectives in Care. *The Journal of Practise and Development*, 7.

Desai, S. and Bevan, D. (2002) Race and Culture, in Thompson, N. (Ed.) (2002) *Loss and Grief: A Guide for Human Services Practitioners*. London: Palgrave.

Desai, S. and Garib, A. (1998) Anti-racist Practice: The Role of The Social Worker in Managing Different Perspectives in Care. *The Journal of Practice and Development*, 7.

DHSS (1975) *Better Services for The Mentally Ill*, CMND 6233, London, HMSO.

Dickens, P. and Gilbert, P. (1979) *The State and The Housing Question*. University of Sussex.

Dinham, A. and Lowndes, V. (2009) Faith and The Public Realm, in Dinham, A., Furby, R. and Lowndes, V. (2009) *Faith in The Public Realm: Controversies, Policies and Practices*. Bristol: Policy Press.

Doel, M. et al. (2009) *Professional Boundaries Research Report for The General Social Care Council*. Centre for Health and Social Care Research, Sheffield Hallam University.

DoH (1998a) *Modernising Health and Social Services*, London, DoH.

DoH (1998b) *Modernising Social Services*. London, DoH.

DoH (1998c) *Modernising Mental Health Services*. London, DoH.

DoH (1999) *Modern Standards and Service Models: National Service Framework For Mental Health*. London: HMSO.

DoH (2001) *The Journey to Recovery*. London: DoH.

DoH (2001) *The Road to Recovery: The Government's Vision for Mental Health Care*. London: HMSO.

DoH (2002a) *Mental Health Policy Implementation Guide: Community Mental Health Teams*. London, DoH.

DoH (2002b) *Mental Health Policy Implementation Guide: Adult Acute Inpatient Care Provision*. London, HMSO.

DoH (2002c) *Developing Services for Carers and Families of People With Mental Illness*, London: DoH.

DoH (2005d) *Delivering Race Equality in Mental Health Care: an Action Plan for Reform Inside and Outside Services and The Government's Response to The Independent Enquiry Into The Death of David Bennett*. London: DoH.

DoH (2006) *Sharing Mental Health Information With Carers: Points to Good Practice for Service Providers*. London: NCCSDO.

DoH (2007) *Mental Health: New Ways of Working for Everyone: Developing and Sustaining a Capable and Flexible Workforce*. DoH.

DoH (2008a) *Safeguarding Adults: A Consultation on The Review of The 'No Secrets' Guidance*. London: DoH.

DoH (2008b) *High Quality Care for All: NHS Next Stage Review Final Report*. London: DoH.

DoH (2008c) *Refocusing The Care Programme Approach: Policy and Positive Practice Guidance*. London: DoH.

DoH (2008d) *Mental Health (Approved Mental Health Professionals) (England) Regulations*, Statutory Instrument 2008/1206.

DoH (2008e) *Mental Health Act 1983: Code of Practice*. London: DoH.

DoH (2008f) *Mental Capacity Act 2005: Deprivation of Liberty Safeguards Code of Practice*. London: DoH.

DoH (2009a) *New Horizons: Towards A Shared Vision for Mental Health*. Consultation document, London: DoH.

DoH (2009b) *High Quality Care for All: Our Journey So Far*. London: DoH.

DoH (2009c) *Living Well With Dementia: A National Dementia Strategy*. London: DoH.

DoH (2009d) *Tackling Health Inequalities: 10 Years On*. London: DoH.

DoH (2009e) *Religion or Belief: A Practical Guide for The NHS*. London: DoH.

DoH (2009f) *Shaping the Future of Care Together. (Green Paper)*. London: DoH.

DoH/DCSF (2009) *Building a Safe, Confident Future: The final report of the Social Work TaskForce*, London: DoH/DCSF.

DoH (Forthcoming) *Policy Document on Mental Health and Public Health*, London: DoH.

Dhanda, M. (2008) What Does The Hatred/Fear of The Veil Hide? *Ethnicity and Equalities in Health and Social Care*, 1: 2.

Double, D. (2002) Redressing The Imbalance. *Mental Health Today*, Sep.

Double, D. (2005) Beyond Biomedical Models: A Perspective From Critical Psychiatry, in Tew, J. (Ed.) *Social Perspectives in Mental Health.* London: Jessica Kingsley.

Dowson, S. and Greig, R. (2009) The Emergence of The Independent Support Broker Role. *Journal of Integrated Care*, 17: 4.

Duggan, M. (2002) *What is The Knowledge Base and Where Does It Come From? Thoughts From The Social Perspectives Network Study Day.* SPN.

Duggan, M. With Cooper, A. and Foster, J. (2002) *Modernising The Social Model in Mental Health: A Discussion Paper.* Social Perspectives Network.

Durrell, L. (1945/1962) *Prospero's Cell: Guide to The Landscape and Manners of The Island of Corfu.* London: Faber and Faber (See Nicholls and Gilbert, 2007).

Edwards, and Gilbert, P. (2007) Spiritual Assessment: Narratives and Responses, in Coyte, M., Gilbert, P. and Nicholls, V. (Eds) *Op Cit.*

Egan, G. (1975) *The Skilled Helper.* CA: Brooks/Cole.

Egan, G. (2002) *The Skilled Helper.* 7th edn. CA: Brooks/Cole.

England, H. (1986) *Social Work as Art: Making Sense for Good Practice.* London: Allen and Unwin.

Faulkner, A. and Bassett, T. (2002) Bringing The Framework to Life. *Mental Health Today*, March.

Faulks, S. (2005) *Human Traces.* London: Vintage.

Fenwick, P. (2009) Neuroscience of The Spirit, in Cook, C., Powell, A. and Sims, A. (2009) *Spirituality and Psychiatry.* London: Royal College of Psychiatrists.

Ferguson, I. (2007) Increasing User Choice or Privatising Risk? The Antimonies of Personalisation. *British Journal of Social Work*, 37, 387–403.

Fernando, S. (2002) *Mental Health, Race and Culture.* 2nd edn. Basingstoke: Palgrave.

Fernando, S. (2007) Spirituality and Mental Health Across Cultures, in Coyte, M.E., Gilbert, P. and Nicholls, V. eds (2007) *Op. cit.*

Fernando, S. (Ed.) (1995) *Mental Health in a Multi-Ethnic Society: A Multi-Disciplinary Handbook.* London, Routledge.

Finkelstein, S. (2004) *Why Smart Executives Fail: and What You Can Learn From Their Mistakes.* New York: Portfolio Books.

Firth, M.T. (1999) Conversing With Clients: A Generic Approach to Mental Health Needs Assessment. *Practice*, 11: 2.

Firth, M.T. (2000) *MANCAS Guide and Schedule.* Central Manchester Health Care NHS Trust.

Fisher, D.B. (2008) Promoting Recovery, in Stickley, T. and Bassett, T. (Eds) (2008) *Learning About Mental Health Practice.* Chichester: Wiley.

Fisher, M. (2002) The Role of Service Users in Problem Formulation and Technical Aspects of Social Research. *Social Work Education*, 21: 3, 305–12.

Flamholtz, E. and Randle, Y. (1989) *The Inner Game of Management.* London: Hutchinson.

Forster, E.M. (1927) *Aspects of the Novel.* The Clark Lectures.

Frankl, V.E. (1946/1984) *Man's Search for Meaning.* New York: Simon and Schuster.

Friedli, L. (2009) *Mental Health, Resilience and Inequalities.* Denmark: WHO, Europe With NIMHE, CPAG, FPH and The Mental Health Foundation.

Freud, S. and Krug, S. (2002) Beyond The Code of Ethics, Part II: Dual Relationships Revisited. *Families in Society*, 83:5/6, 483-92.

Fulford, K.W.M. and Woodbridge, K. (2007) Values-Based Practice: Help and Healing Within a Shared Theology of Diversity, in Coyte, M.E., Gilbert, P. and Nicholls, V. *Op Cit.*

Furness, S. and Gilligan, P. (2009) *Religion, Belief and Social Work: Making A Difference.* Bristol: Policy Press.

Future Vision Coalition (2008) *A New Vision for Mental Health.* Discussion paper. London: Mental Health Foundation, Mind, NHS Confederation, Rethink, Sainsbury Centre for Mental Health, Together, Association of Directors of Adult Social Services.

Gabriel, L. (2005) *Speaking The Unspeakable: The Ethics of Dual Relationships in Counselling and Psychotherapy.* London: Routledge.

Galbreath, W. (2005) Dual Relationships in Rural Communities, in Lohmann, N. and Lohmann, R. (Eds) *Rural Social Work Practice.* New York: Columbia University Press.

Gannon, Z. and Lawson, N. (2008) *Co-Production: The Modernisation of Public Services by Staff and Service Users.* London: Compass.

General Social Care Council (2002) *Codes of Practice for Social Care Workers and Employers.* London: GSCC.

General Social Care Council (2008) *Social Work at Its Best: A Statement of Social Work Roles and Tasks for The 21st Century.* London: GSCC.

George, M. (2002) Take Your Partners. *Mental Health Today*, April.

Gilbert, P. (1985) *Mental Handicap: A Practical Guide for Social Workers*. London, Business Press International.

Gilbert, P. (1992) *Cultural Change in a Public Welfare Agency: Antecedents, Process and Consequences*. Unpublished MBA Thesis, Roffey Park Institute/Sussex University.

Gilbert, P. (2005) Keep Up Your Spirits. *Open Mind*, 135, Sep/Oct. 6–8.

Gilbert, P. (2005) *Leadership: Being Effective and Remaining Human*. Lyme Regis: Russell House Publishing.

Gilbert, P. (2006) Social Care Services and The Social Perspective. *Psychiatry*, Edition on Learning Disability, July, 2006.

Gilbert, P. (2008) *From The Cradle: to Beyond The Grave?* DVD, Proceedings of The Second National Multi-Faith Conference, Stafford: Staffordshire University.

Gilbert, P. (2008) *Guidelines on Spirituality for Staff in Acute Care Services*, Stafford: Staffordshire University/CSIP/NIMHE

Gilbert, P. (2009) Leading to Well-Being, in Thompson, N. and Bates, J., ed *Promoting Workplace Well-Being*. Basingstoke: Palgrave Macmillan.

Gilbert, P. and Thompson, N. (Forthcoming) *Developing Leadership: A Learning and Development Manual*. Learning for Practice Series, Lyme Regis: Russell House Publishing.

Gilbert, P. (2010a, Forthcoming) in Stickley, T. and Basset, T. (Eds) *Voices of Experience*. Oxford: Wiley/Blackwell.

Gilbert, P. (2010b, Forthcoming) Mental Health, Spirituality and Religion, in Atherton, J., Graham, E. and Steadman, I. *The Practices of Happiness: Political Economy, Religion and Well-Being*. London: Routledge.

Gilbert, P. and Kalaga, H. (2007) *Nurturing Heart and Spirit: Papers From The Multi-Faith*.

Gilbert, P. and Nicholls, V. (2003) *Inspiring Hope: Recognising The Importance of Spirituality in a Whole Person Approach to Mental Health*. Leeds: NIMHE.

Gilbert, P. and Parkes, M. with Deuchar, N., Thomas, S. and Barber, J. (Forthcoming) Faith in One City. *BASS*, Forthcoming.

Gilbert, P. and Scragg, T. (1992) *Managing to Care*. Sutton: Reed Business Publishing.

Gilbert, P. and Spooner, B. (1982) Strength in Unity. *Community Care*, 28th Oct.

Gilbert, P. and Thompson, N. (2002) *Supervision and Leadership Skills: A Training Resource*. Wrexham, Learning Curve Publishing.

Gilbert, P. with Hayes, L., Merchant, R. and Moss, B. (2008) *Guidelines on Spirituality for Staff in Acute Care Services: Booklet, Evidence Base and Other Resources*. Stafford: Staffordshire University/CSIP.

Gilbert, P., Boodhoo, J. and Carr, S. (2008) Pilgrimage. *Openmind*, l: 151, May/Jun.

Gilbert, P., Vickery, M., Sewell, H., and Allen, R. (2010) *Making Mental Health Work for People and Communities*. Mental Health Social Care Strategic Network (SCSN).

Gilbert. P. (2009) *Being and Doing Human*. BSMHNHSFT Conference, 6th Nov.

Gilbert, P. ed (2011, forthcoming) *Spirituality and Mental Health*, Brighton: Pavilion.

Gilbert, P., Gilbert, J. and Sanghera, J. (2004) A Focus Group Exploration of The Importance of Izzat, Shame, Subordination and Entrapment on Mental Health and Services in South Asian Women Living in Derby. *Mental Health, Religion and Culture*, 7: 2, 109–30.

Glasby, J. (2009) A Matter of Perception? *Community Care*, 28th May, 28-9.

Glasby, J. and Littlechild, R. (2009) *Direct Payments and Personal Budgets: Putting Personalisation Into Practice*. 2nd edn. Bristol: Policy Press.

Glendinning, C. et al. (2008) *Evaluation of The Individual Budgets Pilot Programme: Final Report*. York: Social Policy Research Unit, University of York.

Glover, H. and Allott, P. (2002) *Developing a Recovery Platform for Mental Health Service Delivery for People With Mental Illness/Distress in England*. NIMHE Connections Conference, Newcastle-Upon-Tyne, June.

Goffee, R. and Jones, G. (2006) *Why Should Anyone Be Led by You? What it Takes to Be an Authentic Leader*. Boston: Harvard Business School.

Goffman, E. (1963/1990) *Stigma: Notes on The Management of Spoiled Identity*. London: Penguin.

Goffman, E. (1970) *Stigma: Notes on The Management of Spoiled Identity*. Harmondsworth, Penguin.

Goleman, D. (1996) *Emotional Intelligence*. London: Bloomsbury.

Goleman, D. (1998) What Makes A Leader? *Harvard Business Review*, Nov-Dec.

Goleman, D., Boyatzis, R. and Mckee, A. (2002) *The New Leaders: Transforming The Art of*

Leadership Into The Science of Results. Boston, Harvard Business School.

Golightley, M. (2008) *Social Work and Mental Health.* 3rd edn. Exeter: Learning Matters.

Gould, N. (2006) An Inclusive Approach to Knowledge for Mental Health Social Work Practice and Policy. *British Journal of Social Work,* 36, 109–25.

Gould, N. (2008) Mental Health History: Taking Over The Asylum. *Health Services Journal,* 6th May, www.Hsj.Co.Uk/Mental-Health-History-Taking-Over-The-Asylum/1136349.Article .

Gould, N. (2008) Research, in Davies, M. (Ed.) *The Blackwell Companion to Social Work.* Oxford: Blackwell.

Gould, N. (2009) *Mental Health Social Work in Context.* Abingdon: Routledge.

Gould, N. and Kendall, T. (2007) Developing The NICE/SCIE Guidelines for Dementia Care: The Challenges of Enhancing the Evidence Base for Social and Health Care. *British Journal of Social Work,* 37, 475-90.

Gould, N. and Richardson, J. (2006) Parent Training/Education Programmes in the Management of Children with Conduct Disorders: Developing an Integrated Evidence Base for Health and Social Care. *Journal of Children's Services,* 1: 4, 47–60.

Gould, N., Huxley, P. and Tew, J. (2007) Finding a Direction for Social Research in Mental Health: Establishing Priorities and Developing Capacity. *Journal of Social Work,* 7: 2, 177-94.

Government Office for Science (2008) *Foresight Mental Capital and Wellbeing Project Final Report.* London: GOS.

Granello, D., Pauley, P. and Carmichael, A. (1999) The Relationship of The Media to Attitudes Towards People With Mental Illness. *Journal of Humanistic Counselling, Education and Development,* 38, 98–110.

Gray, J. (2007) *Black Mass: Apocalyptic Religion and The Death of Utopia.* London: Allen Lane.

Green, H. et al. (2005) *Mental Health of Children and Young People in Great Britain (2004).* London: Office of National Statistics.

Griffiths, R. (1988) *Community Care: Agenda for Action.* London, HMSO.

Griffiths, J. (2010) 'Healthy Relations?, *Community Care,* 11 February, 2010.

Gulliver, P., Peck, E. and Towell, D. (2000) Evaluation of The Implementation of The Mental Health Review in Somerset: Methodology. *Managing Community Care,* 8: 3, June.

Gulliver, P., Peck, E. and Towell, D. (2000) Evaluation of The Implementation of The Mental Health Review in Somerset: Baseline Data. *Managing Community Care,* 8: 4, August.

Gulliver, P., Peck, E. and Towell, D. (2001) Evaluation of The Implementation of The Mental Health Review in Somerset: Results After Fifteen Months of Data Collection. *Managing Community Care,* 9: 1.

Gulliver, P., Peck, E. and Towell, D. (2002) *Modernising Partnerships: Evaluation of The Implementation of The Mental Health Review in Somerset: Final Report.* Institute for Applied Health and Social Policy, Kings College, London.

Gulliver,P., Peck,E., and Towell, D.(2002) Evaluation of The Integration of Health and Social Services in Somerset: Part 2 Lessons for Other Localities. *M.C.C.,* 10: 3, June.

Gupta. S, and Bhugra, D. Assessment Across Cultures. *Psychiatry,* 8: 9, Sep.

Hafford-Letchfield, T. (2006) *Management and Organisations in Social Work.* Exeter: Learning Matters.

Haidt, J. (2006) *The Happiness Hypothesis: Putting Ancient Wisdom and Philosophy to The Test of Modern Science.* London: William Heinemann.

Halmos, P. (1965) *The Faith of The Counsellors.* London: Constable.

Hamer, M. (2006) *The Barefoot Helper: Mindfulness and Creativity in Social Work.* Lyme Regis: Russell House Publishing.

Hammarskjold, D. (1964/2006) *Markings.* London: Vintage Spiritual Classics.

Hampden-Turner, C. (1990) *Corporate Culture: From Vicious to Virtuous Circles.* London, Hutchinson.

Hampson, M. (2005) *Head Versus Heart and Our Gut Reactions: The 21st Century Enneagram.* Ropley: O Books.

Handy, C. (1979) *Gods of Management.* London, Pan.

Handy, C. (1985) *Understanding Organisations.* 3rd edn. London, Penguin Books.

Hanvey, C. and Philpot, T. (1994) *Practising Social Work.* London, Routledge.

Harding, T. and Beresford, P. (1996) *The Standards We Expect: What Service Users Want From Social Services Workers.*London: NISW.

Harris. P. (2009) Whistle Blower Tells of America's Hidden Nightmare for The Sick. *The Observer,* 26th July.

Harrison, R. and Stokes, H. (1990) *Diagnosing Organisational Culture.* Sussex, Roffey Park Management Institute.

Hart, L. (1997) *Phone at Nine Just to Say You're Alive.* London: Pan Books.

Harvey, D. (1990) *The Condition of Postmodernity: an Enquiry Into The Origin of Cultural Change.* Oxford, Blackwell

Harvey-Jones, J. (1986) *Making it Happen: Reflections on Leadership.* Glasgow, William Collins.

Hatfield, B. (2008) Powers to Detain Under Mental Health Legislation and The Role of The Approved Social Worker: an Analysis *of* Patterns and Trends Under The 1983 Mental Health Act in Six Local Authorities. *British Journal of Social Work,* 38, 1553–71.

Hay Group (2009) *Leadership Competences for Foundation Trusts.* London: Hay Group.

Hay, D. (2006) *Something There: The Biology of The Human Spirit.* London: Darton, Longman & Todd.

Health Education Authority, *Promoting Mental Health: The Role of Faith Communities. Jewish and Christian Perspectives.* London: HEA.

Healy, K. (2005) *Social Work Theories in Context: Creating Frameworks for Practice.* Basingstoke: Palgrave Macmillan.

Heimler, E. (1967) *Mental Illness and Social Work.* Middlesex: Penguin.

Heller, T. et al. (Eds) (1996) *Mental Health Matters: A Reader.* London: Open University Press.

Hennessey, R. (2004) Focus on The States: Implementing Recovery-Based Care From East to West, *NASMHPD/NTAC E-Report on Recovery*, National Association of State Mental Health Program Directors and National Technical Assistance Center for State Mental Health Planning.

Hetherington, R. et al. (2001) *The Welfare of Children With Mentally Ill Parents: Learning From Inter-Country Comparisons.* Chichester: John Wiley.

Hewitt, P. (2001) *So You Think You're Mad: Seven Practical Steps to Mental Health.* Handsell.

Hick, S.F. (2009) *Mindfulness and Social Work.* Chicago: Lyceum.

Hill, C. (1972) *The World Turned Upside Down: Radical Ideas During The English Revolution.* London: Temple Smith.

HM Government (2007) *Putting People First: A Shared Vision and Commitment to The Transformation of Adult Social Care.* London: HM Government.

Hoffman, E. (1989) *Lost in Translation: A Life in A New Language.* London: Heinemann.

Hofstede, G. (1980) *Cultures Consequences.* Beverley Hills: SAGE.

Hoggett, B. (1984) *Mental Health Law.* 2nd edn. London: Sweet and Maxwell.

Holloway, M. and Moss, B. (Forthcoming) *Social Work and Spirituality.* Basingstoke: Palgrave Macmillan.

Holt, S. (2009) *Psychotic Interlude*, Brentwood: Chipmunkapublishing.

Home Office (2004) *Working Together: Cooperation Between Government and Faith Communities.* London: Home Office.

Home Office (2008) *Learning Disability Hate Crime: Good Practice Guidance for Crime & Disorder Reduction Partnerships and Learning Disability Partnership Boards.* Home Office.

Hope, R. (2008) The Ten Essential Shared Capabilities: Their Background, Development and Implementation, in Stickley, T. and Basset, T. (2008) *Learning About Mental Health Practice.* Chichester: Wiley.

House of Commons Social Services Committee (1985) *Second Report of The House of Commons Social Services Committee: Community Care,* London: HMSO.

House of Lords European Union Committee (2007*) Improving The Mental Health of The Population: Can The European Union Help?* HL Papers 73-I and 73-II. London: The Stationery Office.

Hudson, B. (2002) Ten Reasons Not to Trust Care Trusts. *M.C.C.,* 10: 2, April.

Hughes, L. (2001) New Culture, New Territory, New Professions? in Allen, I. (Ed.) *Social Care and Health: A New Deal?* London, Policy Studies Institute/University of Westminster.

Huxley, P. and Kerfoot, M. (1994) A Survey of Approved Social Work in England and Wales. *British Journal of Social Work,* 24: 3, 311–4.

Inge, J. (2003) *A Christian Theology of Place.* Aldershot: Ashgate.

International Federation of Social Workers (2004) *Ethics in Social Work, Statement of Principles.* Bern: IFSW.

Jackson, C. and Hill, K. (Eds.) (2006) *Mental Health Today: A Handbook.* Brighton: Pavilion.

Jacques, M. (2006) We Are Globalised, But Have No Real Intimacy With The Rest of The World. *The Guardian,* 17th April.

James, A. (2009) Ten Years After. *Mental Health Today,* Sept.

Jamison, C. (2006) *Finding Sanctuary.* London: Weidenfeld and Nicholson.

Jamison, K.R. (1997) An *Unquiet Mind: A Memoir of Moods and Madness.* London: Macmillan/Picador.

Jaynes, J. (1977) *The Origins of Consciousness in The Breakdown of The Bicameral Mind.* Boston: Haughton Mifflin.

Jenkins, R. et al. (2002) *Developing A National Mental Health Policy.* Hove Psychology Press/Maudsley Monographs.

Jenkins, S. (1995) *Accountable to None: The Tory Nationalisation of Britain.* London, Hamish Hamilton.

Johnson, G. and Scholes, K. (1989) *Exploring Corporate Strategy: Text and Cases.* 3rd edn. Hemel Hempstead: Prentice Hall.

Johnston, D. and Mayers, C. (2005) Spirituality: A Review of How Occupational Therapists Acknowledge, Assess and Meet Spiritual Needs. *British Journal of Occupational Therapy,* 68: 9.

Johnston, D. and Mayers, C. (2008) Spirituality: The Emergence of a Working Definition for Use Within Healthcare. *Implicit Religion,* 11: 3, 265–75.

Johnstone, L. (2000) *Users and Abusers of Psychiatry.* 2nd edn. London: Routledge.

Jones, K. (1972) *A History of The Mental Health Services,* London: Routledge and Kegan Paul.

Jones, K. (1988) *Experience in Mental Health: Community Care and Social Policy.* London: Sage.

Jones, K. (1993) *Asylums and After.* London: Athlone Press.

Jones, K. (2002) *The Making of Social Policy in Britain: From the Poor Law to New Labour.* London: Continuum.

Jones, P. (2002) Statement at Regional Conference Organised by NIMHE on 11th September, In: Gilbert, P. (2003) *The Value of Everything: Social Work and Its Importance in The Field of Mental Health.* Lyme Regis: Russell House Publishing.

Jones, R. (2001) *Mental Health Act Manual,* 7th edn. London: Sweet and Maxwell.

Jones, R. (2008) *Mental Health Act Manual.* 11th edn. London: Sweet and Maxwell.

Jordan, B. (1976) *Freedom and The Welfare State.* London, Routledge and Kegan Paul.

Jordan, B. (1984) *Invitation to Social Work.* Oxford, Martin Robertson.

Kardong, T. (1988) *The Benedictines.* Dublin, Dominican Publications.

Keating, F. (2009) African and Caribbean Men and Mental Health. *Ethnicity and Inequalities in Health and Social Care,* 2, July 41–53.

Kedward. R. (2006) *La Vie En Bleu: France and The French Since 1900.* London: Penguin.

Keedwell. P. (2008) *How Sadness Survived: The Evolutionary Basis of Depression,.*Oxford: Radcliffe.

Kelley, R. (1988) In Praise of Followers. *Havard Business Review,* November.

Kermode, F. (Ed.) (1975) *Selected Prose of T.S. Eliot.* London: Faber.

Kerr, S. (1983) *Making Ends Meet.* London: Bedford Square Press.

Kershaw, I. (2008) *Hitler, The Germans, and The Final Solution.* Yale: Yale University Press.

Keyes CLM (2007) Promoting and Protecting Mental Health as Flourishing: A Complementary Strategy for Improving National Mental Health. *American Psychologist,* 62: 2, 95–108.

Khan, F. and Waheed, W. (2009) Suicide and Self-Harm in South Asian Immigrants.*Psychiatry,* 8, 261–4.

King. M., Weich, S., Nazroo, J. and Blizard, B. (2006) Religion, Mental Health and Ethnicity. EMPIRIC – A National Survey of England. *Journal of Mental Health,* 15: 2, 153–62.

King, U. (2009) *The Search for Spirituality: Our Global Quest for Meaning.* London: Canterbury Press.

Kluger, J. (2009) The Biology of Beliefs. *Time,* 23rd February.

Knight, T. (2004) You'd Better Believe It. *Open Mind,* 128, July.

Koenig, H.G., McCullough, M.E. and Larson, D.B. (2001) *Handbook of Religion and Health.* Oxford: Oxford University Press.

Kohen, D. (Ed.) (2000) *Women and Mental Health.* London: Routledge.

Kotter, J.P. (1995) Leading Change: Why Transformation Efforts Fail.*Harvard Business Review,* March.

Kotter, J.P. (1996) *Leading Change.* Boston, Harvard Business School Press.

Kouzes, J. and Posner, B. (1990) The Credibility Factor: What Followers Expect From Their Leaders. *Management Review,* January.

Kouzes, J. and Posner, B. (2007) *The Leadership Challenge.* 4th edn. San Francisco: Jossey-Bass.

Kuhn, T. (1962) *The Structure of Scientific Revolutions.* Chicago: Chicago University Press.

Lawrence, S. et al. (Eds) (2009) *Introducing International Social Work.* Exeter: Learning Matters.

Layard, R. (2005) *Mental Health: Britain's Biggest Social Problem.* London: PM's Strategy Unit.

Layard, R. and Dunn, F. (2009) *A Good Childhood: Searching for Values in A Competitive Age.* London: Penguin With The Children's Society.

Lazarus, A.A. and Zur, O. (Eds) (2002) *Dual Relationships and Psychotherapy.* New York: Springer.

Le Guin, U.K. (1971) *The Lathe of Heaven*. London: Victor Gollancz.

Le Guin, U.K. (1973) *The Farthest Shore*. London: Victor Gollancz.

Le Guin, U.K. (1974/2002) *The Dispossessed*. London: Millennium Press.

Le Guin, U.K. (1984) S.Q., in *The Compass Rose*. London: Panther.

Le Mesurier, N. and Cumella, S. (2001) The Rough Road and The Smooth Road. *Managing Community Care*, 9: 1.

Lea, L. (2008) Providing Service User Centred Care, in Stickley, T. and Basset, T. (2008) *Learning About Mental Health Practice*. Chichester: Wiley.

Leadbeater, C. (2009) State of Loneliness. *Society Guardian*, 1st July.

Leader, D. (2008) *The New Black: Mourning, Melancholia and Depression*. London: Hamish Hamilton.

Leece, J. and Bornat, J. (Eds) (2006) *Developments in Direct Payments*. London: Policy Press.

Leeds Mental Health Unit (1997) *A Little More Time, Too*: *A Consumer Survey of The Leeds Mental Health Social Work Services*. Leeds Social Services.

Leff, J. (1997) The Downside of Reprovision, in Leff, J. (Ed.) *Care in The Community: Illusion or Reality?* Chichester: Wiley.

Leff, J.P. et al. (1982) A Controlled Trial of Social Interventions in The Families of Schizophrenic Patients. *British Journal of Psychiatry*, 141, 121–34.

Leggatt, A. (2001) *Tribunals for Users: One System, One Service*. London: The Stationery Office.

Lester, H. and Gask, L. (2006) Delivering Medical Care for Patients With Serious Mental Illness or Promoting A Collaborative Model of Recovery? *British Journal of Psychiatry*, 188, 401–2.

Lewis, J. and Glennerster, H. (1996) *Implementing The New Community Care*. Buckingham: Open University Press.

Lynch, G. (2007) *The New Spirituality: An Introduction to Progressive Belief in Twenty-First Century*. London: I.B.Tauris.

Lyons, J. (2005) A Systems Approach to Direct Payments: A Response to 'Friend or Foe? Towards a Critical Assessment of Direct Payments. *Critical Social Policy*, 25: 2, 240–52.

Macdonald, G. and Sheldon, B. (1997) Community Care Services for the Mentally Ill: Consumers Views. *International Journal of Social Psychiatry*. 43: 1, 35–55.

Mackay, R. et al. (2001) *Report of The Independent Enquiry Into The Care and Treatment Afforded to Benjamin Rathbone*. Leicestershire Health Authority.

Magee, B. (1973) *Popper*. London: Fontana.

Mannion, R., Davies, H.T. and Marshall, M.N. (2004) *Cultures for Performance in Health Care*. Maidenhead: Open University Press.

Mantel, H. (2004) *Giving Up The Ghost: A Memoir*. London: Harper Perennial.

Manthorpe, J. et al. (2008) Safeguarding and System Change: Early Perceptions of The Implications for Adult Protection Services of The English Individual Budgets Pilots: A Qualitative Study. *British Journal of Social Work*, 1–16.

Mari, J. and Streiner, D. (1999) Family Intervention for Schizophrenia (Cochrane Review). *Cochrane Library, Issue 1*, Oxford: Update Software.

Markham, E. (1915) *The Shoes of Happiness and Other Poems*. New York: Doubleday.

Marmot (2007) Achieving Health Equity: From Root Causes to Fair Outcomes. *Lancet*, 370, 1153–63.

Marshall, S. (2006) *Mendip Hospital: an Appreciation*. Ely: Melrose Books.

Maslow, A.H. (1965) *Eupsychiam Management*. Homewood, Il: Irwin-Dorsey.

Maslow, A.H. (1968) *Toward A Psychology of Being*. New York: Von Norstrand.

Matthews, T.H. (2009) *Social Work and Spirituality*. Exeter: Learning Matters.

Mcallister, S. (2009) A Pastoral Heart. *The Tablet*, 13th June, 8-98.

McCulloch (2006) Understanding Mental Health and Mental Illness, in Jackson, C. and Hill, K. (Eds) *Mental Health Today: A Handbook*. Brighton: Pavilion/Mental Health Foundation.

McGonagle, I. et al. (2008) The Ten Essential Shared Capabilities in Practice, in Stickley, T. and Basset, T. (Eds) *Learning About Mental Health Practice*. Chichester: Wiley.

McKenzie, K. (2007) Being Black in Britain is Bad for Your Mental Health. *The Guardian*, 2nd April, 32.

McLean, A. and Marshall, J. (1988) *Cultures at Work*. London: LGMB.

McSherry, W. (2007) *The Meaning of Spirituality and Spiritual Care Within Nursing and Health Care Practice*. Wiltshire: Quay Books.

Means, R. and Smith, R. (1994) *Community Care Policy and Practice*, London, Macmillan.

Meltzer, H. et al. (2002) *The Social and Economic Circumstances of Adults With Mental Disorders*. London: HMSO.

Mental Health Act Commission (2001) *The Mental Health Act Commission 9th Biennial Report 1999–2001.* London: HMSO.

Mental Health Foundation (1997) *Knowing Our Own Minds: A Survey of How People in Emotional Distress Take Control of Their Lives.* London: Mental Health Foundation.

Mental Health Foundation (1999) *The Fundamental Facts.* London: Mental Health Foundation.

Mental Health Foundation (2000) *Pull Yourself Together! A Survey of The Stigma and Discrimination Faced by People Who Experience Mental Distress.* London: Mental Health Foundation.

Mental Health Foundation (2000) *Strategies for Living.* London: Mental Health Foundation.

Mental Health Foundation (2002) *Taken Seriously: The Somerset Spirituality Project.* London: Mental Health Foundation.

Merchant, R. and Gilbert, P. (2007) The Modern Workplace: Surfing The Wave or Surviving The Straightjacket? *Crucible,* January, 39–46.

Midwinter, E. (1994) *The Development of Social Welfare in Britain.* Buckingham: Open University Press.

Miller, G. (2009) *Spent: Sex, Evolution and The Secrets of Consumerism.* London: William Heinemann.

MIND (2009) *Personalisation in Mental Health: Creating A Vision. Views of Personalisation From People Who Use Mental Health Services.* London: MIND.

Ministry of Health (1975) *Better Services for the Mentally Ill.* London: HMSO.

Modood, T. (2007) *Multiculturalism: A Civic Idea.* Cambridge, Polity Press.

Morrell, M. and Capparell, S. (2001) *Shackleton's Way: Leadership Lessons From The Great Antarctic Explorer.* London: Nicholas Brealey.

Morris, D. (2001) Citizenship and Community in Mental Health: A Joint National Programme for Social Inclusion and Community Partnership. *The Mental Health Review,* 6: 3.

Moss, B. (2005) *Religion and Spirituality.* Lyme Regis: Russell House Publishing.

Moss, B. (2008) *Communication Skills for Health and Social Care.* London: Sage.

Moss, B. et al. (2009) The Fount of All Knowledge: Training Required to Involve Service Users and Carers in Health and Social Care Education and Training. *Social Work Education,* 28: 5.

Moussavi, S. et al. (2007) Depression, Chronic Diseases and Decrements in Health: Results From The World Health Surveys. *The Lancet,* 370: 9590.

Mulholland, H. (2005) Counting on Change. *Society Guardian,* 7th December.

Murphy, J. (2007) A Greater Role for Faith Based Groups in UK Welfare. Speech in East London, 11th January.

Murray, A. et al. (1997) *More Than a Friend: The Role of Support Workers in Community Mental Health Services.* London: Sainsbury Centre for Mental Health.

Mursell, G. (2005) *Praying in Exile.* London: Darton, Longman and Todd.

Myss, C. (1997) *Anatomy of The Spirit.* New York: Bantam Press.

National Consumer Council (2004) *Making Public Services Personal: A New Compact for Public Services.* London: NCC.

National Health Services Scotland (2002) *Spiritual Care in NHS National Services Scotland.* Edinburgh: NHS Scotland.

National Health Services Scotland (2006) *Spiritual Care in NHS National Services, Scotland: Statement of Intent.* Edinburgh: NHS Scotland.

National Institute for Mental Health in England (2001) *The National Institute for Mental Health in England: Role and Function.* London: HMSO.

National Institute for Mental Health in England (2002) *First Year Strategy for NIMHE: Meeting The Implementation Challenge in Mental Health.* DoH.

National Social Inclusion Programme (2007) *Capabilities for Inclusive Practice.* DoH.

Needham, C. (2006) Realising The Potential of Co-Production: Negotiating Improvements in Public Services. *Social Policy & Society,* 7: 2, 221–31.

Needham, C. and Carr, S. (2009) *SCIE Research Briefing 31: Co-Production: an Emerging Evidence Base for Adult Social Care.* London: SCIE.

New Economics Foundation (2008) *Co-Production: A Manifesto for Growing The Core Economy.* London: NEF.

Newbiggin, K. and Lowe, J. (2005) *Direct Payments and Mental Health: New Directions.* York: Joseph Rowntree Foundation.

Newman, J. (1996) *Shaping Organisational Cultures in Local Government.* London: Pitman.

Neyroud, P. and Beckley, A. (2001) *Policing, Ethics and Human Rights.* Devon: Willan.

NHS Confederation (2009) Fact sheet: key facts and trends in mental health. London: NHSC, November, 2009.

Nicholls, V. (2002) *Taken Seriously: Report of The Somerset Spirituality Project.* London: Mental Health Foundation.

Nicholls, V. and Gilbert, P. (2007) The Sea, Me and God. *Open Mind,* 144, March.

Nocon, A. and Qureshi, H. (1996) *Outcomes of Community Care for Users and Carers.* Buckingham, Open University Press.

O'Hara, M. (2008) Doctors Orders. Interview With Dr Liz Miller, *Society Guardian*, 11th June.

O'Hara, M. (2009) Voice of Experience. Interview With Dr Ian Mcpherson, *Society Guardian*, 24th June.

O'Leary, P. and Gould, N. (2009) Men Who Were Sexually Abused in Childhood and Subsequent Suicidal Ideation: Community Comparison, Explanations and Practice Implications. *British Journal of Social Work*, 39, 950–68.

O'Neill, G. (1997) In *The Context of a Multi-Disciplinary Duty System, Are There Differences in The Practice and Division of Labour Between Community Psychiatric Nurses and Mental Health Social Workers?* Unpublished M.A. Thesis, University of Lancaster.

Office for Disability Issues (2008) *Independent Living: A Cross-Government Strategy About Independent Living for Disabled People.* London: HM Government Office for Disability Issues.

Okasha, A. (2007) The Individual Versus The Family: An Islamic and Traditional Society's Perspective. In Cox, J., Campbell, A.V. and Fulford, K.W. (Eds.) *Medicine of the Person: Faith, Science and Values in Health Care Provision.* London: Jessica Kingsley.

Oldham Social Services and Oldham NHS Trust (2002) *Mental Health Social Work in Oldham.* Oldham Social Services/Oldham NHS Trust.

Olsen, M.R. (Ed.) (1984) *Social Work and Mental Health.* London: Tavistock.

Onyett, S., Pillinger, T. and Muijen, M. (1995) *Making Community Mental Health Teams Work.* London: Sainsbury Centre for Mental Health.

Pagett, N. and Swannell, G. (1997) *Diamonds Behind My Eyes.* London: Victor Gollancz.

Pargament, K.I. (2002) The Bitter and The Sweet: an Evaluation of The Costs and Benefits of Religiousness. *Psychological Enquiry*, 13: 3, 168–81.

Parkes, M., Milner, K. and Gilbert, P. (2010) Vocation, Vocation, Vocation: Staff Attitudes to Spiritual Care. *The International Journal of Leadership in Public Services*, forthcoming issue.

Parkes, M. and Gilbert, P., With Deuchar, N., Thomas, S. and Barber, J. (Forthcoming) Of Gods and Gudwaras: The Birmingham and Solihull Spirituality Research Programme. *Mental Health, Religion and Culture*, Forthcoming Issue.

Parry-Jones, W. (1972) *The Trade in Lunacy.* London: Routledge and Kegan Paul.

Parsons, T. (1951) Illness and The Role of The Physician: A Sociological Perspective. *American Journal of Orthopsychiatry*, 21, 452–60.

Parton, N. and O'Byrne, P. (2000) *Constructive Social Work: Towards a New Practice.* London: Macmillan.

Payne, C. (1988) When Management Skills Are Part of Basic Practice. *Social Work Today*, 23rd June.

Payne, M. (1982) *Working in Teams.* London: Macmillan.

Payne, M. (2002) Balancing The Equation. *Professional Social Work*, January.

Peck, E., Gulliver, P. and Towell, D. (2002) *Modernising Partnerships: an Evaluation of Somerset's Innovations in The Commissioning and Organisation of Mental Health Services, Final Report.* London: Institute for Applied Health and Social Policy.

Peck, E., Towell, D. and Gulliver, P. (2001) The Meanings of Culture in Health and Social Care: A Case Study of The Combined Trust in Somerset. *Journal of Interprofessional Care*, 15: 4, 319–27.

Pendegarth, Y. (2002) *Woman Speak Out: Women's Experiences of Using Mental Health Services and Proposals for Change.* Resisters, Leeds Women's and Mental Health Action Group.

Perkins, R (2002) Are You (Really) Being Served? *Mental Health Today*, September.

Perkins, R. (2008) The Professionalisation of Pain. *Open Mind*, 149, January.

Peters, T. (1989) *Thriving on Chaos.* London: Pan.

Peters, T. and Austin, N. (1986) *A Passion for Excellence: The Leadership Difference.* Glasgow,:William Collins/Fontana Paperbacks.

Phillips, C., Palfrey, C. and Thomas, P. (1994) *Evaluating Health and Social Care.* London: Macmillan.

Philpot, T. (Ed.) (1986) *Social Work: A Christian Perspective.* Tring: Lion Publishing.

Pierson, J. (2002) *Tackling Social Exclusion.* Sutton: Community Care.

Pierson, J. (2009) *Tackling Social Exclusion.* 2nd edn. London: Routledge.

Pilgrim, D. (2005) Protest and Co-Option: The Voice of Mental Health Service Users, in Bell, A. and Lindley, S. (Eds) *Beyond The Water Towers: The Unfinished Revolution in Mental Health Services, 1985–2005.* London: Sainsbury Centre for Mental Health.

Pointon, B. (2007) Who Am I? – The Search for Spirituality in Dementia. A Family Carer's Perspective', in Coyte, M.E., Gilbert. P. and Nicholls, V. *Op. Cit.*

Poll. C., Duffy, S. et al. (2006) *A Report of in Control's First Phase: 2003–2005.* London: In Control.

Pope, K.S. and Keith-Spiegel, P. (2008) A Practical Approach to Boundaries in Psychotherapy: Making Decisions, Bypassing Blunders, and Mending Fences. *Journal of Clinical Psychology,* 64: 5, 638–52.

Porter, R. (2002) *Madness: A Brief History.* Oxford: Oxford University Press.

Pratchett, T. (1993) *Small Gods.* London: Corgi Paperbacks.

Preston-Shoot, M. (1996) Wither Social Work? Social Work, Social Policy and Law at an Interface: Confronting The Challenges and Realising The Potential in Work With People Needing Care or Services. *The Liverpool Law Review,* XVIII.

Priebe, S. and Slade, M. (2002) *Evidence in Mental Health Care.* London: Routledge.

Proehl, R.A. (2001) *Organisational Change in The Human Services.* Thousand Oaks, CA: Sage.

Psychopathology Committee of The Group for The Advancement of Psychiatry (2001) Reexamination of Therapist Self-Disclosure. *Psychiatric Services.* 52: 11, 1489-93.

Pugh, R. (2007) Dual Relationships: Personal and Professional Boundaries in Rural Social Work. *British Journal of Social Work,* 37: 1405–23.

Putnam. R.D. (2000) *Bowling Alone: The Collapse and Revival of American Community.* New York: Simon and Schuster.

Ramon, S. (2001) *Options and Dilemmas Facing British Mental Health Social Work.* Paper for The Conference on Reducing The Biomedical Dominance of Psychiatry, 27th April.

Ramsay, R. et al. (Eds) (2001) *Mental Illness: A Handbook for Carers.* London: Jessica Kingsley.

Rankin, J. (2005) *Mental Health in The Mainstream.* London: IPPR / Rethink.

Reddie, R.S. (2009) *Black Muslims in Britain: Why Are a Growing Number of Black People Converting to Islam.* Oxford: Lion.

Reed, J., Mosher, L.R. and Bentall, R.P. (2004) *Models of Madness: Psychological, Social and Biological Approaches to Schizophrenia.* Hove: Routledge.

Reed, M. (2002) The Practitioner's Perspective. *Professional Social Work,* April.

Reith, M. and Payne, M. (2009) *Social Work in End-of-Life and Palliative Care.* Bristol: The Policy Press.

Repper, J. (2009) Carers of People With Mental Health Problems, in Brooker, C and Repper, J (2009) *Op. Cit.*

Repper, J. and Perkins, R. (2009) Recovery and Social Inclusion: The Changing Mental Health Agenda, in Brooker, C. and Repper, J. (2009) *Mental Health: From Policy to Practice.* London: Churchill Livingstone/Elsevier.

Repper, J. et al. (2008) Carer's Experiences of Mental Health Services and Views About Assessments: Lessons From The Partnership in Carer Assessments Project, in Stickley, T. and Basset, T. (Eds) *Learning About Mental Health Practice.* Chichester: Wiley.

Rethink/CSIP/UCLAN (2007) *Our Voice: The Pakistani Community's View of Mental Health and Mental Health Services in Birmingham – Report From The Aap Ki Awaz Project.* London: Rethink.

Ritchie, J.H., Dick and Lingham, R. (1994) *The Report of The Enquiry Into The Care and Treatment of Christopher Clunis.* London: HMSO.

Robb, J. and Gilbert, P. (2007) Leadership Lessons in Health and Social Care: Integration and Mental Health. *The International Journal of Leadership in Public Services,* 3: 1, 19–25.

Rogers, A., Pilgrim, D. and Lacey, R. (1993) *Experiencing Psychiatry: Users' Views of Services.* London: Macmillan/MIND.

Rogers, C. (1961) *Client-Centred Therapy: It's Current Practice, Theory and Implications.* London: Constable.

Rolheiser, R. (1998) *Seeking Spirituality.* London: Hodder and Stoughton.

Romme, M. and Escher, S. (1993) *Accepting Voices.* London: MIND.

Romme, M. and Escher, S. (2002) *Making Sense of Voices: A Guide of Mental Health Professionals Working With Voice-Hearers.* London: MIND.

Rose, D. (2001) Users' Voices: *The Perspectives of Mental Health Service Users on Community and Hospital Care.* London: The Sainsbury Centre for Mental Health.

Ross, L. (1997) *Nurses' Perceptions of Spiritual Care.* Aldershot: Averbury.

Rushton, A. and Davies, P. (1984) *Social Work and Health Care.* London: Heinemann Educational.

Russell, A., Haldane, J. and Russell, T. (2001) *Positive Practice in Mental Health.* 4th edn. Breakthrough.

Rutherford, S. (2008) *The Victorian Asylum.* Oxford: Shire Library Publications.

Sacks, J. (2002) *The Dignity of Difference: How to Avoid The Clash of Civilisations.* London: Continuum.

Sacks, J. (2005) *To Heal a Fractured World: The Ethics of Responsibility.* London: Continuum.

Sacks, J. (2007) *The Home We Build Together: Recreating Society*. London: Continuum.

Sainsbury Centre for Mental Health (1998) *Acute Problems: A Survey of The Quality of Care in Acute Psychiatric Wards: Briefing Paper 4*. London: SCMH.

Sainsbury Centre for Mental Health (2000) *An Executive Briefing on The Implications of The Human Rights Act 1998 for Mental Health Services: Briefing Paper 12*. London: SCMH.

Sainsbury Centre for Mental Health (2000) *On Your Doorstep: Community Organisations and Mental Health*. London: SCMH.

Sainsbury Centre for Mental Health (2000) *Taking Your Partners: Using Opportunities for Inter-Agency Partnership in Mental Health*. London: SCMH.

Sainsbury Centre for Mental Health (2001) *An Executive Briefing on the White Paper Reforming The Mental Health Act: Briefing Paper 14*. London: SCMH.

Sainsbury Centre for Mental Health (2002) *An Executive Briefing on 'Working for Inclusion': Briefing Paper 15*. London: SCMH.

Sainsbury Centre for Mental Health (2002) *Breaking The Circles of Fear: A Review of The Relationship Between Mental Health Services and African and Caribbean Communities*. London: SCMH.

Sainsbury Centre for Mental Health (2003) *The Economic and Social Costs of Mental Illness*. Policy paper 3, London: SCMH.

Sainsbury Centre for Mental Health/LGA/NHS Confederation/ADSS (2006) *The Future of Mental Health: A Vision for 2015*. London: SCMH.

Sandel, M. (2009) A New Politics of The Common Good. BBC *Reith Lectures*, 30th June.

Schein, E. (1985) *Organisational Culture and Leadership*. San Francisco: Jossey-Bass.

Scott, M.C. (2000) *Re-Inspiring The Corporation*. Chichester: John Wiley.

Scragg, T. (2009) *Managing at The Front Line: A Handbook for Manager in Social Care*, 2nd edn. Brighton: Pavilion.

Scull, A. (1984) *Decarceration: Community Treatment and The Devian: A Radical View*. 2nd edn. Cambridge: Polity Press.

Seebohm Report (1968) *Report by the Committee on Local Authority and Allied Social Services*. London: HMSO.

Seebohm, P. and Grove, B. (2006) *Leading by Example: Making The NHS A Good Corporate Citizen and Exemplar Employer of People With Mental Health Problems*. Disability Rights Commission and SCMH.

Sen, A. (2006) *Identity and Violence: The Illusion of Destiny*. London: Allen Lane.

Sewell, H. (2009) *Working With Ethnicity, Race and Culture in Mental Health*. London: Jessica Kingsley.

Shaping Our Lives/National Centre for Independent Living/University of Leeds Centre for Disability Studies (2007) *SCIE People Management Knowledge Review 17: Developing Social Care: Service Users Driving Culture Change*. London: SCIE.

Shaw, I. and Gould, N. (2001) *Qualitative Research in Social Work*. London: Sage.

Shaw, I. and Middleton, H. (2001) Recognising Depression in Primary Care. *Primary Care Mental Health*, 5: 2.

Shaw, P. (2002) *Changing Conversations in Organisations*. London: Routledge.

Shepherd, S., Boardman, J. and Slade, M. (2008) *Making Recovery a Reality*. London: SCMH.

Sheppard, D. (1996) *Learning The Lessons: Mental Health Inquiries Published in England and Wales Between 1969 and 1996 and Their Recommendations for Improving Practice*. 2nd edn. London: The Zito Trust.

Sheppard, M. (1995) *Care Management and The New Social Work: A Critical Analysis*. London: Whiting and Birch.

Sims, A. (2009) *Is Faith Delusion: Why Religion is Good for Your Health*. London: Continuum.

Singh, M, in Interview With Gilbert, P. (2009) Leadership Interview in *The International Journal of Leadership in Public Services*, 5: 2, July.

Slay, G. (2002) A Question of Judgement. *Professional Social Work*, July.

Slay, G. (2003) What Exactly is It That We Do? *Professional Social Work*, December, 16–7.

Slay, G. (2007) Let's Get Spiritual. *Mental Health Practice*, 11, 4, 27-9.

Smale, G. et al. (1994) *Negotiating Care in The Commmunity*. London: HMSO.

Smale, G., Tuson, G. and Statham, D. (2000) *Social Work and Social Problems: Working Towards Social Inclusion and Social Change*. London: Palgrave.

Small, H. (1998) *Florence Nightingale: Avenging Angel*. London: Constable.

Smith, P. and Peterson, M. (1988) *Leadership, Organisations and Culture*. London: Sage.

Social Care Institute for Excellence (2005) *SCIE Resource Guide 5: Direct Payments: Answering Frequently Asked Questions*. London/Bristol: SCIE/Policy Press.

Social Perspectives Network (2006) *Reaching The Spirit*. SPN Study Paper No9, London: SPN.

Social Perspectives Network (2007) *Whose Recovery is It Anyway?* London: SPN/SCIE/NIMHE.

Social Services Inspectorate (2002) *Modernising Mental Health Services*. London: HMSO.

Social Work, 39, 950–68.

Spandler, H. (2007) Individualised Funding, Social Inclusion and The Politics of Mental Health *Journal of Critical Psychological Counselling*, 7: 1, 18–27.

Spandler, H. and Vick, N. (2005) Enabling Access to Direct Payments: an Exploration of Care Co-Ordinators Decision-Making Practices. *Journal of Mental Health*, 14: 2, 145–55.

Spandler, H. and Vick, N. (2006) Opportunities for Independent Living Using Direct Payments in Mental Health. *Health and Social Care in The Community*, 14: 2, 107–15.

Spicker, P. (1995) *Social Policy: Themes and Approaches*. Hemel Hempstead: Prentice Hall.

SSI (2001) *Inspection of Mental Health Services, London Borough of Hounslow*. London: HMSO.

SSI (2001) *Inspection of Mental Health Services, Southend-On-Sea Borough Council*. London: HMSO.

Stanley, N. and Manthorpe, J. (2001) Reading Mental Health Enquiries: Messages for Social Work. *Journal of Social Work*, 1: 1.

Stevenson, O. (1971) Knowledge for Social Work. *British Journal of Social Work*, 1: 2, Summer.

Stickley, T. and Bassett, T. (Eds) (2008) *Learning About Mental Health Practice*. Chichester: John Wiley.

Styron, W. (1990/2004) *Darkness Visible*. London: Vintage Books.

Survivors History Group (2008) Your History in Your Hands. *Openmind*, 154, 16–7, November.

Sweeney, A. and Woodward, L. (2006) *Values and Methodologies For Social Research in Mental Health*, Bristol: Policy Press and Social Care Institute for Excellence.

Swinton, J. (2001) *Spirituality and Mental Health Care: Rediscovering A 'Forgotten' Dimension*. London: Jessica Kingsley.

Swinton, J. (2007) A Search for Spirituality and Mental Health: A Perspective From The Research, in Coyte, M., Gilbert, P. and Nicholls, V. (Eds) *Op. Cit*.

Sykes, B. (2006) *The Blood of The Isles*. London: Bantam Press.

Tacey, D. (2004) *The Spirituality Revolution: The Emergence of Contemporary Spirituality*. Hove: Brunner-Routledge.

Tadros, G. (2004) *Suicide in Birmingham and Solihull*. Birmingham: BSMHNHSFT.

Taylor, C. and White, S. (2000) *Practising Reflexivity in Health and Welfare: Making Knowledge*. Buckingham: Open University Press.

Taylor, P. and Gunn, J. (1999) Homicides by People With Mental Illness. *British Journal of Psychiatry*, 174, 9–14.

Tew, J. (2002) Going Social: Championing an Holistic Model of Mental Distress Within Professional Education. *Social Work Education*, 1: 2, April.

Tew, J. (2005) Social Perspectives: Towards A Framework for Practice. in Tew, J. (Ed.) *Social Perspectives in Mental Health: Developing Social Models to Understand and Work With Mental Distress*. London: Jessica Kingsley.

Tew, J. (2008) Researching in Partnership: Reflecting on a Collaborative Study With Mental Health Service Users Into The Impact of Compulsion. *Qualitative Social Work*, 7: 3, 271–87.

Tew, J. et al. (2006) *Values and Methodologies For Social Research in Mental Health*. Bristol: Policy Press and SCIE.

The Future Vision Coalition (2008) *A New Vision for Mental Health: Discussion Paper*. London: The Future Vision Coalition.

Thompson, N. (1992) *Existentialism and Social Work* Aldershot: Avebury.

Thompson, N. (1996) *People Skills: A Guide to Effective Practice in the Human Services*. London: Macmillan.

Thompson, N. (1998) *Promoting Equality*. London: Macmillan.

Thompson, N. (2000) *Theory and Practice in Human Services*. Buckingham: Open University Press.

Thompson, N. (2001) Working Together Across Disciplines. *N.T. Research*, 6: 5.

Thompson, N. (2006) *Anti-Discriminatory Practice*. 4th edn. Basingstoke: Palgrave Macmillan.

Thompson, N. (2009) *Understanding Social Work*. 3rd edn. Basingstoke: Palgrave Macmillan.

Thompson, N. and Gilbert, P. (Forthcoming) *Supervision: A Learning and Development Manual. Learning for Practice Series*, Lyme Regis: Russell House Publishing.

Thompson, N. and Bates, J. (2009) *Promoting Workplace Well-Being*. Basingstoke: Palgrave Macmillan.

Timms, N. and Timms, R. (1977) *Perspectives in Social Work*. London: Routledge & Kegan Paul.

Titmuss, R.M. (1961) Paper at The Annual Conference of The National Association for

182   *Social Work and Mental Health*

Mental Health, Reproduced in Titmuss, R.M. (1968) *Commitment to Welfare*. London: Allen & Unwin.

Topor, A. (2000) *Chronic Illness and Recovery*. Unpublished Paper, November.

Trevillion, S. (2000) Social Work Research: What Kind of Knowledge? *British Journal of Social Work*, 30: 429–32.

Ulas, M. and Connor, A. (Eds) (1999) *Mental Health and Social Work*. London: Jessica Kingsley.

Union of Physically Impaired Against Segregation (1975) *Fundamental Principles of Disability*. London: UPIAS.

US Department of Health and Human Services (2005) *National Consensus Statement of Mental Health Recovery*. Rockville, MD.

Utting, W. (2002) Preaching What We Practise. *Professional Social Work*, June.

Wallace Hadrill, J.M. (1971) *Early Germanic Kingship in England and on The Continent*. London: Oxford University Press.

Wallcraft, J. (2005) Recovery From Mental Breakdown, in Tew, J. *Op. Cit.*

Waller, J. (2009) *A Time to Dance, A Time to Die*. London: Icon Books.

Wanless, D. (2002) *Securing Our Future Health: Taking a Long-Term View*. London: DoH.

Watkins, P. (2009) *Mental Health Practice: A Guide to Compassionate Care*. 2nd edn. London: Elsevier.

Weaver (1998) Case Management Conference in Oklahoma Quoted in Allott, P. and Loganathan, L. (2002) *Discovering Hope for Recovery From a British Perspective: A Review of a Sample of Recovery Literature, Implications for Practice and Systems Change*.

Webber, J. (2009) Nobody Can Look The Other Way. *Health Service Journal*, 13th August.

Webber, M. (2008) *Evidence-Based Policy and Practice in Mental Health Social Work*. Exeter: Learning Matters.

Webster, A. (2001) Embodied Leadership. *Ministry*, Summer.

Webster, C. (2002) *The National Health Service: A Political History*. 2nd edn. Oxford: Oxford University Press.

Welch, J. with Byrne, J. (2001) *Jack: What I've Learned Leading a Great Company and Great People*. New York: Headline Press.

Westwood, S. et al. (1989) *Sadness in My Heart: Racism and Mental Health*. Leicester Black Mental Health Group, Leicester University.

WHO Europe (2005) *Mental Health Declaration for Europe: Facing The Challenges, Building Solutions*. WHO European Ministerial Conference on Mental Health: Helsinki.

Wield, C. (2006) *Life After Darkness: A Doctors Journey Through Severe Depression*. Oxford: Radcliffe.

Wilder. T. (1927) *The Bridge of San Luis Rey*. New York: Harperperennial.

Williams, J. and Scott, S. (2002) Service Responses to Women With Mental Health Needs. *The Mental Health Review*, 7: 1.

Williams, R. (2000) *Lost Icons: Reflections on Cultural Bereavement*. Edinburgh: Continuum Books.

Wilson, C. et al. (2000) How Mental Illness is Portrayed in Children's Television. *British Journal of Psychiatry*, 176, 440–3.

Winnicott, D. (1965) *The Mentally Ill on Your Caseload. The Maturational Processes of The Facilitating Environment*. London: Hogarth Press (Reprinted Karnac Books, 1990)

Winterson, J. (2000) *The Power Book*. London: Jonathan Cape.

Wolpert, L. (2006) *Malignant Sadness: The Anatomy of Depression* 3rd edn. London: Faber & Faber.

Woodward, A. and Kohli, M. (2001) *Inclusions and Exclusions in European Societies*. London: Routledge.

Younghusband, E. (1959) *Report of The Working Party on Social Workers in The Local Authority Health and Welfare Services*. London: HMSO.

Younghusband, E. (1978) *Social Work in Britain: 1950–1975*. London: Unwin.

Zohar, D. and Marshall, I. (2000) *S.Q: Spiritual Intelligence, The Ultimate Intelligence*. London: Bloomsbury.

Subject Index

Leadership
Being effective and remaining human

By Peter Gilbert

'Asserts a powerful and clear image of the human services leader.' *The International Journal of Leadership in Public Service*

'Reminds us that leadership occurs at all levels . . . impressive.' *Nursing Standard.*

'The chapter on the use – and potential abuse – of personal power and authority is essential reading . . . suitable for anyone practicing leadership at whatever level and provides excellent scope for reflection on personal aspirations and performance.' *Social Caring*

'An immense amount of useful material.' *Youth & Policy.*

978-1-903855-76-8

Developing leadership
A learning and development manual

By Peter Gilbert and Neil Thompson

The quality of leadership is often the key difference between:
- organisational success and failure
- a positive, energising, place to work, and a negative, stressful environment

This new manual will be especially useful to anyone who wants to move away from managerialist approaches to the workplace, towards cultures and environments that promote **'remaining human' as well as 'being effective'** . . . through enlightened leadership.

'Managerialism' puts the emphasis on targets and the accompanying unavoidable bureaucracy; and can be seen to be trying to squeeze as much out of people as possible. It has a negative impact on morale and a tendency to produce disaffection and stress.

On the other hand, the holistic approach in *Developing Leadership* will help you to:
- get the best out of people
- create cultures and working environments that motivate – and inspire – because they are genuinely supportive of staff and appreciative of their efforts
- develop the skills of actual and aspiring leaders
- help others learn how to train and support leaders.

978-1-905541-61-4